CONTENTS

Editors

David R. Brown, PhD, FACSM
Research Behavioral Scientist
Physical Activity and Health Branch
Division of Nutrition, Physical Activity and Obesity
National Center for Chronic Disease Prevention and Health Promotion
Centers for Disease Control and Prevention

Gregory W. Heath, DHSc, MPH, FACSM, FAHA*
Guerry Professor and Head
Department of Health and Human Performance
Director of Research, College of Medicine
University of Tennessee Chattanooga

Sarah Levin Martin, PhD*
Healthy Maine Partnerships Evaluation Team Leader
Maine Center for Public Health

Contributing Authors

Ross C. Brownson, PhD
Professor and Codirector
Prevention Research Center in St. Louis
Schools of Medicine and Social Work
Washington University in St. Louis

Leigh Ramsey Buchanan, PhD
Epidemiologist
Division of Nutrition, Physical Activity and Obesity
National Center for Chronic Disease Prevention and Health Promotion
Centers for Disease Control and Prevention

David M. Buchner, MD, MPH*
Shahid and Ann Carlson Khan Professor in Applied Health Sciences
Department of Kinesiology and Community Health
University of Illinois at Urbana-Champaign

Tamara Vehige Calise, MEd*
DrPH Candidate
Boston University School of Public Health

Rebeka Cook, MPH
Commission on Ministerial Health
Texas District Lutheran Church-Missouri Synod
Austin, TX

Jacqueline N. Epping, MEd
Team Leader, Guidelines and Recommendations Development Team
Physical Activity and Health Branch
Division of Nutrition, Physical Activity and Obesity
National Center for Chronic Disease Prevention and Health Promotion
Centers for Disease Control and Prevention

Janet E. Fulton, PhD
Team Leader, Epidemiology and Surveillance Team
Physical Activity and Health Branch
Division of Nutrition, Physical Activity and Obesity
National Center for Chronic Disease Prevention and Health Promotion
Centers for Disease Control and Prevention

Sandra A. Ham, MS*
Divinity School
University of Illinois at Chicago

Harold W. Kohl, III, PhD, MSPH[1]
Professor of Epidemiology and Kinesiology
University of Texas School of Public Health, Division of Epidemiology and Disease Control and College of Education, Department of Kinesiology and Health
University of Texas at Austin

Tina J. Lankford, MPH
Public Health Analyst
Physical Activity and Health Branch
Division of Nutrition, Physical Activity and Obesity
National Center for Chronic Disease Prevention and Health Promotion
Centers for Disease Control and Prevention

Sarah M. Lee, PhD
Health Scientist
Division of Adolescent and School Health
National Center for Chronic Disease Prevention and Health Promotion
Centers for Disease Control and Prevention

Refilwe Moeti, MA*
Public Health Educator
Division of Oral Health
National Center for Chronic Disease Prevention and Health Promotion
Centers for Disease Control and Prevention

James H. Rimmer, PhD
Professor
Director, National Center on Physical Activity and Disability
Department of Disability and Human Development
University of Illinois at Chicago

Candace Rutt, PhD
Senior Service Fellow
Physical Activity and Health Branch
Division of Nutrition, Physical Activity and Obesity
National Center for Chronic Disease Prevention and Health Promotion
Centers for Disease Control and Prevention

James F. Sallis, PhD
Professor of Psychology
San Diego State University
Director, Active Living Research

Thomas L. Schmid, PhD
Team Leader, Research and Development Team
Physical Activity and Health Branch
Division of Nutrition, Physical Activity and Obesity
National Center for Chronic Disease Prevention and Health Promotion
Centers for Disease Control and Prevention

Dennis Shepard, MAT, CHES
Senior Project Manager
YMCA of the USA
Leesville, SC

Robin E. Soler, PhD
Coordinating Scientist
The Guide to Community Preventive Services
Division of Health Communication and Marketing Strategy
National Center for Health Marketing
Centers for Disease Control and Prevention

Sara Wilcox, PhD
Associate Professor
Department of Exercise Science
Arnold School of Public Health
Public Health Research Center
University of South Carolina

Lauren M. Workman, MPH
Association of Schools of Public Health Fellow
Division of Nutrition, Physical Activity and Obesity
National Center for Chronic Disease Prevention and Health Promotion
Centers for Disease Control and Prevention

Special thanks to those providing examples of state or local programs
or interventions for the partnership and evaluation chapters

Catherine Costakis, MS
Physical Activity Coordinator
Montana Nutrition and Physical Activity Program
Montana State University
Bozeman, MT

Rebecca Drewette-Card, MSPH
Physical Activity Coordinator
Maine Physical Activity and Nutrition Program
Maine Center for Disease Control and Prevention
Augusta, ME

Amy Jesaitis, MPH, RD, PAPHS
Physical Activity and Nutrition Coordinator
Healthy Heart Program
New York State Department of Health
Albany, NY

Greg Oliver, MS
Health Promotion Director
Missoula City-County Health Department
Missoula, MT

Paula Puntenney, RN, MA
Walk a Hound Lose a Pound Program Director
Indianapolis, IN

Special thanks to those who reviewed preliminary drafts and
provided technical assistance

Susan A. Carlson, MPH
Epidemiologist
Physical Activity and Health Branch
Division of Nutrition, Physical Activity and Obesity
National Center for Chronic Disease Prevention and Health Promotion
Centers for Disease Control and Prevention

Deborah A. Galuska, PhD, MPH
Associate Director of Science
Division of Nutrition, Physical Activity and Obesity
National Center for Chronic Disease Prevention and Health Promotion
Centers for Disease Control and Prevention

Jana S. Wallace, MPH, CHES
Association of Schools of Public Health Fellow
Division of Nutrition, Physical Activity and Obesity
National Center for Chronic Disease Prevention and Health Promotion
Centers for Disease Control and Prevention

Special thanks to the staff at Human Kinetics, including Dr. Michael Bahrke for his encouragement, dedication, and professional guidance over the course of many months; and Melissa Zavala for her editing and creative talents that helped bring this guide to publication.

Special thanks to Division of Nutrition, Physical Activity and Obesity leadership, whose support made this guide possible:

  Director, William H. Dietz, MD, PhD
  Deputy Director, Laurie A. Johnson, MPH
  Physical Activity and Health Branch Chief, Michael Pratt, MD, MPH
  Physical Activity and Health Branch Deputy Chief, Lisa W. Kimbrough, MS

A special thanks to the families and loved ones of all who contributed to this volume, as your support on a day-to-day basis truly helps to make our professional accomplishments possible.

* Formally with the Physical Activity and Health Branch, Division of Nutrition, Physical Activity and Obesity, National Center for Chronic Disease Prevention and Health Promotion, Centers for Disease Control and Prevention, Atlanta, GA

PREFACE

We welcome you to the second edition of *Promoting Physical Activity: A Guide for Community Action*. As with the first edition (USDHHS, 1999), this is a resource for professionals and volunteers who wish to promote physical activity in almost any community setting. The goals of this guide are to provide direction and assistance in program planning and a flexible blueprint for action for professionals who are on the front lines of intervention. Our mission is to help you succeed in getting more Americans physically active! The first edition focused broadly on physical activity promotion at the individual through community levels. This edition introduces you to emerging topics related to physical activity and public health, including evidence-based physical activity community interventions. It further explores the importance of establishing and relying on partnerships during the development and implementation of your interventions, and evaluating your efforts to intervene.

This guide is for you, whether you have just become interested in promoting physical activity but are not sure where to begin, or are experienced in physical activity or health promotion but need new ideas to improve or expand existing programs. Whether you have a staff of one and very few resources or a staff of hundreds with resources to spare, you'll find that this guide includes advice and examples from an array of experiences and perspectives that you can apply to your situation. It's a practical guide to community *action,* fostering physical activity as a pathway to health and quality of life. And you don't have to know a great deal about physical activity to use this book.

Promoting Physical Activity: A Guide for Community Action, Second Edition, is for anyone interested in promoting physical activity behavior change—any professional, in nearly any field. Regardless of your situation, this guide will show you how to intervene to promote and increase physical activity in your community. This guide summarizes the most up-to-date information about physical activity, translates research into practice based on recommended evidenced-based interventions, and includes the basics of program planning and evaluation. Real-life examples are provided along the way. The best-case scenario is that by reading this book you will have found a friend—a user-friendly resource you can turn to again and again for ideas, regardless of which community you find yourself in.

You will discover that there are some things you can do to increase the likelihood that people in your community will change their behavior and become more physically active. And you will have the background information you need to convince others to be on your side. The key is to have the knowledge and the resources at hand, work with your partners, and make it happen. Let's all get Americans moving again!

How to Use This Book

This guide discusses what you need to plan, promote, implement, and evaluate a community-based physical activity intervention or program, yet you need not read the guide from cover to cover. Instead, become familiar with its contents, mark the chapters or pages that interest you most, and start there. Not all chapters apply to everyone. You might need to read some parts of the guide more closely than others. It's a resource tool. Pick it up anytime. Keep it handy on your shelf. Photocopy the pages you like best. Although research findings will certainly change with each passing day, the guide keeps the door open to the future, with endless resource possibilities: places you can turn for continued inspiration, partnership potential, educational resources, or just good advice. The world of physical activity promotion is here at your fingertips. Here's what each part has in store:

- Part I, Foundations for Physical Activity Promotion, explains the scientific basis for promoting physical activity—including the benefits and risks associated with an active lifestyle—and how to meet current physical activity recommendations.

- Part II, Approaches and Interventions for Changing Physical Activity Behavior, takes you through the process of implementing evidence-based interventions found to be effective in promoting physical activity at the community level. These interventions fall within three approaches: (1) informational, (2) behavioral and social, and (3) environmental and policy. Try one, or combine two or more intervention types.

- Part III, Planning, Implementing, and Evaluating Your Intervention or Program, covers the basics of partnerships and shows you how to set program objectives and measure program success. You can apply these principles in any setting.

- Part IV, Resources for Action, is devoted entirely to additional resources for physical activity program planning. You'll find addresses and phone numbers of agencies and organizations across the country that are interested in promoting physical activity, excerpts from the *1996 Surgeon General's Report on Physical Activity and Health* (USDHHS), and many other helpful resources that will make promoting physical activity easier for you.

If you are starting a new program, you may want to work through this guide from the beginning to get the best overview. If you are trying to strengthen an ongoing program, read chapters 3 through 5 to learn valuable keys to successful interventions and chapters 6 and 7 to learn about partners, planning, and evaluation. The glossary will also help you learn and review concepts related to promoting physical activity.

This guide is timely in that it can be used in conjunction with the release of other key initiatives to increase physical activity among Americans. In addition to the 2008 Physical Activity Guidelines for Americans, the first-ever National Physical Activity Plan (www.physicalactivityplan.org) and the State Indicator Report on Physical Activity (www.cdc.gov/nccdphp/dnpa/physical/health_professionals/reports/) are also being released in May 2010. This is truly an exciting time for physical activity, researchers, and practitioners, as these national resources can assist you with your efforts to promote physical activity for all Americans.

What You Won't Find In This Book

Individual behavior change interventions are not ignored in this second edition, but the focus of the book is primarily on interventions used in group or community-based settings. You will most likely recognize that individual behavior change strategies are not discussed from the perspective of individual behavior modification but rather as ways to motivate groups of people (e.g., participants in a community-based exercise class) to increase their physical activity behavior. For readers who are interested in topics such as individual exercise prescription (i.e., the type, frequency, intensity, and duration of physical activity), heart rate monitoring, perceived exertion, or individual risk assessment (e.g., the Physical Activity Readiness Questionnaire), the first edition of this guide (USDHHS, 1999) remains a valuable resource. As individual or joint resources, these guides will prepare and assist you to advance the field of physical activity and public health.

Tips for Additional Resources

This publication is not an all inclusive listing of physical activity promotion programs, interventions, or resources currently available or under development. Although in this guide we attempt to provide most of the basic information you might need to initiate and manage a physical activity intervention, you undoubtedly will have questions that the guide does not answer. For additional assistance see the following:

- Lists of suggested reading and resources at the end of each chapter that will direct you to relevant references if you want more in-depth information on a given topic.
- A comprehensive reference list at the end of the book is separated by chapter to help you locate reference citations easily as you work through an individual chapter.

Best of luck with your physical activity and public health journey!

A National Call to Promote Physical Activity

The human body is designed for daily physical activity. Indeed, with features such as opposable thumbs and bipedal locomotion, humans are designed for physical activity in a manner unlike any other species. As it turns out, daily physical activity does not just help us move and accomplish tasks of everyday life. There is conclusive evidence that regular physical activity improves health and enhances quality of life.

Historically, a life with large amounts of physical activity has been the rule rather than the exception. Yet in the past several hundred years, physical activity has been gradually engineered out of daily life, particularly in economically developed countries. Over the same period, public health organizations made enormous strides in controlling infectious diseases. Consequently, people lived longer lives, but they became afflicted with chronic conditions such as coronary heart disease and stroke, type 2 diabetes, and various forms of cancer.

The link between the steadily increasing prevalence of chronic disease and the steadily decreasing level of physical activity was not immediately obvious. Whereas the first U.S. Surgeon General's report on smoking and health was released in 1964 (U.S. Public Health Service, 1964), the first Surgeon General's report on physical activity and health was not issued until 1996 (USDHHS, 1996). The report announced that the scientific evidence for the health benefits of physical activity was conclusive: Regular physical activity reduces the risk of several major chronic diseases and reduces premature mortality. That is, lack of physical activity is a major preventable cause of the burden of chronic disease in our society.

The Surgeon General's report on physical activity reviewed studies on the amount of physical activity required for health and issued a remarkable finding: A moderate amount of physical activity has substantial health benefits. This finding is a fundamental discovery of physical activity and public health, although you may not find it to be intuitive. People are capable of doing hours of physical activity each day. Elite athletes can do sustained vigorous aerobic activity of 15.0 metabolic equivalents (METS) or more. Yet doing 30 minutes of moderate-intensity aerobic activity in the 3.0- to 6.0-MET range will lead to meaningful benefits. More physical activity—greater frequency, longer duration, or higher intensity—produces substantially greater health benefits, although there are diminishing returns with very high levels of activity.

So we have an indisputable need to engineer physical activity back into daily life. We recognize that the physical activity required for life in the past involved repetitive tasks, hard manual labor, and substantial risk of injury. We have the opportunity to selectively engineer into daily life safe forms of physical activity that enhance quality of life and improve health. This approach does not minimize the importance of individual choice, but it seeks to make the healthy choice the easy choice. The objective is to increase the attractiveness and breadth of choices in a community so as to provide opportunities for sports, active recreation, active transportation, and active tasks around the home (such as gardening). We seek to retain some physical activity opportunities from the past but also to add new opportunities not commonly available in the past. The need to add activity to daily life illustrates the aphorism that challenges are opportunities (and vice versa). The fabric of life has been altered in many ways that have resulted in greater challenges and fewer opportunities for physical activity. To address the challenges and opportunities for promoting physical activity, the Centers for Disease Control and Prevention selected a group of experts to write the second edition of *Promoting Physical Activity: A Guide for Community Action.*

Since the publication of the first edition of the book in 1999, numerous advances in community-based physical activity interventions and programs have occurred and the scientific knowledge base regarding physical activity and public health has grown substantially. This advancement was led by the development of the *Guide to Community Preventive Services* (Zaza et al., 2005), also known as the *Community Guide.* Included in the *Community Guide* is a chapter identifying evidenced-based physical activity interventions. Physical activity interventions published in the scientific literature were systematically evaluated by an independent, nonfederal task force to identify effective physical activity interventions. Considering the strength of the scientific evidence, the task force determined that interventions should be either recommended because of strong or sufficient evidence of effectiveness or not recommended because of insufficient evidence. The *Community Guide,* combined with a growing body of physical activity policy and environmental research, a strong need for evaluation methods to guide public health practice, and an ongoing need to develop and maintain partnerships to promote community-based physical activity interventions, forms the basis of this second edition.

One MET is the energy expenditure needed to rest or sit quietly, which, for the average adult, requires approximately 3.5 milliliters of oxygen uptake per kilogram of body weight per minute (U.S. Department of Health and Human Services, 1999). If you do an activity such as walking at a 4-MET level, this requires four times the metabolic energy expenditure required when sitting quietly.

This book is written for public health practitioners; persons working in the parks and recreation, urban planning, and transportation sectors; and other stakeholders (e.g., elected officials, advocates, and community residents) involved in promoting physical activity in communities. The breadth of content in the book mirrors the breadth of readers, who will find it an easy-to-use and essential resource.

The motifs of the book relate to evidence-based public health. Wagnerian operas can have leitmotivs that infuse the symphonic accompaniment with specific musical motifs for important characters, ideas, and events of the opera. The leitmotivs of this book are the various strains of scientific evidence that stem from fields such as epidemiology, behavioral science, exercise science, and medical science. These form a medley of evidence-based community approaches and best practices to create the public health science of promoting physical activity.

Increasing physical activity is a national health objective for the United States (USDHHS, 2000), and physical activity among Americans is a leading health indicator. As shown in the following list, *Healthy People 2010* has major objectives to reduce sedentary lifestyles and increase the percentage of adults and children who meet physical activity recommendations. The goal of *Healthy People 2010* to "eliminate health disparities" applies to physical activity, because physical activity levels vary by race, ethnic background, and socioeconomic status in the United States.

Healthy People 2010 Physical Activity and Fitness Objectives

Objective 22-1: Reduce the proportion of adults who engage in no leisure-time physical activity.

Objective 22-2: Increase the proportion of adults who engage regularly, preferably daily, in moderate physical activity for at least 30 minutes per day.

Objective 22-3: Increase the proportion of adults who engage in vigorous physical activity that promotes the development and maintenance of cardiovascular fitness 3 or more days per week for 20 or more minutes per occasion.

Muscular Strength/Endurance and Flexibility

Objective 22-4: Increase the proportion of adults who perform physical activities that enhance and maintain muscular strength and endurance.

Objective 22-5: Increase the proportion of adults who perform physical activities that enhance and maintain flexibility.

Physical Activity in Children and Adolescents

Objective 22-6: Increase the proportion of adolescents who engage in moderate physical activity for at least 30 minutes on 5 or more of the previous 7 days.

Objective 22-7: Increase the proportion of adolescents who engage in vigorous physical activity that promotes cardiorespiratory fitness 3 or more days per week for 20 or more minutes per occasion.

Objective 22-8: Increase the proportion of the nation's public and private schools that require daily physical education for all students.

Objective 22-9: Increase the proportion of adolescents who participate in daily school physical education.

(continued)

Healthy People 2010 Physical Activity and Fitness Objectives *(continued)*

Objective 22-10: Increase the proportion of adolescents who spend at least 50 percent of school physical education class time being physically active.

Objective 22-11: Increase the proportion of adolescents who view television 2 or fewer hours on a school day.

Access

Objective 22-12: (Developmental) Increase the proportion of the nation's public and private schools that provide access to their physical activity spaces and facilities for all persons outside of normal school hours (that is, before and after the school day, on weekends, and during summer and other vacations).

Objective 22-13: Increase the proportion of worksites offering employer-sponsored physical activity and fitness programs.

Objective 22-14: Increase the proportion of trips made by walking.

Objective 22-15: Increase the proportion of trips made by bicycling.

U.S. Department of Health and Human Services, 2000.

At the time of the release of this book, the *Healthy People 2020* objectives were not published, but will soon be available to guide national, state, and local efforts towards meeting national objectives to increase physical activity. Community-based approaches to promoting physical activity have been shown to be effective. Following the approaches discussed in this book will result in substantial progress toward meeting national health objectives. A community that has the political will and resources to implement evidence-based approaches will increase the level of physical activity, and consequently the health, of its residents.

Suggested Reading

Sallis JF, Cervero R, Ascher WW, Henderson K, Kraft MK, Kerr J. 2006. An ecological approach to creating more physically active communities. *Annual Review of Public Health* 27:297-322. (doi:10.1146/annurev.publhealth.27.021405.102100). First posted online on September 30, 2005.

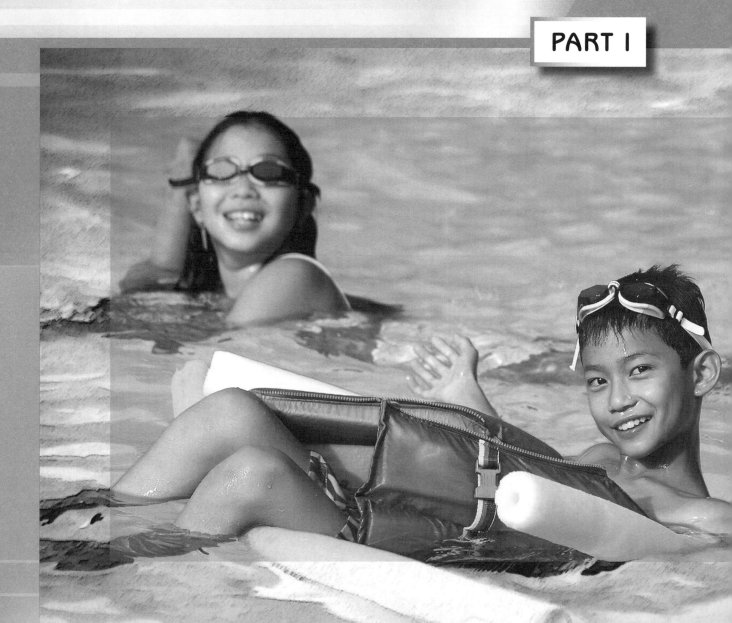

© iStockphoto/Edwin Verin

Foundations for Physical Activity Promotion

People young and old, large and small, of all racial and ethnic groups, with and without disabilities simply need to move more. We all know that physical activity is good for us, but that is not enough to convince many people and communities to make it happen. As promoters of physical activity, we need to arm ourselves with the best information possible to justify our stance and help create the demand for change that will support physically active lifestyles.

In Part I, you will be given the foundation to make the case for physical activity. Chapter 1 highlights all of the positive benefits of physical activity. Not only does regular physical activity help prevent obesity, an array of chronic disease conditions, and premature death, it also helps manage or improve chronic conditions; furthermore, physical activity confers positive mental benefits.

Chapter 2 reviews existing health goals for physical activity that make up national health policies in the United States and provides the most up-to-date information on physical activity recommendations for both youth and adults. These recommendations are an invaluable resource for professionals who want to help people improve their health. The chapter also highlights the national health objectives, which you can adopt or adapt for your community. These recommendations and objectives can serve as the basis for your programs.

CHAPTER 1

Health Benefits of Physical Activity

David M. Buchner

Regular physical activity provides numerous and substantial health benefits. Regular physical activity reduces the risk of premature mortality and the risk of many chronic diseases. It improves our mood and psychological well-being. It is effective treatment for many chronic diseases and reduces the risk of disability. It enhances our ability to perform the tasks of everyday life and thereby promotes independent living. The health benefits associated with physical activity are highlighted in this chapter, but for a very detailed and comprehensive, evidence-based review of these health benefits, see the *Physical Activity Guidelines Advisory Committee (PAGAC) Report* released in 2008 by the U.S. Department of Health & Human Services (Physical Activity Guidelines Advisory Committee [PAGAC], 2008). Before we consider the benefits in greater detail, let's first define some terms, identify the attributes of physical activity related to health benefits, and discuss measurement related to physical activity and energy expenditure.

What Is Physical Activity?

Broadly speaking, physical activity is movement of the body caused by skeletal muscle contractions (USDHHS, 2008). However, in public health, physical activity refers to the types of movement that have health benefits. These movements usually involve the large muscle groups of the body and substantial energy expenditure. In other words, *physical activity* is shorthand for *health-enhancing physical activity*. As discussed later, the evidence of health benefits is strongest for aerobic activity. So when context makes it clear, physical activity sometimes refers to only health-enhancing aerobic activity.

Physical activity belongs to the group of behavioral risk factors affecting health that include tobacco use, diet, drug and alcohol use, and sexual behavior. These risk factors are also referred to as lifestyle factors.

What Is Physical Fitness?

Physical fitness refers to the physiologic capacity of systems of the body that are affected by physical activity. For example, maximal **aerobic capacity** is a fitness measure of maximal ability to perform aerobic work. Other common measures of physical fitness are muscle strength and endurance, range of motion around a joint (flexibility), and **body composition** measures such as percent **body fat** (USDHHS, 2008).

Public health scientists usually use **exercise** to refer to the subset of physical activity done for the purpose of increasing physical fitness (USDHHS, 2008). However, the public does not make this distinction. When developing messages about physical activity for the public, the terminology should be guided by how words like *exercise* or *active lifestyle* are interpreted by members of the **community.**

Physical Activity and Energy Expenditure

A well-known physiologic effect of physical activity is that it expends energy. Scientists measure energy expenditure in units like kilocalories and kilojoules. In popular usage, the term **kilocalorie** is abbreviated as **calorie.** Besides physical activity, the body expends some energy when we eat, called the thermic effect of food. Some energy is used just to keep the body alive, and this basal energy expenditure is measured using the basal metabolic rate. The sum of these three sources of energy expenditure is called total energy expenditure, or TEE.

So if you walk on a treadmill for a mile, and the LED displays 100 calories expended, what does this mean? Most likely, this is the gross energy expenditure during the walk, which is the sum of basal expenditure and activity expenditure. If so, the net caloric expenditure due to the physical activity alone is fewer than 100 calories. Generic formulas are also used to estimate the number of calories

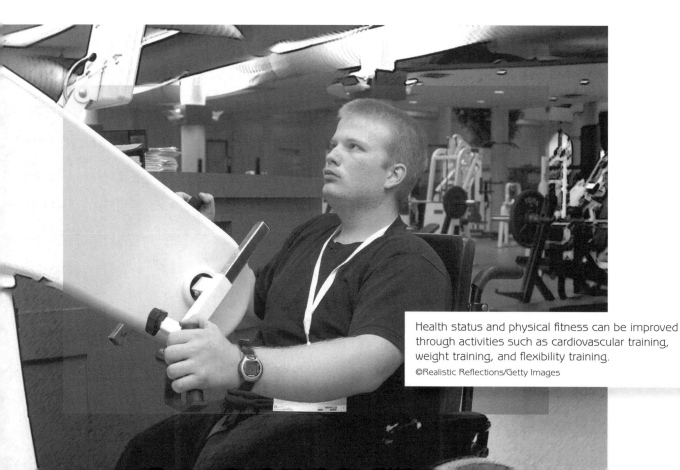

Health status and physical fitness can be improved through activities such as cardiovascular training, weight training, and flexibility training.
©Realistic Reflections/Getty Images

expended while using exercise equipment, and these rarely take into account age, sex, and body weight, so these formulas may not accurately estimate calories expended during exercise.

Determinants of the Health Benefits of Physical Activity

The health benefits of physical activity depend on the type of activity, as described subsequently. There is evidence of the health benefits of activities that increase and maintain muscle strength, although there is much more evidence of the health benefits of aerobic activity. (For information on health benefits of flexibility activities and balance activities, see the sidebars on pages 7-8).

The amount of physical activity (or volume of activity) is strongly related to the health benefits. Higher volumes of physical activity produce greater health benefits. The volume of aerobic activity can be thought of as the product of **frequency** (number of sessions or days per week), **duration** (≥10 minutes of activity per session per day per week), and **intensity** (the MET value of the activity). Volume (particularly of aerobic activity) can be measured as either gross or net energy expenditure during physical activity, total minutes, or as MET-minutes (see the sidebar on page 14).

It is unclear how the **frequency** of physical activity (USDHHS, 2008), or number of days per week of activity, is related to health benefits. There is insufficient evidence to conclude that the benefits of 50 minutes of activity on 3 days differ from the benefits of 30 minutes on 5 days a week. On the other hand, aerobic fitness is strongly related to risk of chronic disease, and aerobic training for fitness is more effective if performed on 3 or more days per week. Most people who are regularly active perform activity on several days a week. When observational studies of physical activity report health benefits from regular activity, the regularly active people in the study are probably performing activity on several days each week. Although there is insufficient evidence on how frequency affects injury risk, it is likely that people who perform large volumes of physical activity on only 1 or 2 days each week have increased risk of activity-related injuries compared to people who spread activity throughout the week.

The **intensity** of aerobic activity (USDHHS, 2008) affects health benefits (the intensity of an activity is the level of effort). Moderate-intensity aerobic activity and vigorous-intensity activity clearly provide substantial health benefits, whereas light-intensity activity does not. Current physical activity guidelines define moderate-intensity aerobic activity as 3.0 to 5.9 METs. Light-intensity activity is 1.1 to 2.9 METs, and vigorous-intensity activity is 6.0 METs and above. Given a set volume of activity, there is limited evidence that achieving this volume of activity with vigorous-intensity aerobic activities (as opposed to moderate-intensity activities) has greater health benefit. The following list provides examples of light-intensity, moderate-intensity, and vigorous-intensity activities.

Light-Intensity Activities (less than 3.0 METs)

- Walking at less than 3 miles per hour
- Bicycling less than 5 miles per hour
- Performing stretching exercises
- Playing golf at a driving range
- Participating in lawn bowling
- Playing horseshoes
- Riding a horse at the horse's walking pace
- Performing light housework

Moderate-Intensity Activities (3.0-5.9 METs)

- Walking at 3.0 to 4.5 miles per hour
- Bicycling on level terrain at 5 to 9 miles per hour
- Performing yoga
- Participating in recreational dancing, such as square dancing
- Walking a golf course
- Playing badminton
- Participating in recreational swimming
- Kayaking on calm water

Vigorous-Intensity Activities (6.0 METs and above)

- Racewalking
- Jogging and running
- Bicycling at 10 miles per hour or higher or bicycling uphill
- Jumping rope
- Playing most competitive sports (e.g., soccer, basketball)
- Swimming steady, paced laps
- Participating in whitewater kayaking
- Shoveling heavy snow

Additional Readings:

For the complete table listing of light, moderate, and vigorous intensity activities see the first edition of this textbook:

U.S. Department of Health and Human Services, Public Health Service, Centers for Disease Control and Prevention, National Center for Chronic Disease Prevention and Health Promotion, Division of Nutrition and Physical Activity. *Promoting Physical Activity: A Guide for Community Action*. Champaign, IL: Human Kinetics, 1999, pp.20-28.

For a compendium of physical activities and their intensities see:

Ainsworth, BE, Haskell, WL, Whitt, MC, Irwin, ML, Swartz, AM, Strath, SJ, et al. Compendium of physical activities: an update of activity codes and MET intensities. *Medicine and Science in Sports and Exercise* 2000;32(9 Suppl.):s498-504.

The **duration** of an individual bout of aerobic physical activity (USDHHS, 2008) also affects health benefits. According to the *Physical Activity Guidelines Advisory Committee Report* released by the USDHHS, bouts (or episodes or sessions) of moderate- to vigorous-intensity aerobic activity of 10 minutes or longer have health benefits (PAGAC, 2008; USDHHS, 2008). For example, it is known that bouts of physical activity that are 10 minutes or longer improve aerobic fitness and some indicators of cardiovascular disease risk.

Chapter 2 discusses how the attributes of physical activity related to health benefits become the basis for public health physical activity recommendations. Physical activity recommendations specify the recommended minimum volume of physical activity in minutes per week, and this volume may be attained by a variety of combinations of frequency × duration × intensity of physical activity per week.

Do Flexibility Activities Have Health Benefits?

Flexibility activities like stretching do not have well-documented, preventive health benefits. In particular, there is insufficient evidence to conclude stretching prevents musculoskeletal injuries due to physical activity (PAGAC, 2008). But properly performed flexibility activities do increase flexibility, and adequate flexibility is necessary to perform physical activity. Some activities, like gymnastics, require high degrees of flexibility. Because arthritis causes stiffness of joints and muscles, flexibility activities are regarded as effective therapy for medical conditions such as arthritis. Many experts regard flexibility activities as an appropriate part of regular physical activity, particularly in older adults, who are at risk for age-related loss of flexibility.

Types of Physical Activity

Specific types of physical activity (e.g., walking, swimming, lifting weights) are grouped into well-known categories according to their main physiologic effects (USDHHS, 2008). **Aerobic** exercise or cardiovascular activities increase the body's ability to use oxygen as a source of fuel for sustained work. Activities to increase muscular strength, which include weight training and resistance training, increase the size and strength of muscle tissue. **Flexibility** activities increase range of motion of joints and the distance a muscle can be stretched. Balance activities increase the stability of the body as it adopts various positions and does tasks, such as standing and walking.

Other Attributes of Physical Activity

The purpose of the physical activity does not influence health benefits. For example, the health benefits of a 30-minute walk at 3.5 miles per hour are the same for walking around a track to increase fitness and walking through the city to get to a grocery store. Similarly, the domain of the activity does not influence health benefits. Domain indicates the context of the physical activity and is usually classified as recreational (or leisure-time), occupational, domestic, and transportation related. Domains have historically been important to understanding measurement of physical activity by questionnaires, because various questionnaires measure different domains.

Preventive Health Benefits of Physical Activity

Before considering the major preventive benefits of physical activity individually, let's consider some general features of the benefits.

Balance Exercise Can Prevent Falls

Fall-related injuries are a major problem for older adults. There are many risk factors for falls, but a common risk factor is impaired balance. Randomized trials show that falls can be prevented by exercise **interventions** that include balance exercise (Robertson et al., 2002). In older adults with gait problems or who are at increased risk of falls, balance exercises are recommended to prevent falls. These exercises include standing on a narrow base of support and more difficult forms of walking (walking backward, or heel-to-toe walking).

- Substantial health benefits result from a medium amount of aerobic physical activity. In scientific terms, this amount of activity is in the range of 500 to 1,000 MET-minutes per week (PAGAC, 2008). In terms of minutes of moderate-intensity physical activity (such as a brisk walk), a medium amount is about 150 to 300 minutes per week (USDHHS, 2008). Accordingly, recent recommendations have consistently advised adults to perform at least 150 minutes of moderate-intensity activity each week (Haskell et al., 2007; Pate et al., 1995). Although there are risks to physical activity, there is conclusive scientific evidence that the benefits of physical activity far outweigh the risks.

- As noted earlier, the evidence of the health benefits of physical activity is strongest for aerobic activity. But for many of the diseases discussed in this section, there is some evidence that muscle-strengthening activities also reduce risk.

- Greater amounts of physical activity produce greater overall health benefits. That is, there is a dose–response relationship. Although this relationship is incompletely understood, the overall dose–response curve appears to be nonlinear. (PAGAC, 2008; USDHHS, 2008). Larger health benefits accrue from increasing physical activity from inactive levels to a minimum recommended amount (e.g., 150 minutes of moderate-intensity activity each week) than accrue from increasing physical activity from a minimum recommended amount to a higher amount (e.g., exceeding 300 minutes a week). Furthermore, obtaining even less than recommended amounts of physical activity provides some health benefits compared with remaining inactive (PAGAC, 2008; USDHHS, 2008). The benefits of physical activity are independent of other risk factors. For example, an active person who smokes has a lower risk of heart disease than an inactive person who smokes (Paffenbarger et al., 1978). An obese, inactive adult who initiates regular physical activity and gains the fitness benefits of that activity, whether or not he loses weight, is at lower risk of all-cause mortality compared with an obese adult who remains inactive (Xuemei et al., 2007).

- Regular physical activity has benefits for both physical health and mental health. The physical health benefits are better known and better documented, but growing evidence links physical activity to mental health, both emotional and cognitive (Morgan, 1997; PAGAC, 2008).

- Obtaining health benefits of physical activity requires regular physical activity over time. But acute beneficial effects of physical activity occur with a single bout of aerobic activity, such as favorable changes in blood lipids (Yiannis et al., 2007; Zhang et al., 2004), reductions in muscle tension (electromyographic activity) (deVries, 1987; deVries and Adams, 1972), and decreases in blood pressure and anxiety (Brown et al., 1993; Raglin and Morgan, 1987).

■ The benefits of physical activity extend to all age groups, all ethnic groups studied so far, and both men and women.

Premature Mortality

Humans have a natural life span, although life span clearly varies from person to person. Regular aerobic physical activity is not believed to extend the natural life span. Rather, physical activity reduces the risk of dying prematurely. Physical activity has a dose–response effect, with higher levels of physical activity producing a greater reduction in risk of premature mortality. For example, in the Harvard Alumni Study, expending 1,000 to 1,499 calories per week reduced risk of mortality by 27 percent, 2,000 to 2,499 calories per week by 38 percent, and 3,000 to 3,499 calories per week by 54 percent (Paffenbarger et al., 1986).

Regular aerobic physical activity increases aerobic fitness, and so aerobically fit people should have lower risk of premature mortality, and this is indeed the case. The exercise capacity of men has been found to be inversely associated with mortality from any cause (Myers et al., 2002). Figure 1.1 shows the relationship

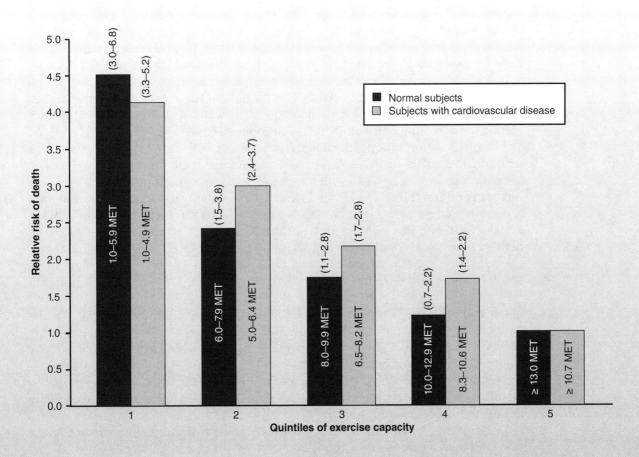

Figure 1.1 Risk of death in men according to exercise capacity.

between maximal exercise (aerobic) capacity in METs, a measure of aerobic fitness, and mortality. There is a dose–response effect, with greater reductions in risk at higher levels of fitness (Myers et al., 2002). As discussed next, physical activity reduces the risk of the most common cause of death in developed countries—cardiovascular disease (CVD). Figure 1.1 demonstrates that the beneficial effect on mortality occurs both in people with CVD and those without CVD. The data in figure 1.1 come from a study that used a treadmill exercise test to assess maximal exercise capacity, a measure of fitness, in METs in older men. The data show a clear dose–response effect: As fitness increases, age-adjusted risk of death decreases. The dose–response relationship was seen in men with and without cardiovascular disease. The subgroup of subjects with the highest exercise capacity (quintile 5) was used as the reference category. For each quintile, the range of values for exercise capacity represented appears within each bar; 95 percent confidence intervals for the relative risks appear above each bar.

Cardiovascular Disease and Stroke

Cardiovascular disease is the name given to a group of diseases of the heart and blood vessels. This group includes coronary heart disease or ischemic heart disease, which causes and is composed of angina and myocardial infarction (heart attack). It includes cerebrovascular disease and stroke. A stroke due to ischemia caused by thrombosis (a blood clot forms within an artery supplying blood to the brain) and embolism (a blood clot or some other particles form away from the brain and lodge in an artery leading to or located in the brain) is called an ischemic stroke, whereas a stroke due to bleeding of a blood vessel in the brain is called a hemorrhagic stroke. The group also includes peripheral arterial disease, which is narrowing of the arteries supplying the arms and legs with blood, which commonly causes pain on walking. The pathogenesis of this group of diseases involves atherosclerosis, which is damage to the walls of an artery that ultimately results in narrowing of its diameter and reduced blood flow.

The observation that physical activity protects against heart disease was first made in the 1950s by Jeremy Morris in a famous study comparing drivers (a sedentary occupation) with conductors (an active occupation) on double-decker buses in London (Morris et al., 1953). Since then, many studies have documented a dose–response protective effect of physical activity on CVD (PAGAC, 2008). Physical activity also reduces risk of thromboembolic stroke (PAGAC, 2008). Inactivity increases risk of stroke by about 60 percent (table 1.1). Figure 1.2 shows the relationship between walking and CVD risk in the Women's Health Initiative study (Manson et al., 2002). In a dose–response manner, the more MET-hours of walking each week, the greater the reduction in risk of CVD in middle-aged and older women. In the Women's Health Initiative observational study, physical activity levels were measured in MET-hours per week. A clear dose–response effect is seen in all age groups. Women obtaining 2.6 to 5.0 MET-hours per week of activity were insufficiently active and did not meet recommended levels of aerobic activity. Yet when compared with the inactive women (0.0 MET-hours per week), even insufficiently active women still had significant reduction in risk of CVD, especially in the 50- to 59-year-old group.

Using principles of epidemiology, it is possible to calculate an estimate of the percentage of a disease in a population that is directly attributable to a risk factor, called the population attributable risk percentage (PAR%). A study applied the relative risks from table 1.1 and estimated that about 19 percent of coronary artery disease and about 24 percent of strokes in Canada were attributable to lack of physical activity (Katzmarzyk and Janssen, 2004).

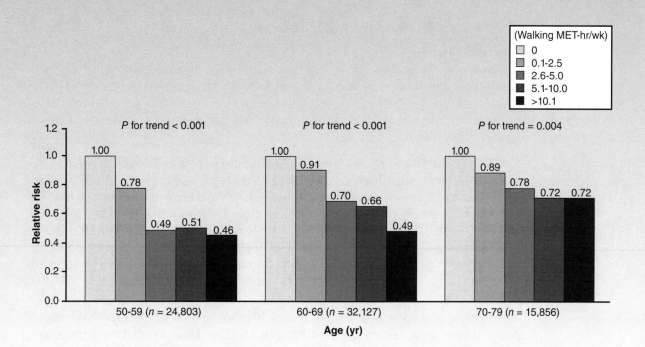

Figure 1.2 The risk of cardiovascular disease in women according to age and level of physical activity

Reprinted, by permission, from J.E. Manson et al., 2002, "Walking compared with vigorous exercise for the prevention of cardiovascular events in women," *New England Journal of Medicine* 347:716-25. © Massachusetts Medical Society. All rights reserved.

Table 1.1. Summary Relative Risk Estimates for the Effect of Physical Inactivity on Risk of Common Diseases

Disease	Summary Relative Risk	95% Confidence Interval
Coronary artery disease	1.45	1.38-1.54
Stroke	1.60	1.42-1.80
Hypertension	1.30	1.16-1.46
Colon cancer	1.41	1.31-1.53
Breast cancer	1.31	1.23-1.38
Type 2 diabetes	1.50	1.37-1.63
Osteoporosis	1.59	1.40-1.80

These relative risks were estimated from a systematic evidence review, which used meta-analysis to derive summary relative risks. Relative risks measure the influence of a factor on overall risk of having a disease. For example, if 10 per 1,000 active adults develop heart disease in a year, and 15 per 1,000 inactive adults develop heart disease in a year, then the relative risk of heart disease due to inactivity is 15/1,000 divided by 10/1,000 = 1.50. A relative risk of 1.5 thus indicates a 50% higher risk of a disease. If a factor (such as physical activity) has no influence on the risk of disease, the relative risk = 1.0. The size of the 95% confidence interval indicates the precision of the estimate of relative risk. When confidence intervals do not include 1.0, the factor is regarded as having a statistically significant association with the risk of a disease.

Adapted from P.R. Katzmarzyk and I. Janssen, 2004, "The economic costs associated with physical activity and obesity in Canada: An update," *Canadian Journal of Applied Physiology* 29(1): 90-115.

Risk Factors for Cardiovascular Disease

Although hypertension (high blood pressure) is a cardiovascular disease, it is also properly regarded as a risk for coronary heart disease and for stroke. Inactive adults have about a 30 percent increased risk of hypertension (table 1.1). The effect of aerobic activity on blood pressure is an exception to the general rule of a dose–response effect, with most of the benefit occurring at relatively low doses of physical activity.

■ Triglycerides and cholesterol are essential components of the body, but too much of either is unhealthy. These substances are carried in the blood by lipoproteins. Too much low-density lipoprotein (LDL) cholesterol increases risk of CVD, whereas high levels of high-density lipoprotein (HDL) cholesterol decrease risk of CVD. Regular aerobic physical activity elevates HDL cholesterol and reduces total cholesterol (Butcher et al., 2008), LDL cholesterol (Woolf-May et al., 1999), and triglycerides (Wong et al., 2008). The findings that physical activity positively influences HDL cholesterol and triglyceride levels are especially consistent (PAGAC, 2008).

■ Stress is regarded as a risk factor for CVD (Rozanski et al., 1999). Work-related stress is the most widely studied type of stress related to CVD. For example, stress at work can be produced by increased responsibility for productivity with decreased control over the processes that influence productivity. Chronic stress appears to cause changes in the circulating hormones and blood pressure. Several reviews conclude that physical activity effectively reduces stress, with the size of the effect ranging between small and medium (Taylor, 2000). As noted previously, physical activity has been found to reduce muscle tension, blood pressure, and anxiety; known markers of stress.

Diabetes and Abnormal Glucose Tolerance

The hallmark of diabetes mellitus is chronic elevation in blood glucose (sugar), called hyperglycemia. Hyperglycemia damages blood vessels and leads to a variety of complications including certain forms of eye disease, kidney disease, and nerve disease. Diabetes increases risk of CVD, which is the most common cause of death in people with diabetes. By far, type 2 diabetes is the most common form of diabetes. In this form, the body produces the hormone insulin that regulates blood sugar, but the body is resistant to the effects of insulin. Regular physical activity reduces insulin resistance. Lack of physical activity increases risk of type 2 diabetes by about 50 percent (table 1.1).

Abnormal glucose tolerance describes people who have some insulin resistance and some hyperglycemia but not enough to meet criteria for a diagnosis of diabetes. This condition clearly increases risk of developing type 2 diabetes. Randomized trials show that physical activity prevents progression from abnormal glucose tolerance to diabetes (PAGAC, 2008). In the Diabetes Prevention Project study of people with abnormal glucose tolerance, regular physical activity (without any weight loss) reduced risk of advancing to diabetes by 44 percent (Hamman et al., 2006), whereas physical activity and weight loss reduced risk by 58 percent (Knowler et al., 2002).

Physical activity effectively reduces stress, a risk factor for cardiovascular disease.

Obesity

When energy intake from food chronically exceeds energy expenditure, the body stores excess energy in the form of fat. Excess body fat has adverse health effects, such as contributing to insulin resistance and type 2 diabetes and increasing the risk of osteoarthritis, gall bladder disease, and postmenopausal breast cancer (USDHHS, 1998). Obesity is usually defined as a **body mass index (BMI)** of 30.0 or greater (USDHHS, 1998), where BMI is defined as weight (in kilograms) divided by height (in meters) squared.

Most adults gain weight from young adulthood into middle age. Observational studies report that regular physical activity and greater aerobic fitness do not entirely prevent this weight gain but do reduce it and thereby reduce a person's risk of reaching a BMI of 30 or more (DiPietro et al., 1998; Lewis et al., 1997; Williams and Wood, 2006). For persons who are obese who wish to achieve weight loss, a dietary intervention also is needed, as the rate of weight loss due to physical activity and caloric restriction is substantially faster than that caused by increasing physical activity only (PAGAC, 2008).

A calorie expended is a calorie expended, so logically there is a dose–response preventive effect between volume of physical activity and obesity risk. From an energy balance standpoint, it does not matter whether caloric expenditure is achieved by performing light, moderate, or vigorous activity. But vigorous activity burns calories at a faster rate. So practically speaking, it is more time efficient to attain the volumes of activity necessary to achieve or maintain a healthy weight through vigorous activity.

Bone Health

Osteoporosis is a condition characterized by reduced bone mass and bone strength. It increases risk of bone fractures, particularly of the femoral neck (hip), radius

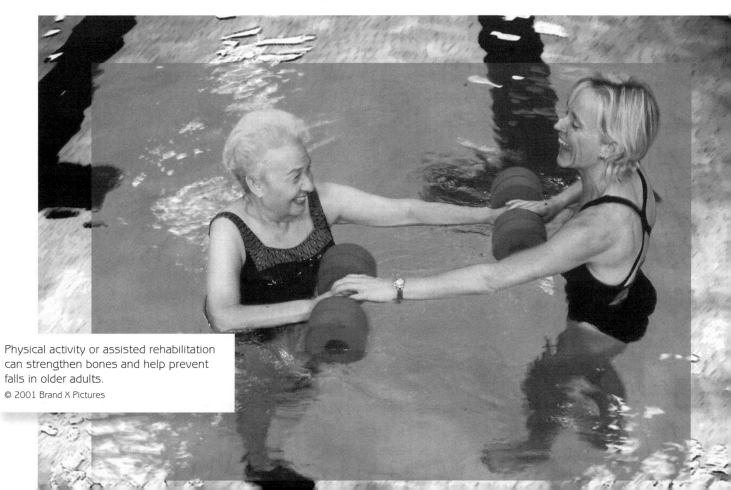

Physical activity or assisted rehabilitation can strengthen bones and help prevent falls in older adults.
© 2001 Brand X Pictures

Measuring the Volume of Physical Activity

The greater the volume of aerobic physical activity, the greater the health benefits. Measures of volume include these:

▶ Energy expenditure due to physical activity (in kilocalories or kilojoules). This measure depends on body weight, because it takes more energy to move a heavier weight. But it is a useful measure to describe individual bouts of activity as well as average levels of activity over time.

▶ Physical activity level, or PAL. PAL is defined as total energy expenditure (TEE) divided by basal metabolic rate (BMR). Although body weight influences TEE and BMR, dividing one by the other minimizes the effect of body weight on PAL. PAL is useful for describing average physical activity over time but not individual bouts. (Note that people do not live a 24-hour day totally at rest without eating [a PAL of 1.0], so an inactive lifestyle has a PAL of 1.3-1.5).

▶ MET-minutes (or MET-hours). A MET (metabolic equivalent) is the ratio of the work metabolic rate to the BMR. So a 4-MET activity expends 4 times the energy used by the body at rest. If you perform a 4-MET activity for 30 minutes, you've done 4 × 30 = 120 MET-minutes of activity. Activities are assigned MET values based on the typical (or average) MET value when people perform the activity. For example, a MET value typically used for walking at 3.0 miles per hour is 3.3 METs. This measure is useful to describe individual bouts of activity and average levels of activity.

(wrist), and vertebra (spine). Incidence of osteoporotic fractures increases with age and is higher in women (USDHHS, 2004). Osteoporotic hip fractures are a major cause of disability in older adults; a fall to the ground is the proximal cause of hip fractures in most cases.

Inactive adults have a 60 percent higher risk of osteoporosis (table 1.1). Because bone is formed according to the stress (load) placed on it, it is not surprising that physical activity can strengthen bone and slow age-related bone loss. Accordingly, the aerobic intensity of an activity is not directly relevant to the beneficial effect of physical activity on bone strength; rather, it is bone-loading effect of the activity. Weight-bearing activity is recommended for the prevention of osteoporosis, as is muscle-strengthening activity (PAGAC, 2008). High-impact activities (such as small jumps) are also effective in increasing bone strength.

Physical activity reduces falls in older adults (USDHHS, 2004). Randomized trials report that in older adults at increased risk of falls, exercise reduces risk as much as 50 percent (Robertson et al., 2002). These exercise programs typically involve aerobic activity like walking, weight lifting, and balance exercises.

Colon Cancer and Breast Cancer

Cancer is a condition characterized by unregulated growth of cells. As cancer cells grow, they invade surrounding tissue and metastasize (spread) to other parts of the body (Centers for Disease Control and Prevention, 2009). Breast cancer in women and colon cancer in adults are two of the most common cancers (Centers for Disease Control and Prevention, n.d.).

Regular physical activity reduces risk of colon cancer by about 30 percent (PAGAC, 2008), with some evidence of a dose–response effect. Physical activity reduces risk of breast cancer by approximately 20 percent (PAGAC, 2008). There are plausible mechanisms for the risk reduction. These include beneficial effects of physical activity on hormones, growth factors, body fat, and immune function (Lee and Oguma, 2006). For example, breast cancer risk is increased by higher exposure of breast tissue to estrogen. There is evidence that physical activity reduces estrogen levels in both premenopausal and postmenopausal women (Lee and Oguma, 2006). It has been further hypothesized that lower rates of colon cancer may be due to an increased intestinal transit time that reduces the risk of exposure to carcinogens in the intestinal track of persons who are physically active compared with those who are not (Lee and Oguma, 2006).

Mental Health

Most of the research on physical activity and mental health deals with the broad categories of depression and anxiety disorders, which contain several subcategories of mental illnesses. Two common and important conditions are major depression and generalized anxiety. Major depression is characterized by a constellation of symptoms that occur for a period of at least two weeks and represent a negative change in functioning, most notably depressed mood and loss of interest or pleasure in life (American Psychiatric Association, 1994). Depression, in its most severe form, can lead to suicide. Symptoms of major depression include increase or decrease in appetite, increase or decrease in sleep, fatigue, weight loss or gain, recurrent thoughts of death, low self-esteem, and difficulty concentrating (American Psychiatric Association, 2000). The cause of depression involves a complex interaction of biological and psychosocial factors and is not completely understood (USDHHS, 1999). Biologically, depression involves alterations in brain neurotransmitters (chemicals that affect how brain cells interrelate), including serotonin. In animal studies, physical activity has been found to alter neurotransmitters that may remediate depression (Dishman et al., 2004). Regular physical activity reduces risk and symptoms of depression in humans (Dishman et al., 2004; Martinsen and Morgan, 1997; PAGAC, 2008; Sjosten and Sivela, 2006).

Generalized anxiety disorder is primarily characterized by excessive worry and anxiety that occur for more days than not in a 6-month period, are difficult to control, and lead to clinically significant distress or impairment in functioning (American Psychiatric Association, 2000). Associated symptoms include restlessness, fatigue, sleep disturbance, and difficulty concentrating (American Psychiatric Association, 2000). Physical activity is associated with reduced symptoms of anxiety (Dishman et al., 2004; Raglin, 1997).

Other mental health benefits of physical activity are improved quality of sleep (Guilleminault et al., 1995; King et al., 1997; King et al., 2002; Tworoger et al., 2003; PAGAC, 2008; Youngstedt et al., 1997), quality of life, psychological well-being, and self-esteem or self-efficacy (Biddle et al., 2000; McAuley et al., 2006; Netz et al., 2005). These benefits are mild to moderate. Physical activity also appears to increase feelings of energy and reduce feelings of fatigue. For example, one meta-analytic review found that physically active adults have increased feelings of energy and decreased feelings of fatigue compared with control subjects (Puetz et al., 2006).

Physical activity reduces risk of colon and breast cancers.

Cognition and Brain Health

Dementia refers to a group of disorders that cause cognitive impairment and mainly occur in older adults. Alzheimer's disease is the most common dementia, characterized by abnormal proteins in brain neurons that lead to death of the neurons. Vascular dementia refers to a group of diseases that cause dementia by affecting blood vessels in the brain.

Several observational studies report that active older adults have reduced risk of cognitive decline (Weuve et al., 2004; Yaffe et al., 2001) and dementia (Abbott et al., 2004; Larson et al., 2006; Taaffe et al., 2008). Some of these studies are specific just to prevention of Alzheimer's disease (Heyn et al., 2004; Lindsay et al., 2002). Studies report that physical activity affects blood flow to the brain and brain mass (Rogers et al., 1990). Increased blood flow and, therefore, oxygen to the brain may be one mechanism leading to improved cognitive functioning, but mechanisms remain unknown (Kramer et al., 2003). Although there is evidence that physical activity prevents or delays cognitive decline associated with aging (PAGAC, 2008), questions remain about the biologic mechanisms that account for the preventive effect (Kramer et al., 2003).

Other Preventive Health Effects

Physical activity may prevent diseases in addition to those already discussed. There is increasing evidence that physical activity is associated with a reduced risk of endometrial cancer and lung cancer (Lee and Oguma, 2006; PAGAC, 2008). There is also evidence that physical activity improves the function of the immune system and thereby reduces risk of infections (Karper and Hopewell, 1998; Kostka et al., 2000; Mackinnon, 2000; Matthews et al., 2002). A few studies suggest that moderate levels of physical activity, particularly walking, may be associated with a reduced risk of knee osteoarthritis (Felson et al., 2007; Hart et al., 1999; Hootman et al., 2003; Rogers et al., 2002). There is less research on the benefits of physical activity on a variety of mental health conditions compared with those discussed previously. However, some studies suggest that future research could prove that physical activity reduces risk of a variety of mental health problems. Consider data from a cross-sectional study of several mental health problems: Currently, for several of these conditions, the causal data are inconclusive as to whether regular physical activity reduces risk of the disease. This study used a survey to assess the presence of mental health problems and level of physical activity (see figure 1.3). The data show a dose–response effect between level of activity and estimated prevalence of mental health conditions.

Health Benefits of Physical Activity in Children

The approach for considering the health benefits of physical activity in children differs from that of adults. Although a few chronic diseases occur in both children and adults (e.g., obesity and type 2 diabetes), children and youth are not at risk for developing most chronic diseases of adulthood. Still, physical activity might delay or prevent the earliest stages and risk factors of some of these diseases during childhood. Also, physical activity provides health benefits to children through promoting healthy growth and development.

A panel of experts recently reviewed the scientific research on the benefits of physical activity in children and youth (Strong et al, 2005; PAGAC, 2008). There was strong evidence that physical activity increases aerobic fitness, muscle strength,

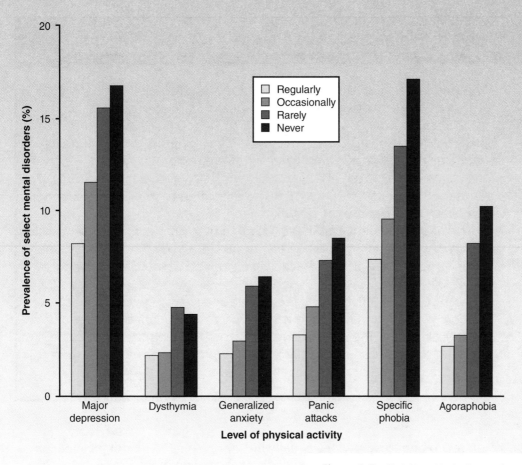

Figure 1.3 Relationship between frequency of physical activity and current mental health problems. The bars indicate the percentage of adults in the United States with select mental disorders by level of physical activity.

Data from R.D. Goodwin, 2003, "Association between physical activity and mental disorders among adults in the United States," *Preventive Medicine* 36:698-703.

and bone strength in children. Physical activity places children on the path of developing higher peak bone mass in young adulthood, which is important to delaying or preventing osteoporosis in later life.

The evidence was adequate for concluding that physical activity improves blood pressure, lipoproteins, adiposity, cardiovascular health, and some aspects of mental health in children (Strong et al., 2005; PAGAC, 2008). The aspects of mental health affected by physical activity include anxiety, depression, and self-concept (how a child perceives herself on attributes such as appearance, social skills, and competence in sports). There was only limited evidence for concluding that physical activity decreased risk of childhood asthma, and there were few data on risk of activity-related injury in young children (Strong et al., 2005).

Prevention of Functional Limitations and Disability

The hallmark of aging is loss of capacity in the physiologic systems of the body. In young and middle-aged adults, physiologic capacity is typically in excess of what

Academic Performance and Physical Activity in Children

There is considerable interest in whether physical activity in children improves academic performance. It is clear that regular physical activity in children improves physical fitness and hence physical performance on tasks like running a race. It is less clear whether physical activity improves mental fitness and hence cognitive performance (e.g., performance on standardized achievement tests). However, a growing body of literature suggests that physically active children have higher academic performance (Strong et al., 2005).

There is no evidence that allocating curricular time to physical education in school has a negative effect on academic performance, even when time allotted to other academic subjects is reduced (Strong et al., 2005; PAGAC, 2008). There is a national health **objective** *Healthy People 2010* objective 22-8 (see the Introduction), to increase the proportion of schools that require daily physical education for all students. Specifically, then, there is no evidence that achieving this objective will have an adverse effect on academic performance in children, and it quite possibly could have a beneficial effect.

is required to perform activities of daily life. As age-related loss of physiologic capacity continues into old age, physiologic capacity commonly drops below levels necessary for performing activities of daily life and living independently, and this change produces limitations or disability. Problems in physical performance in older adults, such as difficulty walking and climbing stairs, are typically described as problems with "functioning." We use the term *physical functional limitations* to refer to loss of ability to perform physical tasks of daily life. Such limitations are considered a disability if the loss also results in an inability to participate in social roles.

We now know that age-related loss of physiologic capacity is due in large part to disease and lifestyle factors instead of normal aging. Observational studies consistently show that physically active older adults are at lower risk of developing physical functional limitations (Hillsdon et al., 2005; Huang et al., 1998; Leveille et al., 1999; Ostbye et al., 2002). For example, a major study called EPESE (Established Populations for Epidemiologic Studies of the Elderly) reported that active older adults who survive to very old age have almost a twofold increase in dying without a disability than sedentary adults who survive to old age (Leveille et al., 1999). Randomized controlled trials of exercise in older adults confirm a beneficial effect of exercise on functional limitations (Binder et al., 2002; Campbell et al., 1997; Lord et al., 2003; Luukinen et al., 2006). Although the size of the effect is modest in some studies, most exercise studies in older adults prescribe a year or less of exercise. It is likely that several years of regular physical activity has a greater effect on functional limitations. Observational studies, which can assess the impact of regular physical activity over many years, report that regular physical activity is associated with a large reduction in risk of functional limitations (PAGAC, 2008).

Therapeutic Exercise

Physical activity has important therapeutic effects (Durstine, 1997; Frontera et al., 2006). Physical activity is recommended as part of treatment for many diseases and conditions, including coronary heart disease, type 2 diabetes, chronic lung disease, osteoporosis, obesity, some lipid disorders, hypertension, osteoarthritis, and stroke rehabilitation. Physical activity is also recommended as part of the management of depressive illness, dementia, pain syndromes, congestive heart failure, back pain, and constipation, conditions that are common in older adults. Thus, the importance of physical activity in older adults relates to both its preventive and its therapeutic effects. Therapeutic exercise is typically individually prescribed to patients by health care providers and administered by exercise physiologists, physical therapists, or athletic trainers. It is not part of a community-wide or population-based public health approach.

Perspective on Physical Activity Risks

Although regular physical activity has numerous health benefits, it also has some risks. Therefore, the promotion of physical activity needs to include risk management strategies to prevent injuries and maximize the net benefit of physical activity.

From a public health standpoint, the most important risk of physical activity is musculoskeletal injury. These are the most common injuries, and every physically active person is at risk for them. These injuries act as barriers to regular physical activity for some people. Common musculoskeletal injuries include overuse injuries (such as tendinitis) and traumatic injuries (such as ankle sprains). Unfortunately, there is not much information on injury rates in people who perform moderate amounts of activity. One study suggested that musculoskeletal injuries affect 20 to 30 percent of active adults in a year (Hootman et al., 2002). However, inactive adults also have musculoskeletal injuries like ankle sprains, and about 15 percent of inactive people in the same study had musculoskeletal injuries. Most activity-related injuries are minor, and the risk of injury is modifiable, demonstrating that the benefits of activity far outweigh the risks.

Three other risks of physical activity are important, but not all active adults are at equal risk. In people with heart disease, heart attacks are more likely to occur during bouts of physical activity, particularly vigorous activity. However, heart attacks during physical activity are rare (Thompson et al., 2007), and overall physical activity protects against heart attack. That is, although people are more likely to have a heart attack during vigorous activity, overall a physically active person is less likely to have a heart attack than an inactive person (Thompson et al. 2007).

Women who perform high levels of physical activity are at risk for menstrual dysfunction, including loss of menses. Sustained disruption of regular menses by exercise produces loss of bone tissue and predisposes a woman to osteoporosis. However, menstrual function can be restored by modest weight gain and reduction in the level of physical activity (Goodman and Warren, 2005; Nattiv et al., 2007).

Finally, upper-respiratory infections are more common in adults with very high levels of physical activity, such as occur during events like marathons (Mackinnon, 2000). The public health significance of this finding is uncertain. Few people perform such high amounts of physical activity, and permanent morbidity from upper-respiratory infections is uncommon.

Conclusion

Regular physical activity is an essential component of a healthy lifestyle. Moderate amounts of physical activity produce substantial health benefits. The benefits of physical activity are extensive and include reductions in the risk of many common chronic diseases, such as cardiovascular disease, colon cancer, breast cancer, osteoporosis, obesity, and type 2 diabetes. Physical activity reduces symptoms of anxiety and depression and reduces risk factors for cardiovascular disease, such as hypertension and high cholesterol. Physical activity promotes healthy growth and development in children, such as improving bone health, increasing physical fitness, and reducing the risk of obesity. Physical activity has important therapeutic benefits and reduces the risk of functional limitations, falls, and disability in older adults. It is likely that all the health benefits of physical activity are not yet known; some health benefits (e.g., prevention of dementia, prevention of prostate cancer) are probable but the evidence is not conclusive. Although there are risks to physical activity, for the most part it is safe and can be promoted in a way to minimize risks by using risk management strategies (PAGAC, 2008; USDHHS, 2008).

Resources

Hardman AE, Stensel DJ. 2003. *Physical Activity and Health: The Evidence Explained.* London & New York: Rutledge.

Kesaniemi YA, Danforth E, Jensen MD, Kopelman PG, Lefebvre P, Reeder BA. 2001. Dose-response issues concerning physical activity and health: an evidence-based symposium. *Medicine and Science in Sports and Exercise* 33(6 suppl): S351-S358.

U.S. Department of Health & Human Services, Physical Activity Guidelines. www.health.gov/PAGuidelines/

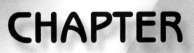
Physical Activity Recommendations

Janet E. Fulton and Harold W. Kohl III

This chapter reviews national health objectives and recommendations for physical activity and presents current information on public health guidelines for physical activity for adults, older adults, and children and adolescents. A large portion of this chapter describes the most current U.S. guidelines for physical activity, contained in the *2008 Physical Activity Guidelines for Americans* (U.S. Department of Health & Human Services [USDHHS], 2008), which is the first document of its kind. After you read this chapter you will be familiar with the background and rationale for developing physical activity recommendations and guidelines as well as with the *2008 Physical Activity Guidelines for Americans* themselves as they pertain to several populations:

Adults

Older adults

Children and adolescents

Healthy People 2010: National Health Promotion and Disease Prevention Objectives Related to Physical Activity and Physical Fitness

Healthy People is the name of the initiative the United States uses to develop and track national health objectives. Health objectives are developed for the entire population and also for subpopulations such as racial or ethnic groups, age groups, or groups differing by level of educational attainment or disability status. As you learned in the introduction, A National Call to Promote Physical Activity, physical activity is one of 28 focus areas that are part of the *Healthy People 2010* objectives (USDHHS, 2000). Physical activity was selected as a leading health indicator, illustrating its public health importance and relevance to population and individual health. Listed in the introduction are five objectives for physical activity and fitness for adults (including one related to muscular strength and one related to flexibility), six objectives for children and adolescents, and four objectives about access to places to be physically active. Next, we explore recommended amounts of physical activity that the *Healthy People 2010* objectives address.

Physical Activity Recommendations for Adults— Historical Considerations

With a large scientific base on which to draw, professional organizations began in the mid-1970s to make official declarations for recommended amounts and types of exercise or physical activity, with separate publications from the American Heart Association (AHA, 1972, 1975) and the American College of Sports Medicine (ACSM, 1978). At the time, more than 20 years had elapsed since the original research publication from Dr. Jeremy Morris on London bus drivers and conductors. In this work, Dr. Morris and colleagues showed that the conductors, who were more occupationally active than the drivers, had a lower risk of fatal and nonfatal heart attack (Morris et al., 1953). A flurry of prospective studies in the interim, including U.S. railroad workers (Taylor et al., 1962), San Francisco longshoremen (Paffenbarger and Hale, 1975), and college alumni (Paffenbarger et al., 1978), started to firmly establish physical inactivity as a risk factor for the development of heart disease.

This rapidly developing science base, as well as clinical practice changes in cardiology and the rehabilitation of patients after a cardiac event, influenced the publication of the first set of exercise guidelines (AHA, 1972). In the mid-1970s these guidelines were clinically oriented and directed specifically toward exercise

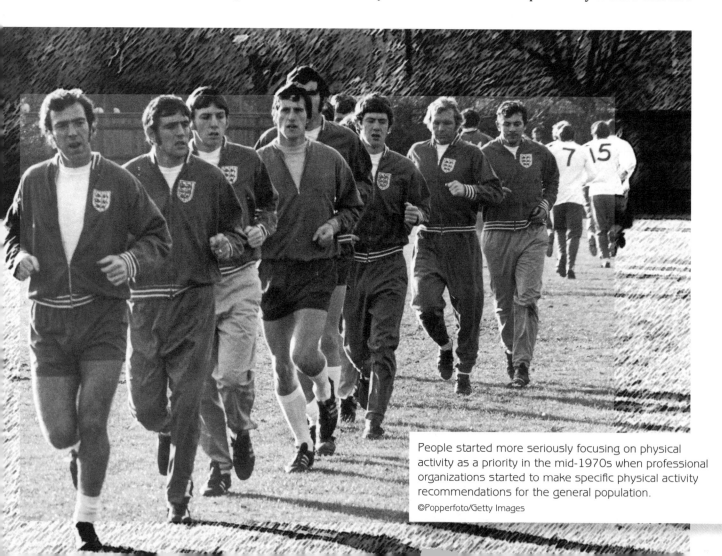

People started more seriously focusing on physical activity as a priority in the mid-1970s when professional organizations started to make specific physical activity recommendations for the general population.
©Popperfoto/Getty Images

specialists and physicians for clinical practice. Here, the idea of the exercise prescription was born. Early sets of exercise recommendations were very precise in terms of type, frequency, intensity, and duration of the exercise. Moreover, they relied largely on the premise that higher levels of exercise training would generally result in higher levels of physical fitness.

In 1978, the American College of Sports Medicine released a position statement on the recommended quantity and quality of exercise for developing and maintaining fitness in healthy adults (ACSM, 1978). These recommendations called for

- a frequency of exercise training of 3 to 5 days per week,
- an intensity of training equivalent to 60 to 90 percent of maximum heart rate,
- a duration of 15 to 60 minutes per training session, and
- the rhythmic and aerobic use of large muscle groups through activities such as running or jogging, walking or hiking, swimming, skating, bicycling, rowing, cross-country skiing, and rope skipping.

As science progressed in the 1980s, the dose–response relationship between physical activity and, in particular, coronary heart disease became clearer (Powell et al., 1987). It was recognized that levels of physical activity that are less intense than recommended by the exercise prescription approach were also related to health and beneficial health outcomes. Continued prospective studies of physical activity in several populations helped lead to the understanding that substantial individual and population health benefits might be realized with physical activity participation at a dose that was lower than the clinical exercise prescription guidelines from the American Heart Association and the American College of Sports Medicine. These emerging data, combined with the existing physical activity **surveillance** data at the time (which suggested that fewer than 10 percent of U.S. adults were active enough to meet the clinical exercise recommendations), led to a union between professionals in exercise science and public health, resulting in the emergence of the field of physical activity and public health.

The foundation on which the field of physical activity and public health was based represented a major shift from the early days of exercise guidelines for clinical practice. Rather than recommending exercise for cardiovascular fitness and performance, the new **model** focused on recommending physical activity for its beneficial relationship with several health outcomes. This new model was fed by ongoing scientific studies, both laboratory based and population based, in the late 1980s and early 1990s. The influence of public health was also very important at the time, with the recognition that population-wide benefits in health might be achieved with relatively small increases in physical activity levels in the population. With such a large proportion of the population sedentary, it was clear this group could benefit from increases in physical activity.

In 1995, physical activity recommendations from the Centers for Disease Control and Prevention (CDC) and the ACSM, written by Pate and colleagues (1995), created a paradigm shift. The recommendations moved away from an emphasis on physical performance and toward an emphasis on promoting physical activity to improve health. The main **goal** of these recommendations was to frame the need for physical activity as a public health issue rather than a solely individual clinical or therapeutic one or even as one related to athleticism. These recommendations stated that "every U.S. adult should accumulate 30 minutes or more of moderate-intensity physical activity on most, preferably all, days of the week" (Pate et al., 1995, p. 402). Achievement of this recommended level of physical activity will substantially improve health and lower the risk of the diseases and conditions discussed in chapter 1. A key part of the recommendations was the acknowledgment of the dose–response **association** between physical activity and several health outcomes; the recommendations stated that higher levels of physical activity were associated with even greater health benefits. The 30-minute recommendation was meant as a minimum amount of physical activity for health benefits.

The *Surgeon General's Report on Physical Activity and Health* (USDHHS, 1996) built on the CDC/ACSM recommendations by providing a thorough scientific review and summary of the physical activity research through 1996. It is an excellent resource for physical activity and public health professionals that includes chapters on the historical background of the field, physiologic responses and **adaptations** to exercise, effects of physical activity on health and disease, patterns and trends in physical activity, and promotion of physical activity.

The CDC/ACSM recommendation was updated in a joint recommendation issued by the ACSM and the AHA (Haskell et al., 2007; Nelson et al., 2007). The CDC/ACSM (Pate et al., 1995) recommendation remained essentially unchanged but was clarified in the new ACSM/AHA recommendation. For example, the CDC/ACSM recommendation encouraged adults to engage in moderate-intensity physical activity on most, preferably all, days of the week. This recommendation raises the question about whether most days of the week means 4 days or 5 days. The ACSM/AHA (Haskell et al., 2007) recommendation specifically states that "adults aged 18 to 65 need moderate-intensity aerobic (endurance) physical activity for a minimum of 30 minutes on five days of each week" (p. 1423). The ACSM/AHA recommendation also places greater emphasis on the benefits of strength (resistance) training than the original 1995 recommendation and encourages adults to engage in a minimum of 2 days a week of resistance training.

Overview of Current Physical Activity Guidelines for Adults

The first comprehensive U.S. physical activity guidelines were released in October 2008 (USDHHS, 2008). The *2008 Physical Activity Guidelines for Americans* provide physical activity-specific guidelines for the U.S. population and are novel in several respects: (1) They are based on a comprehensive, evidence-based review of physical activity and health by a federally appointed expert committee (PAGAC, 2008). (2) They provide physical activity guidance for several population groups: children and adolescents, healthy adults and older adults, pregnant and postpartum women, and people with disabilities and chronic conditions. (3) They identify health benefits, specify the amounts necessary to get the benefits, and provide a bridge to physical activity promotion. (4) Unlike some previous guidelines and recommendations, they provide guidance for nonaerobic activities such as muscle and bone strengthening, flexibility, and balance. (5) They provide a range of physical activity: The more you do, the more benefits you gain. (6) They specify for adults a total amount of activity per week, allowing people the flexibility to design their own way to meet the guidelines.

Current Physical Activity Guidelines for Adults

The four key guidelines for adults are shown in the sidebar on page 25. The first guideline is to avoid being inactive; some health benefits are gained with even small amounts of physical activity. Aerobic and muscle-strengthening activities, however, comprise the key types of activities specified in the guidelines.

Aerobic Physical Activity Guidelines

The guidelines recommend that to achieve substantial health benefits, a person should undertake 150 minutes per week of **moderate-intensity physical activity,**

75 minutes per week of vigorous-intensity physical activity, or an equivalent combination of both. To achieve more extensive health benefits, a person should perform 300 or more minutes per week of moderate-intensity activity, 150 minutes per week of vigorous-intensity activity, or an equivalent combination of both. Although both moderate- and vigorous-intensity activities count toward meeting the aerobic guidelines, time spent in vigorous-intensity activity counts roughly twice that spent in moderate-intensity activity; for example, engaging in 150 minutes of vigorous-intensity activity is equivalent to engaging in 300 minutes of moderate-intensity activity. Healthy adults who find it difficult to meet the guidelines because of time constraints may wish to substitute vigorous-intensity aerobic activity for some moderate-intensity aerobic activity.

Muscle Strengthening Guideline

Muscle-strengthening activities enhance skeletal muscle mass, strength, power, and neuromuscular activation (PAGAC, 2008). For these reasons, muscle strengthening is an important physical activity guideline for adults (sidebar). Adults should strengthen all seven muscle groups (legs, hips, back, chest, abdomen, shoulders, and arms) on at least 2 days of the week. The guidelines do not specify that muscle strengthening be undertaken on nonconsecutive days. Participants should use the overload principle to strengthen muscles, that is, make the muscles do more work

Physical Activity Guidelines for Adults, *2008 Physical Activity Guidelines for Americans*

▸ All adults should avoid inactivity. Some physical activity is better than none, and adults who participate in any amount of physical activity gain some health benefits.

▸ For substantial health benefits, adults should engage in at least 150 minutes (2 hours and 30 minutes) a week of moderate-intensity aerobic physical activity, or 75 minutes (1 hour and 15 minutes) a week of vigorous-intensity aerobic physical activity, or an equivalent combination of moderate- and vigorous-intensity aerobic activity. Aerobic activity should be performed in episodes of at least 10 minutes, preferably spread throughout the week.

▸ For additional and more extensive health benefits, adults should increase their aerobic physical activity to 300 minutes (5 hours) a week of moderate-intensity aerobic physical activity, or 150 minutes a week of vigorous-intensity aerobic physical activity, or an equivalent combination of moderate-and vigorous-intensity activity. Additional health benefits are gained by engaging in physical activity beyond this amount.

▸ Adults should perform muscle-strengthening activities that are moderate or high intensity and involve all major muscle groups on 2 or more days a week, because these activities provide additional health benefits.

Taken from the 2008 Physical Activity Guidelines for Americans (http://health.gov/paguidelines/)

than they are accustomed to doing. To overload the muscle, a person must lift more weight than she is accustomed to and continue lifting until unable to perform another repetition without help. The intensity of muscle strengthening refers to how much weight or force is used relative to how much a person is able to lift.

Scientific evidence shows that muscle strengthening can occur with one set (or series) of 8 to 12 repetitions (number of times a person lifts a weight) per muscle group. One set is sufficient to increase muscular strength, although performing two or three sets may be more effective. There are many ways to strengthen muscles: working with resistance bands, using weight machines, or performing exercises that use one's body weight (such as push-ups, pull-ups, and sit-ups). Increases in the amount of weight lifted or the number of days of training per week will result in stronger muscles.

What's New About the *2008 Physical Activity Guidelines for Americans?*

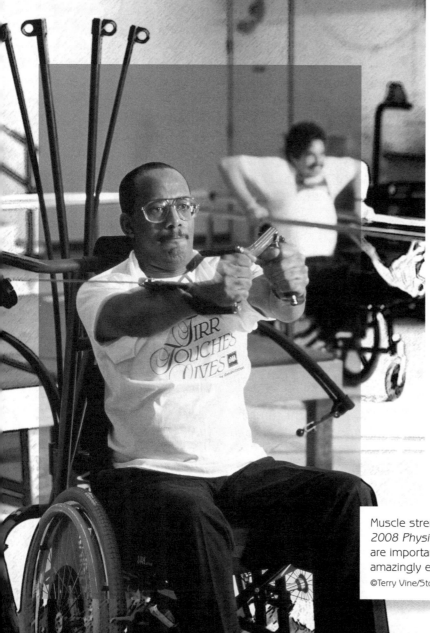

Compared with previous recommendations and guidelines developed over the years (described earlier), the 2008 guidelines offer people flexibility in ways they can meet their activity requirements. For example, the adult guidelines do not specify a minimum number of days per week for aerobic activity, although it is recommended that adults participate in activity that is spread throughout the week. Why is this? Because there is insufficient scientific evidence to recommend a minimum frequency (days per week) of activity associated with health benefits, but, in terms of behavior, it is important to encourage people to develop a habitual pattern of physical activity participation. The guidelines strongly endorse muscle strengthening but not some features typical of training programs; for example, there is no requirement for strength training on nonconsecutive days. There is also a clear statement in the guidelines that *healthy* children and adults do not need physician approval or consultation prior to engaging in physical activity.

Muscle strengthening activities, as explained in the *2008 Physical Activity Guidelines for Americans*, are important for all adults, and weight training is amazingly effective for increasing strength.
©Terry Vine/Stone/Getty Images

Physical Activity Prescription

Some key concepts of the physical activity prescription (frequency, intensity, duration) are important in implementing the guidelines. First, the prescription for aerobic physical activity in the guidelines is based on a total weekly volume of moderate- or vigorous-intensity physical activity. Physical activity volume is the product of frequency (episodes per week—often expressed as days per week), intensity (level of effort—often expressed as an individual's perception of effort as being light, moderate, or vigorous intensity or as a multiple of resting energy expenditure, known as a MET), and duration (time per episode). After reviewing the scientific evidence, a federal advisory committee determined the total volume of aerobic activity to be most related to health—more so than any one component of the physical activity prescription. Next, in the older adult guidelines, intensity is defined in two ways: absolute intensity and relative intensity. Absolute intensity is based on the rate of energy expenditure during the activity, without taking into account a person's **cardiorespiratory fitness**. Absolute intensity is commonly based on the type of activity a person is doing. For example, jogging is generally considered a vigorous-intensity activity, whereas brisk walking is typically considered to be moderate-intensity activity. Relative intensity uses a person's level of cardiorespiratory fitness to assess level of effort. One way to gauge relative intensity is to use a scale of 0 to 10 where sitting is 0 and the highest level of effort possible is 10. On this scale, the level of effort for performing moderate-intensity activity is a 5 or 6 and for vigorous-intensity activity is a 7 or 8. Another way to gauge relative intensity is by using the "talk test." A person engaging in moderate-intensity aerobic activity should be able to talk, but not sing, during the activity. A person undertaking vigorous-intensity activity should not be able to say more than a few words without pausing for a breath. In terms of relative intensity, brisk walking may be a vigorous-intensity activity for an unfit person or may be a moderate-intensity (or lower intensity) activity for a fit person.

More Is Better

The guidelines for aerobic physical activity for adults emphasize that there is not a minimal amount of physical activity for which all health benefits will accrue. Doing some physical activity is better than none. Meeting the minimal aerobic guideline goal of 150 minutes per week of moderate-intensity physical activity (or 75 minutes of vigorous-intensity activity, or the combined equivalent of moderate- and vigorous-intensity activity), however, will provide substantial health benefits like a lower risk of premature death, coronary heart disease, stroke, hypertension, type 2 diabetes, and depression. Achieving 300 minutes per week of moderate-intensity physical activity (or 150 minutes of vigorous-intensity activity, or the combined equivalent of moderate- and vigorous-intensity activity) will provide additional and more extensive health benefits, such as lowering one's risk of colon and breast cancer and preventing unhealthy weight gain.

Overweight and Obesity

Physical activity plays a role (along with intake of food and beverages) in energy balance and is important in maintaining a healthy body weight, losing excess body weight, or maintaining weight loss. There is variability, though, in the amount of physical activity a person needs to achieve and maintain a healthy weight. Some people need more physical activity than others to maintain a healthy body weight, to lose weight, or to keep weight off once it has been lost.

Strong scientific evidence shows that physical activity will help people maintain a stable weight over time; however, the amount of physical activity needed to maintain an optimal weight is unclear. To maintain weight for the long term, many people need more physical activity than the minimal amount recommended to achieve substantial health benefits—that is, the equivalent of 150 minutes per week of moderate-intensity physical activity. Scientific evidence shows over short periods of time (up to 1 year), performing the equivalent of 150 to 300 minutes per week of moderate-intensity physical activity may help a person maintain his weight.

To lose a substantial amount of weight (5 percent or more of body weight) or to keep a significant amount of weight off once it has been lost, many people need to perform more than the equivalent amount of 300 minutes per week of moderate-intensity aerobic activity to meet weight loss or weight control goals. Most of these people will need to reduce caloric intake as well as increase physical activity.

Flexibility

Scientific evidence shows neither a harmful nor a beneficial effect of engaging in flexibility activities. For this reason, undertaking flexibility activities and warm-up or cool-down activities is reasonable and acceptable but is not a specific guideline.

What Counts?

Physical activity must be of at least a moderate intensity to achieve health benefits. Time spent in light-intensity activities (such as light housework) and sedentary behaviors (such as watching TV) do not count toward meeting the aerobic physical activity guidelines. In addition, moderate-intensity activities must be done for at least 10 or more minutes at one time. For example, climbing flights of stairs, although usually of vigorous intensity, is typically done for less than 10 minutes at one time and therefore does not count toward meeting the aerobic guidelines. Efforts have been made to increase stair walking as part of a community-based intervention, as discussed in the Point-of-Decision Prompts subsection of chapter 3 (pp. 57-62), and similar efforts and other types of longer-duration activities are needed to help people achieve recommended amounts of physical activity.

Preventing Injuries and Adverse Events

The guidelines present recommendations for safe participation in physical activity to reduce injuries and to prevent adverse events. The key guidelines for safety emphasize the following: (1) choosing types of physical activity appropriate for one's current fitness level and health goals; (2) increasing physical activity gradually over time, where inactive people should "start low and go slow"; (3) using appropriate gear and sports equipment, locating **safe environments,** following rules and policies, and making sensible choices about when, where, and how to be active; and (4) being under the care of a health care provider if a person has chronic conditions or symptoms. People with chronic conditions and symptoms should consult their health care providers about the types and amounts of activity appropriate for them.

Adults With Disabilities

Adults with disabilities who are able to meet the adult aerobic and muscle-strengthening guidelines should be encouraged to do so. For adults with disabilities who are unable to meet the guidelines, the guidelines state the following:

When adults with disabilities are not able to meet the above Guidelines, they should avoid physical inactivity and be as physically active as their abilities safely allow. Adults with disabilities should consult their health care providers about the amounts and types of physical activity that are appropriate for their abilities.

Physical Activity Recommendations for Older Adults—Historical Considerations

Physical activity at recommended levels will improve and maintain health for all adults, including those age 50 and older. The 1995 CDC and ACSM recommendations (Pate et al., 1995) and the conclusions of the Surgeon General's report (USDHHS, 1996) applied to adults inclusive of older adults. In 1998, the American College of Sports Medicine (ACSM) issued a Position Stand, Exercise and Physical Activity for Older Adults, espousing the benefits of regular physical activity specific to this growing segment of the population.

As with the earlier recommendation for younger adults to promote and maintain health, the ACSM Position Stand indicates that older adults need moderate-intensity aerobic physical activity for a minimum of 30 minutes on 5 or more days each week or vigorous-intensity aerobic physical activity for a minimum of 20 minutes on 3 or more days each week (ACSM, 1998). Moderate-intensity aerobic activity can be accumulated by engaging in physical activity episodes lasting 10 or more minutes to achieve the 30-minute minimum. As is true for younger adults, this recommended amount of aerobic activity is in addition to routine activities of daily living of light intensity or lasting less than 10 minutes.

In 2007 (Nelson et al., 2007), the ACSM and American Heart Association published an additional recommendation for older adults that clarified and built upon earlier pronouncements. This recommendation again confirmed that older adults should obtain at least 30 minutes of moderate-intensity physical activity on 5 days each week or 20 minutes of vigorous-intensity activity on 3 days each week. However, it was also pointed out that persons can obtain the recommended amount of activity by combining both moderate- and vigorous-intensity activities. The recommendation also indicates that older adults should incorporate two or more nonconsecutive days of muscle-strengthening activity into their weekly activities, as well as at least two days of flexibility exercises. Further, it is recommended that older adults having a history of falling or mobility problems do activities that will help improve their balance.

The 1998 ACSM Position Stand was updated and published in 2009. The 2009 Position Stand on Exercise and Physical Activity for Older Adults embraces the above recommendation, as well as Guideline recommendations released in the *2008 Physical Activity Guidelines for Americans* (USDHHS, 2008) that are discussed in more detail below.

Aging brings additional health issues, and the science base regarding physical activity and health for older adults reflects these considerations (ACSM,1998, 2009; Cress et al., 2004; Nelson et al., 2007; PAGAC, 2008; Robert Wood Johnson Foundation, 2001). An important issue in physical activity recommendations for older adults is the definition of intensity. Given the heterogeneity of fitness levels in older adults, a relative intensity level, rather than an absolute intensity level, should be recognized. For example, for some older adults, a walk at a moderate intensity (enough to elicit physiologic responses to exercise) is slow (e.g., less than 3 miles per hour). For those who have a higher fitness level and are more active, walking at this pace would not elicit the same physiologic responses and thus would be classified as less than moderate intensity.

To further promote and maintain health, older adults should perform activities that maintain or increase muscular strength for a minimum of 2 days each week (ACSM, 1998, 2009; Nelson et al., 2007; USDHHS, 2008). Muscle-strengthening activities include a progressive weight training program, weight-bearing calisthenics, stair climbing, and resistance exercises that use the major muscle groups.

Participation in aerobic and muscle-strengthening activities above minimum recommended amounts provides additional health benefits and results in higher levels of physical fitness. For example, the ACSM position stand (ACSM, 1998) states its recommendation this way:

> With increasing muscle strength, increased levels of spontaneous activity have been seen in both healthy, free-living older subjects and very old and frail men and women. Strength training, in addition to its positive effects on insulin action, bone density, energy metabolism, and functional status, is also an important way to increase levels of physical activity in the elderly. (p. 996)

Older adults should exceed the minimum recommended amounts of physical activity if they have no conditions that preclude higher amounts of physical activity and they wish to do one or more of the following: (a) improve their personal fitness, (b) improve management of an existing disease for which it is known that higher levels of physical activity have greater therapeutic benefits, or (c) further reduce their risk of premature mortality and chronic conditions related to physical inactivity. In addition, to help prevent unhealthy weight gain, some older adults may need to exceed minimum recommended amounts of physical activity to a point that is individually effective for energy balance, when considering diet and other factors that affect body weight.

Current Physical Activity Guidelines for Older Adults

The key guidelines for older adults (65 years and older) from the *2008 Physical Activity Guidelines for Americans* are shown in the sidebar. Older adults with no chronic health conditions should follow the adult guidelines. Older adults with one or more chronic conditions should talk with their health care provider to determine whether their condition limits their ability to perform regular physical activity. Such a conversation may help people learn about appropriate types and amounts of physical activity. When older adults cannot meet the guidelines because of health conditions, they should be as physically activity as their condition will allow.

Healthy older adults generally do not need to consult a health care provider before initiating moderate-intensity physical activity. However, health care providers can help people attain and maintain regular physical activity by providing advice on appropriate types of activities and ways to progress at a safe and steady pace.

Intensity

Older adults should use relative intensity to gauge their level of effort while being active, where the level of effort required to perform an activity is relative to a person's level of cardiorespiratory fitness. The physical capacity of older adults

Physical Activity Guidelines for Older Adults, *2008 Physical Activity Guidelines for Americans*

The following guidelines are the same for adults and older adults:

▶ All older adults should avoid inactivity. Some physical activity is better than none, and older adults who participate in any amount of physical activity gain some health benefits.

▶ For substantial health benefits, older adults should perform at least 150 minutes (2 hours and 30 minutes) a week of moderate-intensity aerobic physical activity, or 75 minutes (1 hour and 15 minutes) a week of vigorous-intensity aerobic physical activity, or an equivalent combination of moderate- and vigorous-intensity aerobic activity. Aerobic activity should be performed in episodes of at least 10 minutes and preferably should be spread throughout the week.

▶ For additional and more extensive health benefits, older adults should increase their aerobic physical activity to 300 minutes (5 hours) a week of moderate-intensity aerobic physical activity, or 150 minutes a week of vigorous-intensity aerobic physical activity, or an equivalent combination of moderate-and vigorous-intensity activity. Additional health benefits are gained by engaging in physical activity beyond this amount.

▶ Older adults should also engage in muscle-strengthening activities that are moderate or high intensity and involve all major muscle groups on 2 or more days a week, because these activities provide additional health benefits.

The following guidelines are just for older adults:

▶ When older adults cannot perform 150 minutes of moderate-intensity aerobic activity a week because of chronic conditions, they should be as physically active as their abilities and conditions allow.

▶ Older adults should engage in exercises that maintain or improve balance if they are at risk of falling.

▶ Older adults should determine their level of effort for physical activity relative to their level of fitness.

▶ Older adults with chronic conditions should understand whether and how their conditions affect their ability to engage in regular physical activity safely.

Taken from the 2008 Physical Activity Guidelines for Americans (http://health.gov/paguidelines/)

varies greatly—some older adults are able to jog several miles whereas others are only able to walk a few blocks. To achieve the guidelines, activity of at least a relatively moderate intensity is required (see description of relative intensity on p. 27 of this chapter).

Preventing Falls Through Balance and Flexibility Exercise

With aging comes decreased flexibility and balance and increased risk of falling. Older adults are at risk of falling if they have fallen before or if they have difficulty walking or take certain medications. For older adults at risk of falling, strong evidence shows that regular physical activity is safe and reduces the risk of falling. To help prevent falls and to reduce risk of injury from falls, an older adult should perform activities that maintain or increase flexibility and that maintain or improve balance (Cress et al., 2004; Nelson et al., 2007; USDHHS, 2008a).

Reducing the Risks of Falling

The guidelines recommend that to reduce falls, participants undertake balance and moderate-intensity muscle-strengthening activities for 90 minutes a week plus moderate-intensity walking for about 1 hour a week. Preferably, older adults at risk of falls should engage in balance training 3 or more days a week and do standardized exercises from a program demonstrated to reduce falls. Examples of these exercises include backward walking, sideways walking, heel walking, toe walking, and standing from a sitting position. To increase the difficulty of the exercises, participants progress from holding onto a stable support (like furniture) while performing the exercises to doing them without support. It is not known whether different combinations of type, amount, or frequency of activity can reduce falls to a greater degree. Tai chi exercises also can help prevent falls.

Tracking the Guidelines for Adults

Three health surveillance systems collect data about physical activity on a continual basis among a nationally representative sample of U.S. adults: the National Health Interview Survey (NHIS), the National Health and Nutrition Examination Survey (NHANES), and the Behavioral Risk Factor Surveillance System (BRFSS). Only the NHIS collects information to assess both the aerobic and muscle strengthening guidelines using the same data collection procedure and are collected annually. The BRFSS provides state-specific physical activity information for the 50 U.S. states and territories, which is generally considered to be a representative sample of U.S. adults. The BRFSS and NHANES do not include a question on muscle-strengthening activity and therefore cannot provide U.S. population information about the muscle strengthening guideline. If state-specific data on the proportion of U.S. adults meeting the muscle strengthening guideline are warranted, the BRFSS will need to be modified to include a muscle strengthening question as part of the questionnaire battery. See appendix B for more information on physical activity surveillance.

Physical Activity Recommendations for Children and Adolescents—Historical Considerations

Until recently, physical activity recommendations for youth were issued from several organizations and have generally been written for different audiences. Organizations have developed recommendations for both public health (ACSM, 2000; Byers et al., 2002; Corbin & Pangrazzi, 1998; Health Canada, 2002a, 2002b; NASPE, 2000, 2004; National Academy of Sciences, 2002; NIH, 1996; National Physical Activity Guidelines for Australians, 1999; Pate et al., 1995, 1998; Sallis & Patrick 1994; U.S. Department of Agriculture, 2000) and clinical practice audiences (Agency for Healthcare Research and Quality, 1998; American Academy of Pediatrics, 1994; American Medical Association, 1996; CDC, 1997; Fletcher, 1997; Patrick et al., 2001; Williams et al., 2002; U.S. Preventive Services Task Force, 1996) that offer individuals and groups guidance about assessment and promotion of physical activity. Public health-directed recommendations often address the youth population at large, whereas clinical practice–directed recommendations focus on the individual patient and his or her family.

Fulton and colleagues (2004) examined physical activity recommendations for the youth population for both the public health and clinical communities (see table 2.1). In their review, the authors observed that recommendations written for the public health community were inconsistent, yet explicit, with most organizations (12 of 13; 92 percent) specifying recommended amounts of three of the four physical activity components (frequency, intensity, duration, and type) in their recommendation. Organizations encouraged volumes or amounts of daily moderate- to vigorous-intensity physical activity for youth ranging from 30 to 60 minutes or more.

School-age youth should participate daily in 60 minutes or more of moderate- to vigorous-intensity physical activity.

Fulton and colleagues (2004) found that recommendations written for clinical practice did not generally provide explicit data for physicians to use in assessing and counseling patients and their families. Although the intent of their review (Fulton et al., 2004) was not to select the "best" recommendation, the authors noted that the AHA Committee on Atherosclerosis, Hypertension, and Obesity in the Young (AHOY) recommendation (Williams et al., 2002) provides the clinician with information to assess physical activity and body composition. AHOY also provides the specific components of aerobic physical activity and strength training that physicians can recommend to the patient and family. AHOY recommends that for preschoolers, children, and adolescents, clinicians assess the activity level of the child and any changes in activity level, access to convenient places for activity, and time spent on sedentary behaviors (TV and video games). Psychosocial factors that might influence activity such as familial, socioeconomic, and environmental factors as well as familial attitudes might also be addressed during the patient–clinician encounter. Explicit recommendations, such as those from AHOY, provide the clinician with valuable information to use in conducting the clinical evaluation and counseling the patient and family for health promotion. Although yet to be evaluated, provision of detailed recommendations for the clinician may increase the likelihood of physical activity assessment and counseling in clinical settings (Williams et al., 2002).

In 2003, an expert panel was charged by CDC with reviewing the scientific evidence showing the association between physical activity and key health and functional outcomes among children and adolescents (Strong et al., 2005). The panel's main task was to develop a physical activity recommendation based on current scientific evidence. CDC officials hoped that experts from clinical medicine and public health could together develop recommendations that would harmonize the many different sets of existing recommendations and eventually help to bring clarity and consistency to the field. The experts reviewed the effect of physical activity on several health outcomes: academic performance, adiposity, asthma, cardiovascular health, injury, mental health, and musculoskeletal health. In their review, the panel noted that the majority of intervention studies used supervised programs of moderate- to vigorous-intensity physical activity of 30 to 45 minutes' duration 3 to 5 days per week. The panel, however, believed that a greater amount of physical activity would be necessary to achieve similar beneficial effects on health and behavioral outcomes under ordinary daily circumstances (typically intermittent and unsupervised activity). It was thus concluded that school-age youth should participate daily in 60 minutes or more of moderate- to vigorous-intensity physical activity that is developmentally appropriate, is enjoyable, and involves a variety of activities (Strong et al., 2005). The recommendation from the expert panel is consistent with the youth physical activity recommendation provided in the *2008 Physical Activity Guidelines for Americans* (sidebar on page 37) (USDHHS, 2008).

Table 2.1 Public Health Physical Activity and Physical Fitness Recommendations for Children and Adolescents

Organization and title of recommendation	Age group	Physical activity			Physical fitness		
		Compo-nents	Recommendation	Over-weight	Compo-nents	Recommendation	Over-weight
American Cancer Society American Cancer Society Guidelines on Nutrition and Physical Activity for Cancer Prevention (Byers et al., 2002)	Children, adolescents	Fr/I/D	At least 60 min, moderate to vigorous intensity, at least 5 days/week	NR	NR	NR	NR
American College of Sports Medicine *Guidelines for Exercise Testing and Prescription* (ACSM, 2000)	Children, adolescents	T	Amount and type individualized based on maturity, medical status, skill, and prior exercise	Yes	S	Weight loads allowing at least 8 repetitions/set for 1 or 2 sets Maximum of twice a week 8-10 different exercises including all major muscle groups Not to the point of severe muscular fatigue Avoid powerlifting and bodybuilding	NR
Australia, Common-wealth Department of Health and Aged Care *National Physical Activity Guidelines for Australians* (Common-wealth Department of Health and Aged Care, 1999)	Children, adolescents	Fr/I/T/D	30 min, moderate intensity, most or all days/week Enjoy some regular, vigorous-intensity activity	NR	NR	NR	NR
Health Canada *Canada's Physical Activity Guide for Children* (Health Canada, 2002a) *Canada's Physical Activity Guide for Youth* (Health Canada, 2002b)	Children, adolescents	Fr/I/T/D	Increase daily moderate-intensity activity in progressions of 20-60 min/month Increase daily vigorous intensity activity in progressions of 10-30 min/month Decrease current daily nonactive time in progressions of 30-90 min/month	NR	S/Fl	Combine age-appropriate strength and flexibility activities	NR
Health Education Authority, United Kingdom *Critique of Existing Guidelines for Physical Activity in Young People* (Pate et al., 1998)	Children, adolescents	Fr/I/T/D	60 min, at least moderate intensity (5-8 METs, 40-60% of $\dot{V}O_2$max), nearly every day Types, intensity, and duration of physical activity that are psy-chologically and behav-iorally developmentally appropriate	NR	S	At least twice a week Strength activities emphasizing trunk and upper-extremity activities for young children that involve climbing, gym-nastics, and calisthenics; for adolescents, super-vised resistance training program acceptable	NR

Organization and title of recommendation	Age group	Physical activity		Over-weight	Physical fitness		Over-weight
		Compo-nents	Recommendation		Compo-nents	Recommendation	
International Consensus Conference on Physical Activity Guidelines for Adolescents *Physical Activity Guidelines for Adolescents: Consensus Statement* (Sallis and Patrick, 1994)	Adolescents	Fr/I/T/D	Daily physical activity as part of lifestyle activities At least 20 min, continuous moderate to vigorous intensity, at least 3 sessions/week	Yes	NR	NR	NR
National Association of Sport and Physical Education *Physical Activity for Children: A Statement of Guidelines* (Corbin and Pangrazi, 1998)	Children	Fr/I/T/D	Age and developmentally appropriate activity: ▶ 30-60 min on most or all days ▶ Accumulate ≥60 min/day ▶ At least 10-15 min periods of moderate- to vigorous-intensity activity Discourage long periods of inactivity	NR	S/Fl	Ages 5-9: minimal calisthenics, formal resistance training not recommended; active play activities rather than specific exercises to develop flexibility Ages 10-12: formal weight training acceptable, although other activities are generally better, including activities that require children to move and lift their own body weight; age-appropriate flexibility exercises or activities	NR
National Association of Sport and Physical Education *Physical Activity for Children: A Statement of Guidelines for Children ages 5 - 12* (NASPE, 2004)	Children	Fr/I/T/D	Age and developmentally appropriate activity: ▶ Accumulate at least 60 min, and up to several hours, on all or most days, including moderate- and vigorous-intensity physical activity with majority of time spent in intermittent activity ▶ Several bouts lasting 15 min or more each day ▶ Variety of age-appropriate physical activity to achieve optimal health, wellness, fitness, and performance benefits Discourage extended periods of inactivity (<2 hr)	NR	S/Fl	*Young children:* climbing, jumping, doing stunts, tumbling, and developmentally appropriate calisthenics *Older children:* calisthenics, resistance exercises with exercise bands, resistance training with light equipment, and regular stretching	NR

(continued)

Table 2.1 *(continued)*

Organization and title of recommendation	Age group	Physical activity				Physical fitness		
		Compo-nents	Recommendation	Over-weight	Compo-nents	Recommendation	Over-weight
National Association of Sport and Physical Education *Active Start: A State-ment of Physical Activity Guidelines for Children Birth to Five Years* (NASPE, 2002)	Infants, toddlers, preschool-ers	Fr/T/D	Infants: explore environ-ment, develop move-ment skills, involve large muscle groups Toddlers: at least 30 min of structured physical activity daily Preschoolers: at least 60 min of structured physical activity daily Toddlers and preschool-ers: 60 min to several hours of unstructured physical activity daily; outside of sleeping, no inactivity >60 min	NR	NR	NR	NR
National Institutes of Health *Physical Activity and Cardiovascular Health* (NIH, 1996)	Children, adolescents	Fr/I/T/D	At least 30 min, mod-erate intensity, most or all days	NR	S/Fl	Strength training to im-prove muscular function and provide cardiovascu-lar benefits Activities to improve muscular strength and joint flexibility	NR
Strong et al., 2005 *Evidence Based Physi-cal Activity For School-Age Youth* (Strong et al., 2005)	Children, adolescents	Fr/I/T/D	School-age youth should participate daily in 60 minutes or more of moderate to vigor-ous physical activity that is developmentally appropriate, enjoyable, and involves a variety of activities.	NR	NR	NR	NR
U.S. Department of Agriculture *Nutrition and Your Health: Dietary Guide-lines for Americans* (USDHHS and USDA, 2005)	Children, adolescents	Fr/I/T/D	60 min, moderate intensity, most or all days Limit TV, computer, other inactivity by al-ternating with physical activity periods	NR	S/Fl	Type of physical activity to include aerobic, strength building, and flexibility activities	NR
US Department of Health and Human Ser-vices, *2008 Physical Activity Guidelines for Americans* (USDHHS, 2008)	Children, adolescents	Fr/I/T/D	Children and adoles-cents should perform 60 minutes (1 hour) or more of physical activ-ity daily. Aerobic: Most of the 60 or more minutes a day should be either moder-ate- or vigorous-inten-sity aerobic physical ac-tivity; vigorous-intensity physical activity must be included at least 3 days a week. It is important to en-courage young people to participate in physical activities that are ap-propriate for their age, that are enjoyable, and that offer variety.	NR	BS, S	Bone-strengthening: As part of their 60 or more minutes of daily physical activity, should include bone-strengthening physical activity on at least 3 days of the week. Muscle-strengthening: As part of their 60 or more minutes of daily physical activity, should include muscle-strengthening physical activity on at least 3 days of the week.	NR

BC = body composition; BS = bone strengthening; CR = cardiorespiratory fitness; D = duration; Fl = flexibility; Fr = frequency; I = intensity; NR = not reported; S = strength; T = type.

Reprinted, by permission, from J.E. Fulton et al., 2004, "Public health and clinical recommendations for physical activity and physical fitness: special focus on overweight youth," *Sports Medicine* 34(9): 581-599.

Current Physical Activity Guidelines
for Children and Adolescents

The key guidelines for children and adolescents are shown in the sidebar. Consistent with other recommendations for youth (Strong et al., 2005; USDHHS and USDA, 2005), the guidelines recommend at least 60 minutes each day of moderate- to vigorous-intensity aerobic physical activity for children and adolescents. A unique aspect of the youth guideline is inclusion of a 3-day-per-week goal for children and adolescents to perform muscle-strengthening, bone-strengthening, and vigorous-intensity aerobic physical activities. And, unlike adults, children and adolescents are given no choice about the frequency of aerobic physical activity—daily physical activity is required. Activities that are appropriate for a child's age and that are enjoyable should be encouraged.

There was insufficient information in the scientific literature to specify exact amounts for vigorous-intensity aerobic, muscle-strengthening, and bone-strengthening activities. Similarly, the first chapter of the guidelines affirms the importance of physical activity for children younger than age 6 years, although the science was not comprehensively reviewed by the federal advisory committee (PAGAC, 2008) for children less than 6 years.

Type of Activity

Because the Guidelines apply to children and adolescents, they must be flexible to include types of activities appropriate for this wide age range of school-age

---

Physical Activity Guidelines for Children and Adolescents, *2008 Physical Activity Guidelines for Americans*

- ▸ Children and adolescents should perform 60 minutes (1 hour) or more of physical activity daily.
  - ▪ Aerobic: Most of the 60 or more minutes a day should be either moderate- or vigorous-intensity aerobic physical activity; vigorous-intensity physical activity must be included at least 3 days a week.
  - ▪ Muscle-strengthening: As part of their 60 or more minutes of daily physical activity, children and adolescents should include muscle-strengthening physical activity on at least 3 days of the week.
  - ▪ Bone-strengthening: As part of their 60 or more minutes of daily physical activity, children and adolescents should include bone-strengthening physical activity on at least 3 days of the week.
- ▸ It is important to encourage young people to participate in physical activities that are appropriate for their age, that are enjoyable, and that offer variety.

Taken from the 2008 Physical Activity Guidelines for Americans (http://health.gov/paguidelines/)

youth. To meet the Guidelines, youth can participate in either unstructured (e.g., unorganized playground games) or structured (e.g., organized sports) physical activities. As children age, structured activity often becomes a more preferred way to be physically active.

Muscle- and bone-strengthening activities are recommended for children and adolescents on at least 3 days of the week. Muscle-strengthening activities include playing games such as tug-of-war, doing calisthenics such as push-ups or sit-ups, or doing resistance exercises using one's own body weight, resistance bands, or weights. Bone-strengthening activities include jumping activities like jumping rope or games or sports that involve jumping, like gymnastics, basketball, or volleyball. Some activities (e.g., gymnastics) serve dual purposes and may help build strong muscles and bones.

Intensity

There is strong scientific evidence that a combination of moderate- and vigorous-intensity physical activity improves the cardiorespiratory fitness of school-age youth (USDHHS, 2008). The guidelines for children and adolescents, therefore, require some participation in vigorous-intensity activity—participation in moderate-intensity activity only is not sufficient for youth. Again, the exact amount of vigorous-intensity activity needed could not be ascertained from the available scientific evidence, but it is recommended that children and adolescents participate in vigorous-intensity activity on at least 3 days of the week.

Ensuring Age Appropriateness and Enjoyability

It is imperative that children and adolescents are encouraged to participate in a variety of activities that reflect their developmental stage and are also enjoyable—the latter being key to participation. Participation in a variety of activities allows youth to build a diverse set of skills and reduce the risk of overuse injuries. For children and adolescents, having fun is the critical factor in long-term adherence to physical activity.

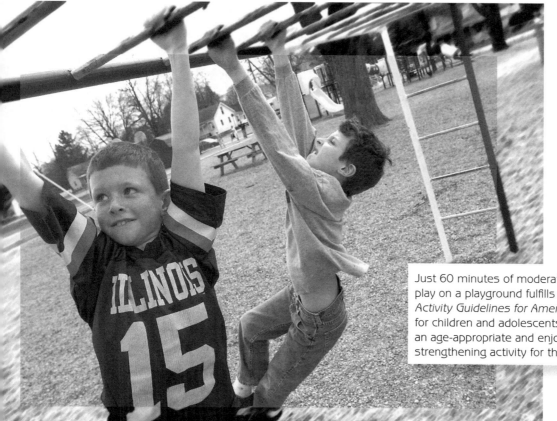

Just 60 minutes of moderate- or vigorous-intensity play on a playground fulfills the *2008 Physical Activity Guidelines for Americans* daily requirement for children and adolescents. The monkey bars is an age-appropriate and enjoyable muscle-strengthening activity for these boys.

Tracking the Guidelines for Youth

One ongoing surveillance system in the United States, the Youth Risk Behavior Surveillance System (YRBSS), is able to track students in grades 9 to 12 who achieve 60 minutes of moderate- to vigorous-intensity daily physical activity. Current U.S. surveillance systems for youth physical activity (to include the YRBSS and NHANES) are unable to track the number of youth who participate in muscle-strengthening or bone-strengthening activities on at least 3 days of the week. Current surveillance systems will need substantial modification to comprehensively assess the physical activity guidelines in U.S. children and adolescents.

Summary

Physical activity is important for all ages. Recommended levels of physical activity are stated either as *Healthy People 2010* objectives or as guidelines. You can use this information to establish goals for people in various age groups for various purposes, such as planning physical activity interventions and programs in your community (see chapter 7 for information on program planning).

Suggested Readings

For an explanation of terms such as *moderate-* and *vigorous-intensity physical activity*, see the glossary.

For more information on adult recommendations

2008 Physical Activity Guidelines for Americans. www.health.gov/paguidelines/default.aspx

American College of Sports Medicine Position Stand. 1998. The recommended quantity and quality of exercise for developing and maintaining cardiorespiratory and muscular fitness, and flexibility in healthy adults. *Medicine and Science in Sports and Exercise* 30(6):975-991.

Blair SN, LaMonte MJ, Nichaman MZ. 2004. The evolution of physical activity recommendations: how much is enough? *American Journal of Clinical Nutrition* 79(5):913S-920S.

Pate RR, Pratt M, Blair SN, et al. 1995. Physical activity and public health: a recommendation from the Centers for Disease Control and Prevention and the American College of Sports Medicine. *Journal of the American Medical Association* 273:402-407.

For more information on youth recommendations

2008 Physical Activity Guidelines for Americans. www.health.gov/paguidelines/default.aspx

Fulton JE, Garg M, Galuska DA, Rattay KT, Caspersen CJ. 2004. Public health and clinical recommendations for physical activity and physical fitness: special focus on overweight youth. *Sports Medicine* 34(9):581-599.

Strong WB, Malina RM, Blimkie CJ, Daniels SR, Dishman RK, Gutin B, Hergenroeder AC, Must A, Nixon PA, Pivarnik JM, Rowland T, Trost S, Trudeau F. 2005. Evidence based physical activity for school-age youth. *Journal of Pediatrics* 146(6):732-737. www.healthysd.gov/Documents/Youth%20PA%20recs.pdf

For more information on older adults

American College of Sports Medicine Position Stand. 1998. Exercise and physical activity for older adults. *Medicine and Science in Sports and Exercise* 30(6):992-1008.

American Council on Exercise. 1998. *Exercise for Older Adults.* www.humankinetics.com/products/showproduct.cfm?isbn=088011942X

Brawley LR, Rejeski WJ, King AC. 2003. Promoting physical activity for older adults: the challenges for changing behavior. *American Journal of Preventive Medicine* 25(3 suppl 2):172-183.

Exercise & Physical Activity: Your Everyday Guide From the National Institute on Aging. 2009. www.nia.nih.gov/HealthInformation/Publications/ExerciseGuide/

The National Blueprint: Increasing Physical Activity Among Adults Age 50 and Older. www.agingblueprint.org

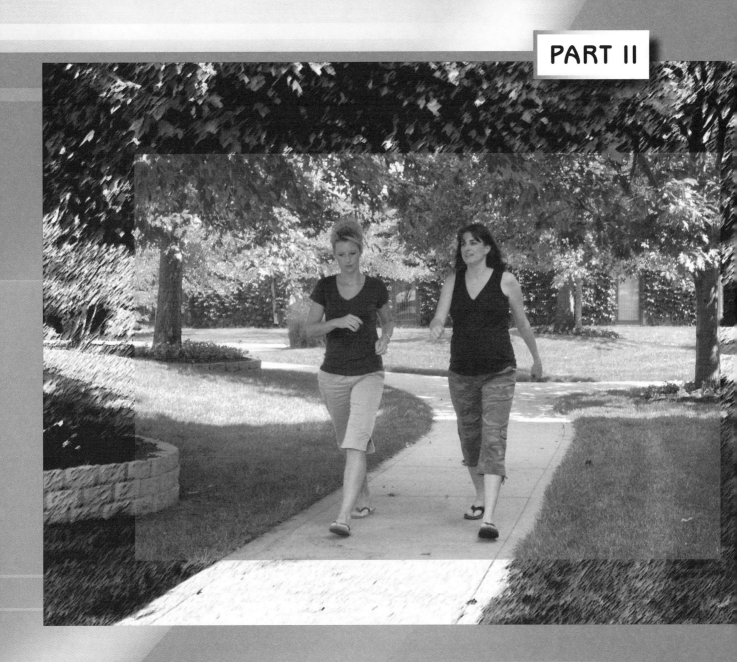

PART II

Approaches and Interventions for Changing Physical Activity Behavior

art II provides you with information about evidenced-based, recommended interventions for increasing physical activity in your community. These interventions are recommended by the *Guide to Community Preventive Services* (i.e., the *Community Guide*) based on an extensive evidence review of what works. These interventions are described in the physical activity chapter of the *Community Guide* (Zaza et al., 2005) and in scientific review articles (Heath et al., 2006; Kahn et al., 2002). The bodies of evidence of intervention effectiveness may be characterized as strong, sufficient, or insufficient according to the *Community Guide* (Zaza et al., 2005) methods for evidenced-based reviews. The chapters in Part II discuss physical activity interventions that were found to have sufficient or strong evidence for their effectiveness. According to the *Community Guide*:

> One can achieve sufficient or strong evidence in a variety of ways. For example, sufficient or strong evidence can be achieved through one or two well designed and executed studies with few threats to validity. Alternatively . . . a group of individually less persuasive studies can provide sufficient or strong evidence taken together, especially if their flaws are not overlapping. (p. 443)

Part II is divided into three chapters, each with subsections that explain the recommended interventions. The broader chapter title describes the type of approach the intervention uses. Chapter 3 covers two interventions using informational approaches to increasing physical activity. Chapter 4 addresses behavioral and social approaches and discusses three interventions for increasing physical activity. Chapter 5 focuses on environmental and policy approaches and discusses three types of interventions to increase physical activity (two interventions, community-scale and street scale urban design and land use, are covered in the same chapter subsection). The subsections in this part use similar formats: (1) an explanation of the intervention, (2) a discussion of what the research has shown (according to the *Community Guide*), (3) practical applications and special considerations for carrying out the interventions in your community, and (4) selected readings.

Informational Approaches (Chapter 3)

The *Community Guide* describes informational approaches as interventions that focus on increasing physical activity by providing information to motivate and enable people to change behavior and to maintain that change over time. According to Kahn and colleagues (2002), these interventions focus on the cognitive processes thought to precede behavior change. The interventions primarily use communication approaches to present general health information, including information about cardiovascular disease prevention and risk reduction and specific information about physical activity (Kahn et al., 2002; Zaza et al., 2005). Information is provided with the intention of changing knowledge about the benefits of physical activity, increasing awareness of opportunities within a community for increasing physical activity, explaining methods to overcome barriers and negative attitudes about physical activity, and increasing participation in community-based activities (Kahn et al., 2002; Zaza et al., 2005).

Behavioral and Social Approaches (Chapter 4)

The *Community Guide* describes behavioral and social approaches as interventions that focus on increasing physical activity by teaching widely applicable behavioral management skills and by structuring the social environment to provide support for people trying to initiate or maintain behavior change (Kahn et al., 2002; Zaza et al., 2005). As noted in the *Community Guide,* these interventions frequently involve behavioral counseling and often include people who constitute a person's social environment. The *Community Guide* further focuses on the skills needed for recognizing cues and opportunities for physical activity and ways to help people initiate physical activity, maintain behavior, and prevent relapse. Interventions typically involve making changes in the home, family, school, and work environments (Kahn et al., 2002; Zaza et al., 2005).

Environmental and Policy Approaches (Chapter 5)

Environmental and policy approaches that promote physical activity in community settings can increase access to programs, create or improve built environment supports for physical activity, and create incentives to be active (Sallis et al., 1998; Schmid et al., 2006). Examples of interventions to increase physical activity include the creation or enhancement of walking and bicycle trails and other public recreation facilities, land use policies that support active transportation to neighborhood destinations, designs for buildings that encourage physical activity, and policies or incentives that promote physical activity during the workday (Frank and Engelke, 2001). There are many environmental and policy interventions that can be used to promote physical activity. Although it is not known which approaches are the most effective, interventions using environmental and policy approaches to promote physical activity are important for several reasons. First, they complement informational approaches to decreasing barriers to places to be physically active (Handy et al., 2002). For example, they can be used to create physical activity opportunities as part of broader community-wide campaigns (an informational approach intervention category), and point-of-decision prompts (also an informational approach intervention category) can be used to call attention to increased physical activity opportunities generated by environmental and policy interventions. Second, they reach all people exposed to an environment, rather than just those who choose to enroll in programs (Brownson et al., 2001; King et al., 2002). Third, they may be especially cost-effective because once created, environmental supports continue to exert their influence over a long period (Frank and Engelke, 2001; Hann et al., 2004; King et al., 2002; Saelens et al., 2003).

The environmental determinants of active transportation behavior differ from the determinants of active recreation behavior. People walk and cycle more for transportation when they live in neighborhoods with nearby destinations (mixed land use), connected streets, and higher residential density (Frank and Engelke, 2001; Handy et al., 2002; Saelens et al., 2003). Recreational activity is related to access to recreational facilities such as parks, trails, and sidewalks, especially when the aesthetics of those places are favorable (Humpel et al., 2002).

Selecting and Implementing Interventions for Your Community

From the menu of options, you may decide that informational approaches best suit your needs to increase physical activity in your community. If so, you could be involved in conducting one or two effective interventions. For example, you may find it valuable to establish point-of-decision prompt interventions in specific settings in your community to encourage people to use stairs rather than elevators or escalators. Or, you may be involved in developing and implementing a large-scale community-wide physical activity campaign. These two interventions can be used simultaneously to enhance your efforts to reach a greater number of people. You will learn more about both interventions in chapter 3.

You may find that behavioral and social approaches best suit your needs to motivate people in your community to become more physically active. If so, the *Community Guide* recommends that you consider school-based physical education, individually adapted health behavior change, and community-based social support interventions as your foundation for effectively increasing physical activity among the sedentary members of your community. These interventions are discussed in chapter 4.

You may also have as one goal to create a built environment that makes it easy, safe, and convenient for people to choose to be physically active. The built environment includes all physical components of human settlements such as buildings, open spaces, transportation infrastructure, and recreation facilities. Changing built environments typically requires modifying policies and laws through participation in political processes with governments and public and private organizations. Accordingly, promoting physical activity in your community will often require involvement from not only health professionals but also professionals from many other sectors, such as urban planners, architects and landscape architects, city and county officials and staff, transportation engineers, recreation department officials, leadership from community organizations, legislators, and the mass media. Thus, if you decide to help your community members be more physically active by relying on interventions using environmental and policy approaches, you will need to join forces with a variety of community partners. For example, a partnership may be needed to create or enhance access to places for physical activity and provide informational outreach promoting these opportunities, or bring to fruition community-scale and street-scale urban design and land use policies and practices to successfully achieve your physical activity objectives. These types of interventions are discussed in chapter 5.

Effective physical activity interventions are important in their own right. They have been found to increase physical activity behaviors and therefore possess the potential to reduce the burden of chronic diseases and disabilities. However, they may also interact with public health initiatives in other ways. For example, the interventions recommended in the *Community Guide* can play a role in your efforts to increase physical activity using an ecological model (Green et al., 1996, McLeroy et al., 1988; Sallis and Owen, 1996) to bring about large-scale behavior change among inactive youth and adults. Ecological models require that you intervene in multiple community sectors that include intrapersonal, interpersonal, organizational, legislative, and policy levels (McLeroy et al., 1988). The *Community Guide*'s recommended interventions collectively address multiple levels of physical activity interventions characteristic of ecological models (Sallis et al., 1998): they include individually adapted behavior change interventions delivered at the community level, interpersonal or social support interventions used in community settings, and the use of legislative or policy initiatives to create urban design and land use practices that favor physically active lifestyles.

Promoting physical activity in your community requires involvement from health professionals and professionals from other sectors.

Community-based health promotion efforts can also rely on the recommended interventions identified in the *Community Guide* to achieve *Healthy People 2010* physical activity objectives for the nation (see objectives listed in the introduction, pp. xvii-xviii). All *Community Guide* interventions can address *Healthy People 2010* physical activity objectives in unique and different ways. For example, increases in stair use in the natural environment, as part of transportation or purposeful activity, can contribute to total amounts of daily physical activity. If used as part of a community-wide physical activity campaign, stair use can add to other types and amounts of daily moderate- to vigorous-intensity physical activity sufficient to address *Healthy People 2010* objectives to reduce the proportion of people who are inactive and to increase the proportion who are physically active at recommended levels (USDHHS, 2000). A number of *Healthy People 2010* physical activity and fitness objectives exist related to school-based physical education and adolescent physical activity (USDHHS, 2000) (objectives 22-6 through 22-11). School-based physical education interventions, such as those recommended by the *Community Guide,* can be used to directly help meet these *Healthy People 2010* objectives. The relationship between the built environment, including community-scale and street-scale urban designs and physical activity, also can address important *Healthy People 2010* objectives, such as increasing the proportion of trips people make by walking (objective 22-14) or by bicycling (objective 22-15). The information in chapters 3, 4, and 5 may serve as the foundation for community partnerships (see chapter 6) to intervene at multiple community levels to both increase physical activity and to meet *Healthy People 2010* objectives.

Suggested Reading for Part II

Zaza S, Briss PA, Harris KW (Eds). 2005. *Physical Activity. The Guide to Community Preventive Services: What Works to Promote Health?* New York, NY: Oxford University Press, 80-113.

Brownson RC, Gurney JG, Land G. 1999. Evidence-based decision making in public health. *Journal of Public Health Management and Practice* 5:86-97.

Brownson RC, Baker EA, Leet TL, Gillespie KN. 2003. *Evidence-Based Public Health.* New York: Oxford University Press.

Briss PA, Brownson RC, Fielding JE, Zaza S. 2004. Developing and using the *Guide to Community Preventive Services*: lessons learned about evidence-based public health. *Annual Review of Public Health* 25:281-302.

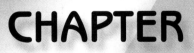

CHAPTER 3

Informational Approaches to Promoting Physical Activity

Sara Wilcox, Dennis Shepard, Sarah Levin Martin, Leigh Ramsey Buchanan, and Robin E. Soler

Informational approaches to promoting physical activity include interventions that increase awareness about physical activity. The approaches strive to increase knowledge about the benefits of physical activity, how to overcome barriers to physical activity, and physical activity opportunities among broad and diverse segments of the population. These approaches typically disseminate information about physical activity to the general population (such as an entire community), or a segment of the population (e.g., youth, older adults) in a variety of settings (e.g., schools, worksites, shopping malls, train and bus stations). Large multi-component interventions might include mass media campaigns, educational materials, and events coordinated among partners in a variety of venues to motivate people to increase physical activity. In other cases, point-of-decision-prompt interventions have been successfully used in community-based settings to educate people about the benefits of physical activity and to increase stair-climbing behavior rather than using elevators or escalators. These types of approaches are described next in greater detail.

Community-Wide Campaigns

A **community-wide campaign** is a concentrated effort to promote physical activity using a variety of methods delivered in multiple **settings.** As you may suspect, community-wide campaigns are not single events, short-term interventions, or small-scale endeavors. According to the Task Force on Community Preventive Services (Kahn, et al., 2002; Zaza, et al., 2005), community-wide campaigns involve many community sectors and partnerships, are large in scale and require high-intensity efforts with sustained high visibility, and use communication techniques to develop the physical activity campaign messages. Characteristics of community-wide campaigns are listed in the sidebar.

Unlike mass-media campaigns, community-wide campaigns have multiple components. Your community-wide campaign may include components such as self-help groups, physical activity counseling support, risk factor screening and education, community events, and policy or environmental changes such as the creation of walking trails (Kahn et al., 2002; Zaza et al., 2005).

Community Guide Task Force on Community Preventive Services Recommendation for Community-Wide Campaigns

The Guide to Community Preventive Services (Zaza et al., 2005), which is usually referred to as the *Community Guide,* included 10 articles that examined the effectiveness of community-wide campaigns (Goodman et al., 1995; Jason et al., 1991; Luepker et al., 1994; Malmgren and Andersson, 1986; Meyer et al., 1980; Osler and Jespersen, 1993; Owen et al., 1987; Tudor-Smith et al., 1998; Wimbush et al., 1998; Young et al., 1996). Of these, all but three studies (Jason et al., 1991; Owen et al., 1987; Wimbush et al., 1998) were interventions designed to decrease cardiovascular disease morbidity and mortality in a community over several years. The fact that these interventions possess the potential to promote physical activity broadly among community members means that they may be used in diverse communities small and large. The *Community Guide* emphasizes that community-wide campaigns will need to be adapted to resonate with community residents who may include both genders, a wide range of age groups and abilities, different racial and ethnic groups, and different levels of socioeconomic status. For example, bilingual or multilingual materials may need to be developed to reach people who have limited abilities to speak and read English, or materials may need to be available to accommodate low reading literacy. Because community-wide campaigns may take place over the course of many months or years, you may also need to consider a wide variety of activities or events to accommodate the seasonal changes in weather. Relative to more targeted interventions, community-wide campaigns may require greater and more creative efforts on your part to reach the large and diverse population subgroups that characterize most communities.

The *Community Guide* reports that in studies that examined the increase in the percentage of physically active people, the median net increase was 4.2 percent. In studies that examined increased energy expenditure, the median net increase was 16.3 percent. Most of the community-wide campaigns also yielded improvements in other cardiovascular disease risk factors and contributed to building

Characteristics of Community-Wide Campaigns

Mass media

Multiple components (variety of methods)

Multiple settings

Individual-level and community-level strategies

High visibility

Plan for sustainability

and strengthening social capital and social networks in the communities where they were implemented (Kahn et al., 2002; Zaza et al., 2005). Given the favorable effects on physical activity participation and energy expenditure, the Task Force on Community Preventive Services concluded that there is strong evidence to recommend community-wide campaigns to increase physical activity in communities (Zaza et al., 2005).

Update on Community-Wide Campaigns Research

Since publication of the *Community Guide,* a number of other relatively large-scale community-wide campaigns to increase physical activity have been published. These include the Stockholm Diabetes Prevention Program (Bjaras et al., 2001), Wheeling Walks (Reger et al., 2002; Reger-Nash et al., 2005), Agita Sao Paulo Program (Matsuda et al., 2002, 2004), 10,000 Steps Ghent (De Cocker et al., 2007, 2008), 10,000 Steps Rockhampton (Brown et al., 2006), Romsås in Motion (Jenum et al., 2006; Lorentzen et al., 2007), Burngreave in Action (Cochrane and Davey, 2008), and the largely mass media and social marketing VERB campaign (Huhman, Heitzler, et al., 2005; Huhman, Potter, et al. 2005; Wong et al., 2005). These campaigns have generally shown positive results, consistent with findings of the *Community Guide.*

Application and Special Considerations

Community-wide campaigns use a range of methods to disseminate information and engage community partners in promotional or educational efforts focused on increasing physical activity. These methods may include several coordinated activities such as establishing walking groups at schools or work sites, building a new trail for walking and biking, or providing health risk appraisals and physical activity counseling at the local mall. Table 3.1 presents examples of activities that may be part of community-wide campaigns. If multiple activities are used as part of a community-wide campaign, they should be part of a comprehensive long-term plan. This type of plan ensures that a variety of methods will be connected by a common theme, such as reducing cardiovascular disease or increasing physical activity among middle-aged and older adults, and will be delivered in multiple settings over a sustained period of time. Community-wide campaigns also typically use a wide range of media as an ongoing part of the campaign. Typically, the campaign messages about physical activity are directed widely to large and relatively undifferentiated audiences through diverse media, including television, radio, newspaper columns and inserts, direct mailings, billboards, advertisements in transit stations, and trailers in movie theaters (Kahn et al., 2002; Zaza et al., 2005). Consider using different media outlets to ensure that your methods reach a broad cross-section of the community.

Across the various methods you and your partners use, consider adopting a logo, theme, or tag line to increase "brand recognition" and the visibility of your campaign. It is best to budget for a creative advertising firm to **pilot test** what is developed. An additional critical ingredient for you to consider during the development of your community-wide campaign is a plan for successfully sustaining as many aspects of the campaign as resources allow.

You will need to evaluate the effect of the campaign on the community. This is especially important because many of the community-wide campaigns that have been evaluated have addressed other cardiovascular disease risk factors in addition to physical inactivity (Pearson et al., 2001). This makes it difficult to tease out the outcomes associated with the different behavioral changes that may occur as a result of a multicomponent community intervention. Asking specific questions

Table 3.1   Examples of Community-Wide Campaign Activities

Activities	Setting	Sustainability
Walk-to-school events or walking groups	Schools, media, work sites, other community settings (e.g., senior centers, health clubs)	Schools endorse policies that promote walking to school.
Parks and recreation physical activity events	Community, work sites, media	Parks and recreation departments include events in annual budget.
Health risk appraisals and physical activity counseling or prescriptions	Health care settings, work sites	Health care providers and employee assistance programs adopt this as standard practice.
Media campaign	Media, work sites, schools, and other community events	Media outlets establish ongoing planned series of media coverage.
Transportation plan for biking and waking	Government, work sites, schools, community organizations	Physical activity advocates become members of local or state transportation-planning committees.
Walking and biking trail development	Government, work sites, schools, community organizations	Physical activity advocates serve in leadership positions in organizations engaged in trail planning and implementation.

about physical activity and other targeted behaviors can provide valuable insight into whether people participate in your physical activity component and what benefits are obtained. For example, does the campaign increase community members' readiness and willingness to become more active? Does it improve their knowledge, attitudes, and beliefs about physical activity? To what extent do community members participate? Does the campaign help community members become more physically active? As part of the evaluation, keep a record of the events you conduct, mass media efforts, and the **reach** of all these activities. For additional discussion on evaluating your physical activity intervention, see chapter 7.

Carrying out community-wide campaigns requires careful planning and coordination, well-trained staff, and usually substantial resources. If you become involved in a community-wide campaign to promote physical activity, you will need to work with many community partners and be adept at forming and sustaining collaborative relationships. The following list, Examples of Potential Partners for Community-Wide Campaigns, suggests partners you can approach in your community to help develop and support a community-wide physical activity campaign. Community-wide campaigns are most likely to succeed when there is substantial community buy-in and ample community resources in terms of time, money, and trained staff. One risk with community-wide campaigns is that the adequate "dose" required for changing knowledge, attitudes, and behaviors may not be delivered because of a lack of resources. The campaigns reviewed in the *Community Guide* were effective but also were expensive and intensive. If your community does not have the resources to deliver an effective dose, there is a risk that the campaign will have no effect and community members may be unwilling to devote time and resources for subsequent physical activity–related events. Thus, community-wide campaigns are not feasible in all communities. To implement successful community-wide campaigns similar to those reviewed in the *Community Guide,* you will need to focus on the characteristics that define a successful community-wide campaign (see sidebar on p. 48) and adopt those characteristics that are important to you and your community.

Examples of Potential Partners for Community-Wide Campaigns

Local and state public
    health agencies

Transportation departments

Local and state government

Schools and colleges

Parks and recreation
    agencies

Media: print, radio, and
    television

Service organizations

Nonprofit organizations:
    health, social, and
    environmental

Faith-based organizations

Professional associations

Chambers of commerce

Business and industry

Hospital-based
    wellness programs

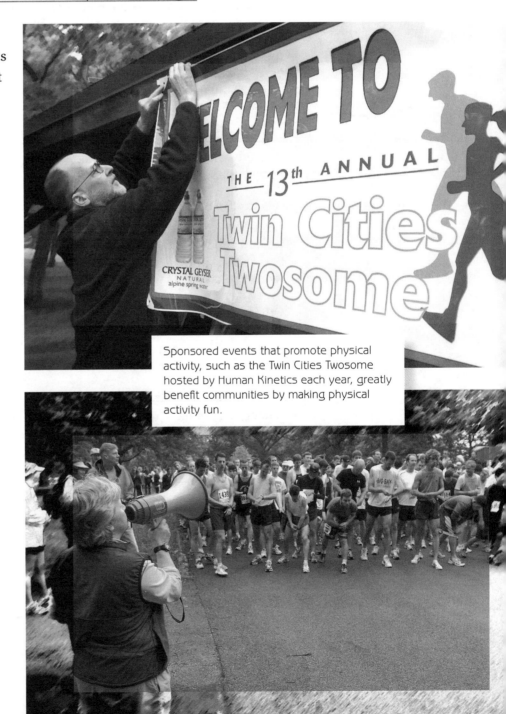

Sponsored events that promote physical activity, such as the Twin Cities Twosome hosted by Human Kinetics each year, greatly benefit communities by making physical activity fun.

Translation Research Examples

The Wheeling Walks campaign (Reger et al., 2002; Reger-Nash et al., 2005) is a good example of a community-wide campaign. It was comprehensive and built on research related to both community-wide campaigns and mass media campaigns. The Wheeling Walks campaign was a **theory**-based intervention designed to directly target and increase walking behavior. It was also unusual in that unlike many of the other community-wide campaigns, it was directed to a specific population segment: sedentary and irregularly active adults, aged 50 to 65 years.

Wheeling Walks promoted 30 minutes or more of moderate-intensity physical activity through daily walking for better health (Reger et al., 2002). The **target audience** was sedentary adults in Wheeling, West Virginia, aged 50 to 65 years. Sedentary adults were those not meeting the 1995 Centers for Disease Control and Prevention (CDC)/American College of Sports Medicine (ACSM) physical activity recommendations (as described in chapter 2, see section titled Physical Activity Recommendations for Adults—Historical Considerations, p. 22). The community-wide campaign ran from April 17, 2001, to June 9, 2001. Parkersburg, West Virginia, was the comparison community and did not conduct a campaign. Wheeling and Parkersburg are 92 miles apart and have separate media markets. The effectiveness of the campaign was determined by telephone surveys at baseline, 3 months, 6 months, and 12 months.

Key Components of the Wheeling Walks Campaign

- Paid advertisements: newspaper, television, radio
- Public relations activities
- Work site program: Work Site Wellness Walking Challenge
- Web site exposure (www.wheelingwalks.org): information about the campaign, events, and celebrity endorsements and space for residents to register and submit minutes walked
- Prescriptions for Walking: a program in which physicians were asked to write prescriptions for their patients to walk 30 minutes or more on almost every day
- Other public health education programs: health professional presentations, church bulletins
- Based on behavioral and communication theories and models: **theory of planned behavior**, elaboration likelihood model, **social marketing**

Major Results From Wheeling Walks

- Wheeling residents reported higher proportions of walkers than Parkersburg residents over time.
- Of the sedentary respondents identified at baseline, 32 percent in Wheeling and 18 percent in Parkersburg reported that they increased physical activity by walking at least 30 minutes for at least 5 days a week.
- Pre- and posttest observations of walkers at five popular walking sites in Wheeling and Parkersburg showed a 23 percent increase in walkers in Wheeling compared with no change in the percentage of walkers in Parkersburg.

In the next section, we highlight three community-wide type campaigns implemented at state or national levels to illustrate the potential generalizability of this intervention category. Two campaigns targeting adults in North Carolina and Utah highlight state efforts, and VERB illustrates a U.S. national campaign to increase physical activity targeting tweens.

Translation Research

For translation research examples that build on the Wheeling Walks campaign, see these articles about Broome County Walks and West Virginia Walks:

Reger-Nash B, Fell P, Spicer D, Fisher B, Cooper L, Chey T, Bauman A. 2006. BC Walks: replication of a community-wide physical activity campaign. *Preventing Chronic Disease* 3(3):A90.

Reger-Nash B, Bauman A, Cooper L, Chey T, Simon KJ, Brann M, Leyden KM. 2008. WV Walks: replication with expanded reach. *Journal of Physical Activity and Health* 5(1):19-27.

The North Carolina Division of Public Health's Physical Activity and Nutrition Branch has engaged in a long-term initiative to increase physical activity throughout North Carolina. The initiative has been highly visible, has used multiple intervention approaches in a wide variety of settings, and has established numerous partnerships to ensure sustainability. Since the beginning of the initiative, statewide efforts have centered on building capacity within communities through training opportunities such as those based on a North Carolina State publication titled Winning With Aces! How You Can Work Toward Active Community Environments—A Policy Guide for Public Health Practitioners and Their Partners (available at www.startwithyour-heart.com/tools/aces.pdf). The overall initiative has established partnerships with various organizations and individuals interested in increasing the number of media events focused on increasing physical activity, training communities on policy and environmental tools for building active communities, and developing community assessment tools. All partnership efforts have been underpinned with a commitment to using evidenced-based approaches and materials as much as possible. By using all these strategies, the partners have maximized their chances of success. This approach is consistent with the *Community Guide*—community-wide campaigns are more likely to succeed if multiple methods are incorporated in a variety of community sectors with a comprehensive long-term approach. For more information on North Carolina's programs, visit www.EatSmartMoveMoreNC.com.

Another community-wide type campaign, A Healthier You, is a collaboration between the Utah Department of Health and various community partners. As part of the Salt Lake City 2002 Winter Olympic Games, the Department of Health and 18 health organizations in Utah worked with the Salt Lake City Olympic Organizing Committee to initiate a program to promote physical activity and good nutrition throughout the state. The program engaged multiple organizations and numerous individuals at the state and local levels in long-term initiatives based in communities, work sites, schools, and college campuses. Olympic themes of bronze, silver, and gold, as well as platinum, are the inspiration for the different levels that communities, schools, work sites, and college campuses could achieve (for additional information see www.health.utah.gov/ahy/ and click on community, school, or worksite links). Approximately 50 Legacy Gold Medal Miles were also marked and mapped around the state. These one-mile long walking trails in communities and locations across Utah were, and still are, used to encourage Utah residents to increase physical activity. For more information on the walking trails see www.utahwalks.org (click on the Maps link for walking trail locations).

Utah schools' participation in this program was exceptional, and it became known as the Gold Medal Schools program (Neiger et al., 2008). This part of the program encourages students and teachers to eat a healthful diet, be active, and avoid tobacco. A study comparing two schools that implemented the program with two schools that did not reported more favorable outcomes in the Gold Medal Schools on body mass index and consumption of soft drinks (Jordan et al., 2008). Children from both schools increased days walked or biked to school, but the increase was larger and more significant in non–Gold Medal Schools. The authors of this paper noted that rates of walking or biking to school were high at baseline, which might have limited increases over time. For more information on this program, see http://health.utah.gov/hearthighway/gms/.

The VERB Campaign, conducted from 2002 to 2006, was a $339 million national physical activity campaign funded by the U.S. Congress (Huhman et al., 2009). It was a multiethnic mass media and social marketing campaign to increase physical activity among United States tweens 9 to 13 years of age (Huhman, Heitzler, et al., 2005; Huhman, Potter, et al., 2005; Huhman et al., 2007; Huhman et al., 2009; Wong et al., 2005). Although the VERB campaign was predominantly a social marketing media campaign, it incorporated some components that may be used as part of successful community-wide campaigns. VERB used diverse media (television, radio, and newspaper advertising), community promotions with distribution of promotional and educational materials, local on-site planned programming, partnerships, and Internet-based promotional and educational information and tools to advertise and market the VERB brand (Wong et al., 2005). Multiple community channels were used, including schools, businesses, and other community groups and organizations (Wong et al., 2005). The national VERB campaign has also been used as a foundation for more traditional community-wide interventions in Lexington, Kentucky and Greeley, Colorado (as described in Bretthauer-Mueller et al., 2008).

After 1 year, 74 percent of children surveyed were aware of the campaign (Huhman, Potter, et al., 2005). Children who were more aware of the campaign were more likely to show increased physical activity in their free time. A significant positive relationship was found between level of awareness of the VERB campaign (no recall of the VERB campaign, recall but no understanding, aided recall with understanding, and unaided recall with understanding) and the median number of weekly free-time physical activity sessions reported by the overall study population of 9- to 13-year old youth and by subgroups of children (e.g., those age 9-10 years, girls, children with parents having less than a high school education, children from families with annual incomes of $25,001-$50,000, those from densely populated urban areas, and children who were low active at baseline). The campaign also led to increased free-time physical activity among children in the subgroups who were aware of VERB, relative to those who were unaware of the campaign (Huhman, Potter, et al., 2005). For the majority of the study population, the VERB campaign had no significant effect on participation in organized physical activities. However, among children categorized as low active at the start of the VERB campaign, a significantly higher percentage who were aware of VERB compared to those unaware of VERB at the one-year intervention time point (39.1 percent vs. 31.9 percent), reported participating in organized physical activity.

Successful community-wide campaigns use a variety of methods to reach people.

After 2 years, there was a significant dose–response relationship between exposure to VERB and two outcomes: physical activity reported on the day before the interview and the median number of weekly sessions of physical activity during free time (Huhman et al., 2007). Also, among children aware of VERB versus unaware of VERB, at the year 2 time point, 61.2 percent versus 45.7 percent reported physical activity on the previous day. Similar differences were seen in the number of weekly sessions of free-time activity (3.9 vs. 3.0, respectively). The results for tweens aware and unaware of VERB at 2 years were even more positive than at year 1, as the findings were significant for the overall study population rather than for select subgroups.

VERB findings at year 4 (Huhman et al., 2009) showed that among a cross-sectional analysis of 2006 data, greater exposure to the campaign was associated with higher percentages of tweens being physically activity the day prior to taking the survey—ranging from 62 percent with no campaign exposure to 68 percent for those who were exposed to campaign advertising every day. Further, a significant positive association was found for frequency of exposure to the VERB campaign and reported sessions of weekly free-time physical activity among a cohort of adolescents evaluated at baseline, in 2002, through 2006 time points.

VERB demonstrated that a national media campaign, combined with activities characteristic of community-wide campaigns to advertise and market the VERB brand, resulted in modest increases in physical activity behavior. However, Huhman and colleagues (2009) note that even modest increases in physical activity may result in important health benefits when multiplied across millions of children at a population level. A 2008 *American Journal of Preventive Medicine Supplement* (Volume 34, Issue 6, Supplement 1) was devoted to describing VERB in detail. For more information on the VERB campaign, see also www.cdc.gov/youthcampaign.

The four campaigns previously described, the community-wide campaign in Wheeling, West Virginia, one each in North Carolina and Utah, and the VERB national campaign, used multiple intervention approaches to encourage individual and environmental changes that support physical activity, and a long-term plan was put in place to ensure each campaign's success. Specific funding sources were identified for these programs, as were built-in mechanisms to ensure sustainability at the state and community levels. Through built-in aspects of the program, individuals and organizations were challenged to identify and commit to long-term interventions that would change physical activity behaviors and environments. This long-term view is needed to bring major and significant improvements in physical activity levels within a community, and also at state and national levels. Ultimately, congressional monetary support of VERB was not continued beyond a five-year funding cycle. Unstable local, state, and national funding is a reality facing community-wide campaigns and should be taken into consideration when developing and implementing community-wide campaigns and how to sustain them over the long term.

Conclusion

The keys to building and implementing successful community-wide campaigns are to select a multicomponent approach using a variety of methods to reach community members, engage a wide variety of organizations, plan carefully, and build the campaign in ways that can be evaluated and sustained. The evidence supporting the selection of a community-wide campaign as an effective way to achieve behavioral change is well documented in the *Community Guide*, but the duration, number of components, and selection of specific components are critical areas you will need to consider as you plan your own community-wide campaign.

Suggested Reading and Resources

Internet Resources Related to Physical Activity Promotion in Communities

Active Living by Design: www.activelivingbydesign.org

This site highlights innovative approaches to increase physical activity through community design, public policies, and communications strategies.

Active Living Research: www.activelivingresearch.org

This site provides the latest research, tools, and information about active community environments and policies.

America on the Move: www.americaonthemove.org

This site provides resources for communities to start walking programs and provides examples of what other communities are doing.

America Walks: The National Coalition of Walking Advocates: www.americawalks.org

This site provides information about coalition building, event planning, advocacy, and examples of community initiatives.

American Association for Physical Activity and Recreation: www.aahperd.org/aapar

This site describes professional activities related to physical activity and recreation and includes links to additional healthy lifestyle sites.

Centers for Disease Control and Prevention Nutrition and Physical Activity: www.cdc.gov/nccdphp/dnpa/dnpalink.htm

This site provides a list of resources for physical activity promotion and other related topics.

In Motion: www.in-motion.ca

This site provides information about resources and events to get your community moving.

North Carolina Prevention Partners: www.ncpreventionpartners.org

This site offers broad-based **primary prevention** information linking physical activity to overall health.

National Center for Bicycling & Walking: www.bikewalk.org

This site includes assessment tools, policies, and media information.

National Recreation and Park Association: www.nrpa.org

This site provides program and partnership information.

Nova Scotia, Canada: Health Promotion and Protection: www.gov.ns.ca/hpp/physicalActivity/index.asp

This site describes community-focused programs and events in Nova Scotia, Canada.

President's Council on Physical Fitness and Sports: www.fitness.gov

This site provides useful physical activity ideas and events.

Canadian Council for Health and Active Living at Work: www.cchalw-ccsvat.ca/english/

This site offers advice for working with businesses and communities.

Rails-to-Trails Conservancy: www.railtrails.org

This site provides community and partnership ideas for promoting rails to trails.

Sports, Play, and Active Recreation for Kids (SPARK): www.sparkpe.org

This site offers ideas for how to help children become more active.

University of South Carolina Prevention Research Center: http://prevention. sph.sc.edu

This site summarizes the latest research, policy and environmental information, and reports on community-focused physical activity. You can sign up for a physical activity newsletter and listserve.

YMCA: www.ymca.net

This site provides information about local YMCAs, Activate America, and potential partnership opportunities.

Suggested Readings

Key References

Luepker RV, Murray DM, Jacobs DR Jr, et al. 1994. Community education for cardiovascular disease prevention: risk factor changes in the Minnesota Heart Health Program. *American Journal of Public Health* 84(9):1383-1393.

Pearson TA, Wall S, Lewis C, et al. 2001. Dissecting the "black box" of community intervention: lessons from community-wide cardiovascular disease prevention programs in the US and Sweden. *Scandinavian Journal of Public Health Supplement* 56:69-78.

Young DR, Haskell WL, Taylor CB, Fortmann SP. 1996. Effect of community health education on physical activity knowledge, attitudes, and behavior: the Stanford Five-City Project. *American Journal of Epidemiology* 144(3):264-274.

Books

Bracht N (Ed). 1999. *Health Promotion at the Community Level 2: New Advances*. Thousand Oaks, CA: Sage. (See especially chapters 1, 4, 5, and 6.)

Kreuter MW, Lezin NA, Kreuter MW, Green LW. 2003. *Community Health Promotion Ideas That Work,* 2nd edition. Sudbury, MA: Jones & Bartlett.

Wurzbach ME (Ed). 2002. *Community Health Education and Promotion: A Guide to Program Design and Evaluation,* 2nd edition. Sudbury, MA: Jones & Bartlett.

Point-of-Decision Prompts

Point-of-decision prompt interventions are one of two informational approaches found to be effective by the *Community Guide* in increasing physical activity (Kahn et al., 2002; Soler et al., 2005; Zaza et al., 2005). This area has been updated in a review by Soler and colleagues to be published in a supplement to the *American Journal of Preventive Medicine*, and a summary of this work can be found at www. thecommunityguide.org/pa/environmental-policy/podp.html.

Point-of-decision prompts are signs posted by elevators and escalators to encourage people to walk using nearby stairs. The signs may inform people about a health or weight loss benefit from using the stairs and remind people already predisposed to becoming more active, for health or other reasons, about the opportunity to use the stairs (Kahn, 2002; Soler et al., 2005; Soler et al., 2010). Point-of-decision prompts can be used alone or with stairwell enhancements in an attempt to improve the effectiveness of the prompt (i.e., by making stairwells more attractive to potential users) (Soler et al., 2005; Soler et al., 2010).

Community Guide Task Force on Community Preventive Services Recommendation on Point-of-Decision Prompts

An updated *Community Guide* review identified 11 studies (one article reported two studies) (Adams and White, 2002; Andersen et al., 1998, 2000; Blamey et al., 1995; Boutelle et al., 2001; Brownell et al., 1980; Coleman and Gonzalez, 2001; Kerr et al., 2001; Marshall et al., 2002; Russell et al., 1999; Russell and Hutchinson, 2000) conducted between 1980 and 2005 that used point-of-decision prompts to promote increased stair use. The studies took place in various settings, including shopping malls (Andersen et al., 1998; Brownell et al., 1980; Kerr et al., 2001), train and bus stations (Andersen et al., 2000, Blamey et al., 1995; Brownell et al., 1980), airports (Coleman and Gonzalez, 2001; Russell et al., 1999), an office building (Coleman and Gonzalez, 2001), a bank (Coleman and Gonzalez, 2001), a health care facility (Marshall et al., 2002), a medical school (Adams and White, 2002), a university (Boutelle et al., 2001), and a university library (Coleman and Gonzalez, 2001; Russell et al., 1999).

In an article summarizing the early *Community Guide* findings, Kahn and colleagues (2002) reported that point-of-decision prompts were effective among both men and women as well as younger and older adults. Although the signs were effective among overweight and non-overweight people, the median increase in the percentage of overweight people using the stairs was greater (Andersen et al., 1998). A sign that linked stair use to the potential for weight loss resulted in a greater increase in stair use among overweight people than a sign linking stair use to general health benefits. Stair use among children was not assessed in the included studies. Taken together, results from point-of-decision prompt interventions suggest that they are likely to be effective across diverse settings and population groups provided that appropriate care is taken to adapt the messages to resonate with the target audiences (Khan et al., 2002; Soler et al., 2005; Soler et al., 2010; Zaza et al., 2005). However, a study conducted in Hong Kong (Eves and Masters, 2006) found that a point-of-decision prompt intervention did not lead to a significant increase in stair climbing. Thus, consistent with good public health practice, taking into account settings, customs,

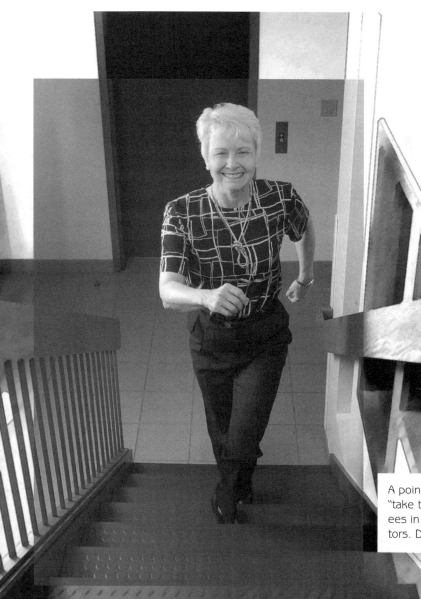

A point-of-decision prompt, such as a sign saying "take the stairs," could encourage more employees in this company to use stairs instead of elevators. Daily lifestyle physical activity adds up!

and languages is a top priority in translating point-of-decision prompt interventions for use in different cross-cultural contexts.

Despite the effectiveness of point-of-decision prompts overall, stair climbing has typically been shown to decrease after signs prompting the use of stairs are removed. However, although stair use diminished fairly rapidly in one study, it did not reach the baseline level of stair use until the 3-month follow-up. The authors noted that the persistence of the findings is surprising given the minimal intervention required to change behavior (Brownell et al., 1980).

To examine effects relative to baseline stair use, 11 qualifying studies that included 21 study arms for stair use were evaluated in terms of relative change. The median absolute increase in stair climbing in 21 study arms of 11 studies was 2.4 percentage points (the interquartile interval for effect sizes was 0.83-6.7 percentage points) (Soler et al., 2005; Soler et al., 2010). The majority of studies reported low baseline stair use (less than 20 percent). The median relative improvement in observed stair use was 50 percent (interquartile interval: 5.4 percent, 90.6 percent) from baseline.

According to the *Community Guide* rules of evidence, there is strong evidence showing that point-of-decision prompts are effective in motivating people to take the stairs rather than an elevator or escalator (Soler et al., 2005). Although taking the stairs may lead to a large increase in relative energy expenditure, this increase in physical activity is of very short duration and does not account for a large proportion of one's absolute total daily expenditure. Thus, point-of-decision prompts may best be considered as only one part of a broader campaign or multicomponent intervention to help people increase their total daily energy expenditure.

Enhancement of stairs or stairwells, an environmental intervention, when combined with point-of-decision prompts was also examined as part of this *Community Guide* review. This intervention includes modifying stairwells by painting walls, laying carpet, adding artwork, and playing music in addition to using point-of-decision prompts. There was not enough evidence in this body of literature to draw conclusions about the effectiveness of the combined physical enhancements and point-of-decision prompts. In one study conducted in an office building, all interventions (paint, carpet, art, signs, and music) together led to a relative increase in stair use of 8.8 percent (baseline use 2.14 mean trips per day per occupant) (Kerr et al., 2004). The other study examined the effectiveness of point-of-decision prompts with artwork and music and reported a 39.6 percent relative increase in stair use (percentage of people using stairs at baseline: 11.1 percent) (Boutelle et al., 2001).

Update on Point-of-Decision Prompts Research

Since the *Community Guide* findings were released, at least two reviews have been published (Dolan et al., 2006; Eves and Webb, 2006). Dolan and colleagues (2006) reviewed eight studies examining the effect of motivational prompts on stair versus escalator use in public settings. Drawing on the findings of their review, the authors estimated that in a hypothetical intervention conducted in a city, stair use would increase 2.8 percent and would result in weight loss or weight gain prevention of 300 grams per person per year among new stair users (Dolan et al., 2006). These authors concluded that point-of-decision prompts may help communities attain small steps; however, the impact of this intervention alone on correcting energy imbalance may be minimal.

Eves and Webb (2006) reviewed evidence of effectiveness for point-of-decision prompts when used in work sites. This review did not find any evidence of effectiveness. The authors suggested that this setting might be different from public buildings because work sites offer a choice between the stairs and an elevator rather than an escalator. They postulate that stair versus elevator choice may be harder to alter than the stair versus escalator choice. The authors caution it would be misleading to conclude that point-of-decision prompts do not have a future in work sites because many of the reviewed studies provide encouragement that increases in stair use can be obtained, particularly with additional enhancements such as improved aesthetics, music, or encouragement from an e-mail (Eves and Webb, 2006).

In addition to these two reviews, nine studies have been published since early 2005 (van den Auweele et al., 2005; Eves and Masters 2006; Eves et al., 2006; Eves et al., 2009; Iversen et al., 2007; Kwak et al., 2007; Olander et al., 2008; Webb and Eves, 2005, 2007). These studies examined point-of-decision prompts in public places such as shopping malls (Webb and Eves, 2005, 2007) and train stations (Eves et al., 2009; Olander et al., 2008; Iversen et al., 2007) and in work sites (van den Auweele et al., 2005; Eves et al., 2006; Kwak et al., 2007). One study examined the use of prompts to encourage stair use instead of travelator (i.e., a moving walkway or escalator without steps) use in Hong Kong (Eves and Masters, 2006). In general, these studies found an increase in stair use when the signs were in place, but the studies examined additional details of signage use, such as the layout of the intervention site, type of signage, and size of posters. The information from these new studies is consistent with the findings of the *Community Guide* review described previously.

Practical Application and Special Considerations

The studies discussed here point to some keys to success in implementing a point-of-decision intervention in a community:

- Do **formative research** to learn what messages might motivate your target audience.
- Consider different messages for different subpopulations.
- Reintroduce new prompts over time to try to maintain stair use.
- Make the stairwell aesthetically pleasing to the eyes and ears:
  - Bright lighting
  - Colorful walls
  - Carpeting
  - Music
- Be aware of barriers to stair use and work to overcome these barriers:
  - Difficult to find stairwells
  - Poorly lit stairwells
  - Poorly maintained stairwells
  - Unsafe stairwells (either structurally or by hidden location)
  - Locked stairwells

 ### Translation Research Example

The following example is taken from the StairWELL to Better Health (CDC, 2007) point-of-decision prompts intervention used by the Centers for Disease Control and Prevention. The StairWELL project was a low-cost, four-stage passive intervention that was implemented over the course of 3 1/2 years that included motivational signs, carpeting and painting, framed artwork, and music. Infrared beams were used to track the number of stair users.

Definition of Formative Research

Research conducted during the developmental stages of a project or campaign. It may include reviews, pretesting messages or materials, and pilot testing programs on a small scale before full implementation. The primary purpose of formative research is to maximize the likelihood of effective intervention; it can suggest improvements in messages or program content and delivery as well as identify potentially misleading or misunderstood messages and intervention strategies before more costly implementation occurs. (USDHHS, 1999, p. 364)

■ Motivational signs, like the one shown, were placed where people have the choice between stair and elevator use. The motivational messages for this intervention were tested in **focus groups** to ensure they were motivating to the audience. Prompt messages can be inspirational, factual, health-related, or humorous; find out what works best with your audience (see figure 3.1).

■ In addition to using point-of-decision prompts, CDC enhanced the targeted stairwells. Carpeting was laid and rubber treading was added to each of the steps to maximize safety. The bare walls were transformed by adding brightly colored paint, with each floor a different color. Framed artwork also was added to each floor, which featured people being active, photos of nutritious foods, and picturesque scenery. Royalty-free clip art was used for many of the pictures to keep the cost of artwork low.

■ Music was added to the targeted stairwells by installing a digital satellite receiver that feeds the incoming signal into an integrated amplifier that, in turn, feeds five stairwell speakers (one on each floor). Digital satellite music systems allows a variety of musical genres (e.g., classical, country, jazz, Latin, oldies, popular contemporary, and urban) to be played.

Walking up stairs burns almost 5 times more calories than riding an elevator.

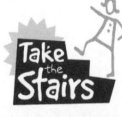

Take the Stairs

Figure 3.1   Motivation sign.
Reprinted from the CDC.

■ Stair use can be tracked before, during, and after the renovation phases. Ways to track include direct observation, video cameras, and infrared sensors. Each method of tracking stair use has its own benefits and limitations, but all of the methods can be used in a way that protects the identity and anonymity of persons being observed or counted. For the StairWELL to Better Health intervention, infrared beam sensors were installed to collect **baseline data** and conduct ongoing data collection of stair traffic.

Note: check with your building manager, safety officer, or lawyer to identify all relevant permits and fire and building codes.

Conclusion

Point-of-decision prompts are a simple way to increase stair use, and although no economic evidence is available, this intervention seems to be a low-cost option to promote overall daily physical activity in some settings. The point-of-decision intervention alone, however, will not increase physical activity enough to obtain recommended amounts of physical activity for health promotion and disease prevention. Point-of-decision-prompts should be used as one component of a multicomponent intervention or in conjunction with other physical activity interventions.

CHAPTER 4

Behavioral and Social Approaches to Promoting Physical Activity

Jacqueline N. Epping, Sarah M. Lee, David R. Brown, Tina J. Lankford, Rebeka Cook, and Ross C. Brownson

Behavioral and social approaches to promoting physical activity include community-based (home-, school-, work-, or health care-based) interventions that 1) teach cognitive and behavior skills and mobilize social support to help people increase their physical activity or 2) make changes to the settings that accommodate greater amounts of physical activity. Although these interventions frequently use principles of behavior modification (e.g., goal setting, monitoring progress, feedback, and reinforcement) that have been used to help individuals change and self manage behaviors, the principles have been adapted for use with groups, including participants in exercise classes or Internet interventions, to increase physical activity behaviors in settings such as work sites. Changes in policies and curricula have also been used in school settings to increase attendance and amount of physical activity participation in school-based physical education classes. These types of approaches are described next in greater detail.

Enhanced School-Based Physical Education

Enhanced school-based physical education interventions, in the context of the recommendations in *The Guide to Community Preventive Services: What Works to Promote Health? (Community Guide),* issued by the Task Force on Community Preventive Services, refers to interventions that included at least one of the following three components: (1) increasing the amount of time students spend in moderate-to vigorous-intensity physical activity (MVPA) during physical education class, (2) adding physical education classes to the school curriculum, and (3) lengthening the time of existing physical education classes (Kahn et al., 2002; Zaza et al., 2005). Whether your role is educator, parent, health professional, business leader, or concerned community member, you may find yourself in a position to support or advocate for school-based physical education policies and programs. You will learn in this chapter that there are many reasons why it is important to do so.

Task Force Recommendation on School-Based Physical Education

Thirteen studies that were included in the *Community Guide* examined the effectiveness of school-based physical education interventions (Kahn et al., 2002; Zaza et al., 2005). These interventions focused on changes to policies, curricula, and teaching practices. Two studies were conducted in high schools, and all other studies were carried out in elementary school settings. The Task Force on Community Preventive Services indicates that findings from these studies should generalize and apply to middle schools (Zaza et al., 2005) as well as to diverse settings and populations (Kahn et al., 2002).

The *Community Guide* (Kahn et al., 2002; Zaza et al., 2005) reports that school-based physical education interventions increased the total amount of time students spent in MVPA in physical education classes by about 10 percent, and percent of class time students spent engaged in MVPA increased by almost 50 percent. Most of the school-based interventions also yielded improvements in other measures, including an 8 percent increase in aerobic capacity, an increase in energy expenditure, and modest increases in flexibility and **muscular endurance.** Also important are findings showing that students increased their knowledge about exercise and fitness and their motivation to exercise (Kahn et al., 2002; Zaza et al., 2005). Considering the favorable effects on increasing participation in physical activity, energy expenditure, and aerobic capacity, the Task Force concluded that there is strong evidence to recommend school-based physical education interventions (Kahn et al., 2002; Zaza et al., 2005).

Practical Application and Special Considerations

School-based physical education is the foundation of a school's physical activity programming, which also includes recess (elementary and middle schools), intramural sports, interscholastic sports, active transport to school initiatives (e.g., walk to school programs), and recreation opportunities for all students. School-based physical education interventions can maximize the amount of time students are physically active in physical education class and contribute to students' overall fitness levels (Kahn et al., 2002; Zaza et al., 2005). School-based physical education interventions also help young people meet physical activity recommendations, as discussed in chapter 2, which call for 60 minutes or more of daily MVPA (U.S. Department of Health & Human Services, 2008). Nationwide, more than 60 percent of students do not meet daily recommendations for physical activity (Center for Disease Control and Prevention, 2006). Physical education also provides a unique opportunity for young people to learn skills that are necessary to lead physically active lifestyles.

However, Lee and colleagues (2007) reported that only a small percentage of schools surveyed (3.8 percent of elementary schools, 7.9 percent of middle and junior high schools, and 2.1 percent of high schools) offered daily physical education or its equivalent for the entire school year for students in all grades. Even if daily physical education is offered, students are not always adequately active during class. For example, McKenzie and colleagues' (1995) observations of elementary school students during physical education indicated that students were not moderately to vigorously physically active for at least 50 percent of class time.

These problems can be addressed by the interventions discussed in the *Community Guide,* which indicate that **policy changes,** physical education curricular changes, or modifications to physical education teaching practices are necessary to enhance school-based physical education programs. The National Association for Sport and Physical Education (2004) also emphasizes that appropriate and effective policies, practices, curricula, and instruction are essential for implementing successful school-based physical education. We next explore these types of modifications in more detail. Keep in mind that such interventions will most likely require that you work in partnership with school health councils, parent–teacher associations, school principals, physical education teachers, or other neighborhood school or school district staff to bring about change.

Policy Changes

Developing new or modifying existing physical education policies assists schools in offering more opportunities for students to be physically active during the school day. This may be accomplished with policies that require lengthening physical education class time or increasing the number of days physical education is offered. For example, the SPARK (Sports, Play, and Active Recreation for Kids) intervention required that physical education classes last 30 minutes and be held three times per week throughout the school year (Sallis et al., 1997). This type of strategy provides regular, ongoing opportunities for students to engage in physical activity. Students who participated in classroom teacher– and physical education teacher–led physical education intervention classes obtained 32.7 and 40.2 minutes per week, respectively, of MVPA. These findings compare with 17.8 minutes of weekly physical activity obtained by students in a control condition consisting of their usual physical education program. A similar strategy was used

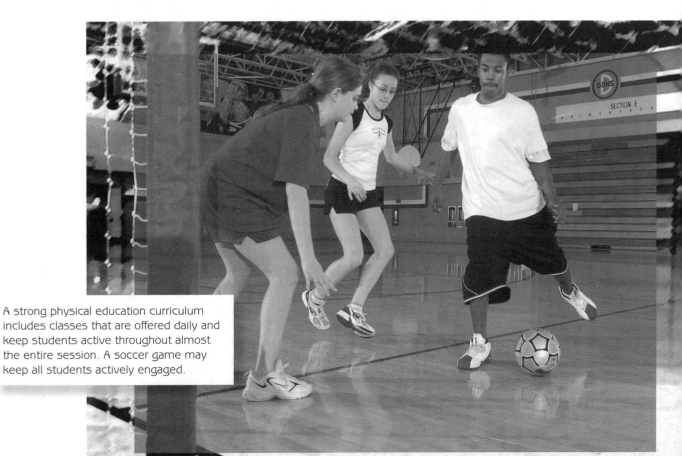

A strong physical education curriculum includes classes that are offered daily and keep students active throughout almost the entire session. A soccer game may keep all students actively engaged.

in the Physical Activity for Teenage Health (PATH) intervention, which required 30-minute physical education classes to be held five times per week (Fardy et al., 1996). Students in the physical education intervention obtained 20 to 25 minutes of physical activity through circuit training and received a 5-minute health behavior lecture each class period. The control participants in this study also were physically active in that they participated in volleyball in physical education class over the course of the study. Both boys and girls in the physical education intervention significantly improved their health knowledge compared with the volleyball control group. Girls in the physical education intervention also improved dietary habits, increased their estimated aerobic capacity, and reduced cholesterol compared with girls in the volleyball control group. The physical education component of the Child and Adolescent Trial for Cardiovascular Health (CATCH) intervention required schools to complete contracts for participation, and part of the contract agreement was the provision of at least 90 minutes of CATCH physical education per week, delivered over at least 3 school days (McKenzie et al., 1996). Compared with students in control classes (i.e., usual physical education classes, which served as the measurement-only condition), students in the CATCH classes engaged in more MVPA during physical education class (52 percent for the CATCH intervention vs. 42 percent for the control condition).

Although school policies often originate from the local level through school boards and districts or even individual schools, legislation at the federal or state level also can play an extremely important role in influencing policy changes. For example, Congress passed legislation within the Child Nutrition and WIC Reauthorization Act of 2004 that requires every school district participating in the federally funded school meals program to develop local wellness policies. This requirement states that wellness policies must include goals for physical activity and nutrition education, among other activities, to promote wellness. Although Congress did not provide funds to create and implement wellness polices and imposed no penalties for a school district's failure to do so, the legislation paved the way for states and school districts to make school-based physical activity or physical education policy changes. For example, in 2005, Kentucky passed Senate Bill 172 that calls for Kentucky school districts to assist schools with assessing their physical activity and nutrition environments, assess K–5 students' levels of physical activity annually, integrate language into their local wellness policies to promote up to 150 minutes per week of MVPA for K–5 students, and abide by nutritional standards for foods and beverages. The bill also requires school districts to develop a report based on the assessment of physical activity and nutrition environments in schools; these reports are to be shared with parents, local school board members, and school council members and must include recommendations to make improvements. To support the implementation of the required activities, the Kentucky Board of Education developed guidance documents, sample policy language, and sample reporting formats for local school districts to use.

Information resulting from tracking state-level legislative activity related to physical education and physical activity in schools indicates that the volume of legislation has increased consistently over the course of legislative session years. In 2001-2002, 316 bills related to physical education were introduced and 60 bills passed in state legislatures, according to the Centers for Disease Control and Prevention, Division of Nutrition, Physical Activity and Obesity State Legislative database (Centers for Disease Control and Prevention, 2007). In 2003-2004, 321 bills were introduced and 57 passed, and in 2005-2006, 410 bills were introduced and 94 passed. The attention state legislatures have given to physical education and physical activity in schools indicates that there is increasing visibility and awareness of the risks of inactivity among youth today. Your efforts to promote physical activity among youth may capitalize on this increasing awareness and the recent legislative and policy initiatives.

Modifications to Physical Education Curriculum

In addition to policy changes, modifications to the written curriculum can increase the amount of physically active time during existing physical education class. One type of curricular change is to modify game rules to make games more active. For example, the SPARK and CATCH interventions modified traditional softball game rules so that the entire team at bat ran the bases and the fielding team had a designated number of fielders to whom the ball was thrown before the batting team could be declared "out" (McKenzie et al., 1996; Sallis et al., 1997).

The attention state legislatures have given to physical education and physical activity in schools indicates that there is increasing visibility and awareness of the risks of inactivity among youth today.

Another example of modifying game rules is to replace a game that requires large teams but allows few players to be active at any given point, such as traditional kickball, with a modification that uses several small teams (e.g., four-on-four or two-on-two). This strategy not only increases students' physical activity but also provides more time for skills practice and development. In addition to modifying game rules, curricula can be changed by replacing games or activities that tend to provide low levels of physical activity with those that are inherently more active. For example, replace traditional softball games, in which only a few students are active at a time, with soccer, in which every member of both teams is active during most of the game (see CATCH PE lesson sidebar later in this chapter).

Another curricular modification that might increase students' MVPA and contribute to improved physical fitness is the incorporation of fitness activities into all physical education lessons. In SPARK, every 30-minute physical education class consisted of 15 minutes of health-related fitness activities and 15 minutes of skill-based activities (Sallis et al., 1997). Games and activities that increase aerobic and muscular fitness, such as fitness stations, jogging, jump rope, and active tag games, also can be included as part of all lessons. The PATH intervention consisted of a variety of circuit training (a combination of resistance and aerobic exercise) stations that enabled students to be consistently active for at least 20 minutes of the 30-minute physical education class (Fardy et al., 1996). Finally, in both the Children's Active Physical Education (CAPE) intervention (the physical education component of a school-based physical activity and healthy diet program) and the physical education component of a 2-year intervention conducted by Donnelly and colleagues (1996), physical education class time was spent on aerobic exercises that could easily be incorporated into students' lifestyles. These aerobic exercises included hopping, skipping, dancing, jumping rope, and noncompetitive aerobic games (Donnelly et al., 1996; Simons-Morton et al., 1991).

Modifications to Physical Education Teaching Practices

Many of the interventions recommended within the *Community Guide* included physical education teacher training that developed teachers' ability to modify instructional strategies to increase time spent in MVPA (Manios et al., 1999; McKenzie et al., 1996; Sallis et al., 1997; Vandongen et al., 1995). One example of a teaching modification is to ensure that all students have manipulative equipment, such as balls and jump ropes. This allows every student to have adequate skill practice and full participation rather than wait in long lines or on the sidelines to practice and participate. Modifying teaching practices also involves providing active instruction and active class management. For example, instead of sitting or standing during activities such as roll call or receiving equipment, students walk or engage in some other form of physical activity.

To increase students' participation in physical activity, teachers can also use strategies to increase students' enjoyment, such as (1) teaching physical activities that include all students; (2) excluding elimination and child-as-target games (e.g., traditional tag and dodge ball, which typically eliminate the less active or athletic students); (3) providing enthusiastic role modeling and positive **reinforcement** for active engagement; and (4) focusing on physical activities that students enjoy. Enjoyment of physical activity was a major goal and focus of the CATCH physical education program and the CAPE intervention. In the CAPE intervention, for example, students were instructed on two or three cardiovascular fitness activities during each physical education class, thus allowing them to experience new and enjoyable movement forms (Simons-Morton et al., 1991). Both SPARK and CATCH programs trained teachers to use appropriate teaching methods and effective role modeling for developing and maintaining an active lifestyle (McKenzie et al., 1996; Sallis et al., 1997).

Effects of Implementing Policy, Curricular, and Teaching Strategies

School-based physical education that uses the strategies discussed here would be characterized by activities that include all students and keep most students moving purposefully most of class time. Students would not wait in long lines to participate, sit or stand still for long periods of instruction, or participate in games and activities from which they would be eliminated or have limited opportunity to participate. The strategies described here are among those used in the studies that the Task Force reviewed before making its recommendation to increase the amount of time in which students are physically active during physical education class and to improve physical fitness levels of students. The CATCH intervention is described in more detail in the sidebar on page 70.

Many of the strategies used in the interventions recommended in the *Community Guide* are related to one or more of the following characteristics or primary components of quality physical education programs overall, as described by the National Association for Sport and Physical Education (2004):

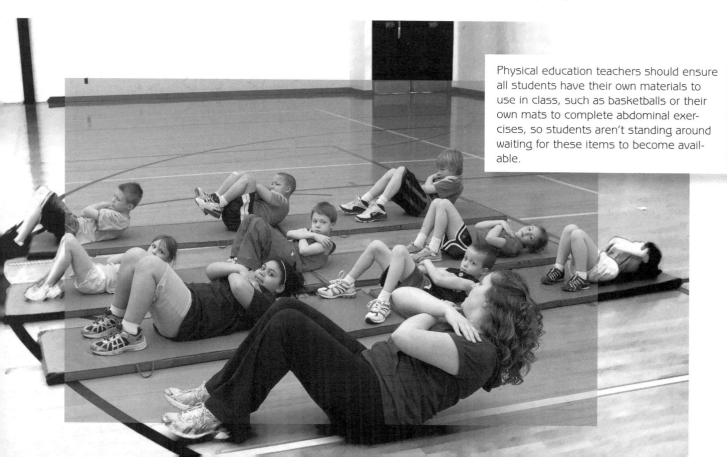

Physical education teachers should ensure all students have their own materials to use in class, such as basketballs or their own mats to complete abdominal exercises, so students aren't standing around waiting for these items to become available.

■ *Opportunity to learn,* which includes certified or credentialed physical education specialists, adequate instructional time (daily physical education for all students), and adequate and age-appropriate facilities and equipment

■ *Meaningful content,* which includes emphasis on motor, fitness, physical activity, social, and cooperative skills; fitness education and assessment; and promotion of physical activity throughout the lifespan

■ *Appropriate instruction,* which includes full inclusion of all students, maximum practice time for students to learn and apply skills, well-designed lessons to facilitate learning, out-of-school assignments to promote learning and student physical activity, a policy that physical activity is not used as punishment, and regular assessment to monitor and reinforce student learning

Many of the interventions that were recommended by the Task Force on Community Preventive Services used multiple components of a comprehensive and coordinated approach to delivering enhanced school-based physical education and integrating it into the school day. School-based physical education needs to be seen as part of the overall learning environment. It is not a luxury add-on that is divorced from the rest of a school's curricular offerings, as we discuss next.

Comprehensive and Coordinated Approaches to Physical Education

A physical education program offered within the context of a coordinated school health program (CSHP) model will optimize a school or school district's intent to improve overall student health and well-being. Physical education is one component of the eight-component CSHP model, which includes (1) physical education; (2) health education; (3) nutrition services; (4) health services; (5) healthy school environment; (6) counseling, psychological, and social services; (7) health promotion for staff; and (8) family and community involvement. All components, working collaboratively, play a vital role in supporting the health and physical activity habits of students, staff, and the community (Fetro, 1998). The effectiveness of school physical education can be enhanced when it is implemented as an integral and collaborative part of CSHP.

The following list provides examples of how school-based physical education interventions might use the CSHP model to develop and deliver intervention activities:

■ *Health education:* The reinforcement of physical activity and nutrition knowledge and concepts within classroom-based health education offered students the opportunity to practice decision making, goal setting, self-assessment, time management, and self-reinforcement skills in CATCH (McKenzie et al., 1996), SPARK (Sallis et al., 1997), CAPE (Simons-Morton et al., 1991), and the Cardiovascular Health in Children studies (Harrell et al., 1996). Including nutrition education in comprehensive interventions enables schools to establish consistent, healthy lifestyle messages related to healthy eating and regular physical activity. Health education lessons also may provide links to physical activity opportunities in and out of the school setting.

■ *Healthy school environment:* Including physical activity and healthy eating messages as part of school communications (e.g., daily intercom messages, school newspaper, bulletin boards) and providing safe indoor and outdoor facilities and equipment for physical education classes are strategies that can create consistently healthy environments for students (McKenzie et al., 1996; Simons-Morton et al., 1991). Active transport to school activities, one component of a school's comprehensive physical activity program, focus on providing safe and enabling environments for being physically active on the commute to school. These initiatives reinforce and complement a school-based physical education program by providing additional opportunities for students to be physically active.

■ *Parent, family, and community involvement:* Hosting parent or family physical activity nights and engaging parents in their child's physical education program may increase their ability to instill healthy habits at home. Partnering with local or community-based organizations, such as parent–teacher associations, health departments, YMCAs, and community recreation centers, to purchase equipment, train staff, and share facilities and program materials allows for greater program dissemination. For example, a health care provider in a Texas community provided funding to implement the Child and Adolescent Trial for Cardiovascular Health in low-income schools (Coleman et al., 2005). The funds allowed the program to purchase necessary equipment, pay for staff training, and promote the program at each school.

■ *Counseling, psychological, and social services:* Manios and colleagues (1999) worked with school counselors to deliver seminars to classroom and physical education teachers about the importance of integrating nutrition and physical fitness messages and lessons into teaching practices. School counselors and psychologists equipped to work with students on improving self-efficacy and self-competence for physical activity can support the efforts of physical education teachers.

■ *Nutrition services:* Improving school meal programs (e.g., lower-fat and lower-sodium food) and training food service staff to promote physical activity (e.g., via messages on table tents or posters in cafeterias) reinforce a school's overall healthy lifestyle approach. Requiring that vending machines, school stores, and fund-raising programs sell healthy food items creates a consistent message about overall healthy habits.

Details of the CATCH Physical Education Intervention

▶ **Intervention goal:** The primary goal of CATCH physical education was for third-, fourth, and fifth-grade students to participate in and enjoy MVPA. Schools provided a minimum of 90 minutes and a minimum of three classes of physical education per week.

▶ **Goal for teachers:** The primary goal for teachers was to engage all students in MVPA for at least 50 percent of class time.

▶ **Goal for students:** The primary goals for students were to enjoy being physically active, to participate in MVPA during physical education classes, and to use their skills to be active outside of physical education class and throughout life.

▶ **Teacher training:** Teachers were provided with initial training and materials—including a guidebook and a set of recommended activities—to help them select appropriate activities and use effective teaching and class management strategies to meet their goals. Schools received equipment as necessary and help in identifying and using available facilities. In addition to receiving the initial training, schools and teachers had regular on-site follow-up technical support and training.

■ *Health services*: School nurses and other health care providers can work with physical education teachers to refer students to physical activity programs in the community, provide physical activity prescriptions, recommend physical activity resources, and deliver lessons in physical education or health education classes on the role of physical activity in health and disease (e.g., blood pressure, cholesterol) (Pate et al., 2005).

■ *Health promotion for staff*: School employee wellness programs that include physical activity can increase teacher morale and improve general well-being and perceived ability to handle job stress (Allegrante & Michela 1990; Cullen et al., 1999). Physical activity clubs or fitness classes, offered as part of a comprehensive staff wellness program, provide school staff with multiple ways to be physically active and become role models for students. Schools or school districts might consider incentives or awards for staff who lead active lives. School staff working with physical education teachers might volunteer after-school time to lead physical activity and sports and recreation clubs.

Developing, implementing, and sustaining the strategies described here may seem to be an overwhelming task. Creating a school health council or enhancing an existing council may help with the ongoing development, monitoring, and sustainability of an enhanced school-based physical education program. The school health council is made up of a diverse group of individuals such as physical educators, health educators, food service staff, parents, community members, school administrators, school counselors, nurses, and students. The role of a school health council is to manage and coordinate school health policies, programs, activities, and resources (American Cancer Society, 1999). A school health council can strengthen the school's capacity to improve and sustain physical education policies, curricula, and instructional strategies and to coordinate efforts across many components of the CSHP model.

Finally, gaining support from school administrators and other school staff is necessary to sustain physical education programming. Providing these stakeholders with regular updates about the district's physical education programs and policies can raise awareness and foster ongoing interest and involvement in physical education.

Translation Research Example

The following physical activity research by Coleman, Heath, and colleagues (Coleman et al., 2005; Heath and Coleman, 2003) is an example of how evidenced-based interventions for school-based physical education have been translated for use to increase physical activity among youth. The El Paso CATCH program (www. catchtexas.org) was designed to use the framework of the national CATCH trial but was translated for use in Hispanic and low-income communities. Schools participating in CATCH in this study had a 95 to 99 percent Hispanic student population; 82 to 92 percent of children were eligible for free or reduced-cost meals or other form of public assistance, and 33 to 72 percent had limited English proficiency.

The process by which El Paso CATCH was able to implement the national program in its community included convening the appropriate stakeholders, leveraging funding, using experts and trained staff, and building sustainable partnerships to institutionalize the program. As part of modifying CATCH for this target population, the CATCH curriculum was adapted to reflect the Mexican descent and heritage of the El Paso population, such as character changes in the video and curriculum materials (e.g., Hearty-Heart and Friends was changed to CATCH Amigos). The

EAT SMART component included the healthier preparation of Mexican dishes as well as more innovative ways to introduce children to vegetables, because this region had the lowest fruit and vegetable consumption of any area in the nation.

The El Paso CATCH program resulted in significant increases in MVPA during physical education (increases ranged from 52 to 59 percent) among participating students (Heath and Coleman, 2003). The program also halted the increase in obesity among the students served. The results of the El Paso program showed no increase in obesity for either girls or boys in the third through fifth grades, whereas comparison schools experienced increases in obesity among girls and boys in these grades from 26 to 40 percent and 39 to 49 percent, respectively (Coleman et al., 2005).

Conclusion

This section provides evidence-based strategies for implementing enhanced school-based physical education. The following features, when implemented, have the potential to create sustainable enhancements to school-based physical education: (1) creation of new physical education policies or modifications to existing policies (e.g., longer physical education classes, additional physical education classes); (2) changes to physical education curriculum (e.g., modifying traditional sports, integrating fitness activities into each physical education lesson); and (3) modifications to teaching practices (e.g., keeping students active during roll call, role modeling during physical education class, offering a variety of new movement forms in physical education class). These changes have great potential for increasing students' active time during physical education class and improving students' overall fitness levels. When changes are complemented, supported, and coordinated by physical education teachers, health education teachers, nutrition services staff, school administrators, school nurses, counselors, and other school staff, it is more likely the changes will be sustained.

Key Resources for Enhanced School-Based Physical Education

The following resources may help you in designing and implementing enhanced school-based physical education programs. This is not intended to be an exhaustive list.

Federal Government

2008 Physical Activity Guidelines for Americans
Author and Publisher: U.S. Department of Health & Human Services
www.health.gov/paguidelines

Guidelines for School and Community Programs to Promote Lifelong Physical Activity Among Young People (1997)
Author and Publisher: Centers for Disease Control and Prevention
www.cdc.gov/healthyyouth/physicalactivity/guidelines/

Healthy People 2010, Volume II, 2nd edition (2000) (chapter 22, Physical Activity and Fitness)
Author and Publisher: U.S. Department of Health & Human Services
www.healthypeople.gov/Document/HTML/Volume2/22Physical.htm

Health Education Curriculum Analysis Tool
Author and Publisher: Centers for Disease Control and Prevention
www.cdc.gov/healthyyouth/hecat

*Physical Education and Physical Activity Fact Sheets: Results from the School
   Health Policies and Programs Study 2006.*
Author and Publisher: Centers for Disease Control and Prevention
www.cdc.gov/healthyyouth/shpps/2006/factsheets/pdf/FS_PhysicalEduca-
   tion_SHPPS2006.pdf
www.cdc.gov/healthyyouth/shpps/2006/factsheets/pdf/FS_PhysicalActivity_
   SHPPS2006.pdf

Physical Education Curriculum Analysis Tool
Author and Publisher: Centers for Disease Control and Prevention
www.cdc.gov/healthyyouth/pecat

*School Health Index for Physical Activity, Healthy Eating, and a Tobacco-Free
   Lifestyle: A Self-Assessment and Planning Guide—Elementary School* (2004),
   Middle/High School (2004)
Author and Publisher: Centers for Disease Control and Prevention
www.cdc.gov/healthyyouth/shi

Physical Education

Appropriate Practices for Elementary School Physical Education (2000)
Appropriate Practices for Middle School Physical Education (2001)
Appropriate Practices for High School Physical Education (2004)
Author and Publisher: National Association for Sport and Physical Education
   (NASPE)
www.aahperd.org/naspe

CATCH: Coordinated Approach to Child Health
The CATCH Program
www.catchinfo.org
Also CATCH Texas: www.catchtexas.org

*Concepts and Principles of Physical Education: What Every Student Needs to
   Know*, 2nd edition (2003)
Author: Mohnsen B
Publisher: National Association for Sport and Physical Education (NASPE)
www.aahperd.org/naspe

Designing the Physical Education Curriculum (2004)
Author: Kelly L, Melograno V
Publisher: Human Kinetics
www.humankinetics.com/products/showproduct.cfm?isbn=9780736041782

Fit, Healthy, and Ready to Learn: A School Health Policy Guide (2000)
Author: Bogden JF
Publisher: National Association of State Boards of Education (NASBE)
www.nasbe.org

Moving Into the Future: National Standards for Physical Education, 2nd edition (2004)
Author and Publisher: National Association for Sport and Physical Education (NASPE)
www.aahperd.org/naspe

National Standards for Beginning Physical Education Teachers, 2nd edition (2003)
Author and Publisher: National Association for Sport and Physical Education (NASPE)
www.aahperd.org/naspe

Opportunity to Learn Standards for Elementary School Physical Education (2000), *Middle School Physical Education* (2004), and *High School Physical Education* (2004)
Author and Publisher: National Association for Sport and Physical Education (NASPE)
www.aahperd.org/naspe

Physical Education for Lifelong Fitness: The Physical Best Teacher's Guide, 2nd edition (2005)
Author: National Association for Sport and Physical Education (NASPE)
Publisher: Human Kinetics
www.humankinetics.com/products/all-products/physical-education-for-life-long-fitness-2nd-edition

Senior Physical Education: An Integrated Approach (1999)
Authors: Kirk D, Burgess-Limerick R, Kiss M, Lahey J, Penney D
Publisher: Human Kinetics
www.humankinetics.com/products/all-products/physical-education-for-life-long-fitness-2nd-edition

SPARK
The SPARK Programs
www.ed.gov/pubs/EPTW/eptw9/eptw9f.html

Teaching Children Physical Education: Becoming a Master Teacher, 2nd edition (2001)
Author: Graham GM
Publisher: Human Kinetics
www.humankinetics.com/products/all-products/teaching-children-physical-education-3rd-edition

Teaching Middle School Physical Education: A Blueprint for Developing an Exemplary Program, 2nd edition (2003)
Author: Mohnsen B
Publisher: Human Kinetics
www.exrx.net/Store/HK/TeachingMiddleSchoolPhysEd.html

Teaching Physical Education for Learning, 4th edition (2002)
Author: Rink J
Publisher: McGraw-Hill
http://books.mcgraw-hill.com

Typical CATCH Physical Education Lesson

▶ A *warm-up* of 3 to 5 minutes, which began immediately upon arriving at the activity area. Often, instructions were given and equipment was distributed during this time, while students were moving.

▶ A *Go Fitness Activity* of 5 to 12 minutes. These activities were aerobic; they engaged all students in continuous MVPA. Examples include walking, jogging, and running games; a category of activities called "fast games"; and specific fitness activities.

▶ A *Go Activity* of 10 to 15 minutes. This was the main activity bout of the lesson and included a wide range of recreation and sports activities such as aerobics, hula hoop, jump rope, and parachute activities and modified basketball, football, flying disc, soccer, and volleyball.

▶ A *cool-down* of 3 to 5 minutes. This tapered the activity intensity down to a level for students to transition back to the classroom. While students were engaged in this activity, teachers often reviewed instructions, reinforced positive behavior, elicited feedback from students, and provided lesson closure.

Results of Intervention

The CATCH intervention increased student MVPA during class from 37 percent to 52 percent of class time, meeting the *Healthy People* objective. Most of the increase in MVPA was the result of teachers' modifying their activities and teaching methods.

Individually-Adapted Health Behavior Change Interventions

As described in the *Community Guide* (Kahn et al., 2002; Zaza et al., 2005), effective individually-adapted health behavior change interventions incorporate the following set of skills:

- Setting physical activity goals and self-monitoring progress toward successfully completing the goals
- Creating social support for becoming more physically active
- Reinforcing physical activity behavior change using self-rewards and positive self-talk
- Problem solving to initiate and maintain increases in physical activity
- Developing skills to prevent relapse to low levels of weekly physical activity

These skills can be used by people who are modifying their behavior to become more active or self-managing to remain active. In this regard, individually-adapted health behavior change interventions can be especially beneficial when used in clinical or laboratory settings, such as cardiac rehabilitation programs, in which individual exercise prescriptions and behaviors are closely monitored and adjusted when necessary. However, individually-adapted health behavior change interventions can also play an important role in community-level efforts to increase physical activity among groups of people and are therefore included here as effective community-based interventions. Such interventions have commonly been used to assist people enrolled in community-based physical activity classes, such as work site or university-based classes, or programs that encourage people to be more active through home-based programming. These types of physical activity opportunities can use individually-adapted health behavior change interventions delivered by program or exercise leaders face-to-face or using mail, telephone, or computer technology.

Task Force Recommendation
on Individually-Adapted Health Behavior Change Interventions

Eighteen studies that evaluated individually-adapted behavior change interventions designed to increase physical activity met the inclusion criteria for review by the Task Force on Community Preventive Services (Blair et al., 1986; Cardinal et al., 1995; Chen et al., 1998; Coleman et al., 1999; Dunn et al., 1999; Foreyt et al., 1993; Jarvis et al., 1997; Jeffry et al., 1998; Jette et al., 1999; Kanders et al., 1994; King et al., 1991; Marcus et al., 1998; Mayer et al., 1994; McAuley et al., 1994; Noland et al., 1989; Owen et al., 1987; Peterson et al., 1999; Wing et al., 1996). The studies rest largely on a foundation of theories or models such as the **social cognitive theory** (Bandura, 1986), the **health belief model** (Rosenstock, 1990), and the **transtheoretical model** (Prochaska and diClemente, 1984). These theories recognize and take into account the individual variability among people, including their physical activity preferences, interests, and readiness to make behavior changes (Kahn et al., 2002). Therefore, the individually-adapted health behavior change interventions have the potential to be used in a variety of settings with diverse population subgroups.

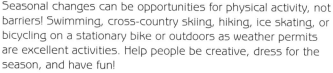

Seasonal changes can be opportunities for physical activity, not barriers! Swimming, cross-country skiing, hiking, ice skating, or bicycling on a stationary bike or outdoors as weather permits are excellent activities. Help people be creative, dress for the season, and have fun!
Photos courtesy of Roxanne C. Brown.

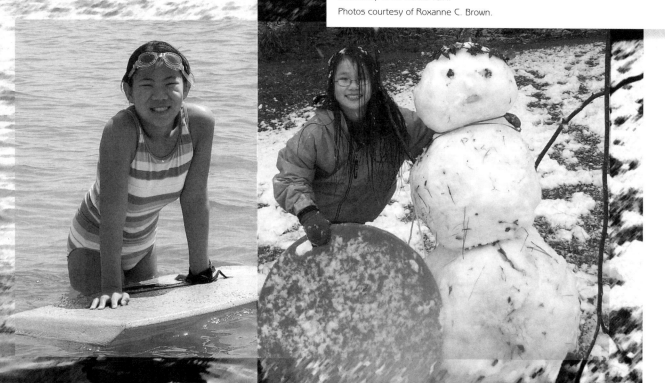

A summary of the effects of these interventions is as follows: There was a median increase of 35.4 percent in the amount of time that study participants were physically active (interquartile range 16.7-83.3 percent) and a 64.3 percent median increase in energy expenditure (interquartile range 31.2-85.5 percent) attributed to the behavior change interventions. Studies that assessed maximal oxygen uptake resulted in a 6.3 percent median increase (interquartile range 5.1-9.8 percent) in this measure of aerobic fitness. The *Community Guide* also reports that individually-adapted health behavior change interventions reduced body weight and percent body fat and increased strength and flexibility of participants in studies that assessed these outcomes. Based on these findings, the Task Force on Preventive Services determined that strong evidence exists to recommend the use of **individually-adapted health behavior change** physical activity interventions (Kahn et al., 2002; Zaza et al., 2005).

Update on Individually-Adapted Health Behavior Change Interventions

Although not defined as a review of individually-adapted health behavior change interventions to increase physical activity per se, a Cochrane review related to this intervention category was conducted and published (Foster et al., 2005) after the *Community Guide* findings were reported. The authors reviewed physical activity interventions that included components related to individually-adapted health behavior change interventions as described in this chapter. The Cochrane review focused on studies that included

- one-to-one counseling, advice, or group counseling;
- self-directed or prescribed physical activity;
- home- or facility-based physical activity;
- ongoing face-to-face support;
- telephone support;
- written educational and motivational support; and
- self-monitoring strategies.

With the exception of one study, there was no overlap between the studies that met inclusion criteria in the *Community Guide* and Cochrane review. Thus, the studies that are part of the Cochrane review further advance the knowledge base about this intervention category through 2005. The inclusion criteria used in the *Community Guide* process were more liberal than those used in the Cochrane review, which focused specifically on randomized controlled trials (RCTs). As a result, the findings reported by the Cochrane review were more conservative than those generated by the *Community Guide;* however, the Cochrane review authors concluded that the physical activity RCTs they reviewed have a positive and moderate effect on increasing self-reported physical activity and cardiorespiratory fitness.

The Cochrane review also points to the value of using telephone and printed educational materials in some interventions to support people in their efforts to initiate and increase physical activity. In the past decade, interventions using mediated approaches such as telephone, print, and Web site interventions to prompt individual behavior change have substantially increased (Castro and King, 2002; Humpel et al., 2004; Marcus et al., 2007; Marcus et al., 2000; Marcus, Owen, et al., 1998; Marshall et al., 2004; Napolitano and Marcus, 2002; Pinto et al., 2002; Vandelanotte et al., 2005, Vandelanotte et al., 2007; Van den Berg et al., 2007). Although it can be argued that these interventions are media-based rather than "classic" individual behavior change interventions, it is clear that theoretical approaches such as behavior theory, social cognitive theory, social learning theory, and the transtheoretical model have been successfully used beyond traditional face-to-face behavior modification and counseling efforts. Mediated approaches certainly can have their place in mass media campaigns or community-wide campaigns to increase physical activity, but they may also overlap with individually-adapted health behavior change interventions. Goal setting, feedback, monitoring of personal efforts to change physical activity behavior, reinforcement, and social support, for example, have been interwoven into a variety of mediated approaches to increase physical activity. Thus, individually-adapted health behavior change interventions have evolved with the evolution of information technology, and these strategies have tremendous potential to increase the prevalence of physical activity on a population level (see, e.g., Marcus et al., 2007).

Practical Application and Special Considerations

You may be involved in increasing physical activity behavior among members of group exercise classes or physical activity programs conducted in community-based settings such as university, work site, or senior centers. If so, you should use effective individually-adapted health behavior change interventions that use health behavior theories to assist the participants in your physical activity program gain the cognitive and behavioral skills to succeed with reaching their physical activity goals. Behavioral theories and individual behavior change interventions will provide you with a framework for guiding and evaluating the progress and success of your program participants. Your efforts in this regard may be guided by resources such as the first edition of this book (USDHHS, 1999), the National Cancer Institute's Theory at a Glance, and a book published by Marcus and Forsyth (2009) (see sidebar).

Because your goal is to help people develop lifestyle skills to initiate and maintain greater physical activity, you may ask, What skills or strategies can I pass on or teach to others to help them manage their own efforts to be physically active? This is an important question, because these interventions, when used in a public health context (typically with people participating in a group physical activity program) are delivered to individuals in person or by mail, computer, or telephone.

Resources

U.S. Department of Health & Human Services, Public Health Service, Centers for Disease Control and Prevention, National Center for Chronic Disease Prevention and health Promotion, Division of Nutrition and Physical Activity. 1999. *Promoting Physical Activity: A Guide for Community Action.* Champaign, IL: Human Kinetics.

Glanz, Karen and Rimer, Barbara K. September 2005. *Theory at a Glance*: A Guide for Health Promotion Practice. National Cancer Institute, National Institutes of Health, U.S. Department of Health and Human Services. NIH Pub. No. 05-3896. Washington, DC: NIH.

Marcus BH, Forsyth LH. 2009. *Motivating People to be Physically Active*. Champaign, IL: Human Kinetics.

Lack of training, planning and coordination, or important materials and resources will be barriers to the success of an intervention.

This part of the chapter describes some individually-adapted health behavior change strategies that have helped people increase their physical activity behavior. Whether people can successfully maintain increases in physical activity as a regular lifestyle behavior will be determined by the interaction between social (e.g., colleague support, a walking group among neighbors) and physical (e.g., opportunities for physical activity: parks and green spaces, facilities, sidewalks, traffic patterns) environmental factors, and the personal characteristics they possess (e.g., health status, motivation, behavioral skills). As a health professional, you can be a major catalyst for physical activity behavior change if you are able to identify barriers to physical activity and further plan and implement a course of action taking into account the interaction between individuals and their social and physical environments.

Although the following discussion focuses on studies that were evaluated as part of the *Community Guide* process, as consistent with the intended purpose of this book, the 12 intervention components described next are also characteristic of individually-adapted health behavior change interventions that have been conducted since the release of the *Community Guide*. Some of these interventions have been systematically evaluated in the Cochrane review (Foster et al., 2005) as described earlier in the section on updating this intervention category.

There is a need in public health to identify which components of physical activity interventions are effective in bringing about behavior change, but the state-of-the-art research indicates only whether multicomponent interventions overall are effective. Thus, it is incorrect to state that the components listed next have alone been effective. However, they are part of theory-based and evidence-based comprehensive interventions described in a few studies selected from the *Community Guide* as representative examples of individually-adapted health behavior change interventions. Review the full articles to learn how the individual components were integrated into broader intervention efforts. The evidence suggests that you should help people do the following:

1. Assess and increase participants' awareness and knowledge about physical activity and the health benefits of physical activity.

   • Distribute written information about physical activity (Chen et al., 1998; King et al., 1991) that may include materials and self-help booklets on starting and maintaining an exercise program (Chen et al., 1998; Marcus, Emmons, et al., 1998), a walking kit (Chen et al., 1998), printed information on the benefits of physical activity (Marcus, Emmons, et al., 1998), or an exercise manual (Coleman, et al., 1999) on walking and how to begin a walking program (Jarvis et al., 1997).

   • Increase knowledge about physical activity opportunities and provide individuals with tips about participating in safe and enjoyable activities (Marcus, Emmons, et al., 1998).

   • Provide participants with information about flexibility, strength, and endurance activities in a health promotion and education class (Mayer, et al., 1994) or teach them about their fitness levels and the physiological adaptations and fitness changes that can occur with exercise (McAuley et al., 1994).

2. Determine participants' readiness or intention to become more physically active.

- Use a computer-generated assessment to determine a participant's stage of motivational readiness (Marcus, Emmons, et al., 1998).

- Assess a participant's stage of change (Jarvis et al., 1997; Marcus, Emmons, et al. 1998) and use motivationally matched manuals (Marcus, Emmons, et al., 1998), or telephone-linked communications (Jarvis, 1997) to target each stage of readiness.

- Encourage participants to obtain their physical activity weekly goal in a way "uniquely adapted to each person's lifestyle" and level of motivational readiness to be physically active (Dunn et al., 1999).

3. Identify barriers to participants' ability to be more physically active and factors that facilitate their attempts to increase physical activity.

- Provide participants with information about perceived barriers to physical activity and decision making that balances the reasons for remaining inactive versus reasons to become more physically active (Marcus, Emmons, et al., 1998).

- Identify obstacles in weekly meetings with an activity counselor that are keeping participants from reaching their walking goals (Coleman et al., 1999).

- Use telephone calls to assess participants' barriers to physical activity (Chen et al., 1998).

4. Explore solutions to barriers to physical activity (e.g., time management, free or low-cost physical activity opportunities, child care options during participation in physical activity, social support) and ways to maximize or increase personal, social, and environmental influences that facilitate physical activity.

- Provide participants with mailings (Owen et. al.,1987) or a booklet (Marcus, Emmons, et al., 1998) that, in part, addresses obstacles to physical activity.

- In weekly meetings with an activity counselor, problem solve and determine solutions to obstacles keeping participants from reaching their walking goals (Coleman et al., 1999).

- Use telephone calls and tip sheets to help participants problem solve and find solutions to barriers (Chen et al., 1998).

- Provide small-group, facilitated discussions on cognitive and behavioral strategies for initiating and maintaining a physically active lifestyle (Dunn et al., 1999).

- Use a videotape or other materials designed to address misconceptions about exercising in later life (Jette et al., 1999).

5. Identify participants' goals and reasons for becoming active.

- Help participants set physical activity and exercise goals (Coleman et al., 1999; Dunn et al., 1999; Mayer et al., 1994). Individualize goals to tailor their physical activity to their different ability levels (Jette et al., 1999).

- Use health risk appraisal assessments and provide feedback of results to help participants with goal setting (Mayer et al., 1994).

- Develop physical activity goals for participants as part of their behavioral contracts (Coleman et al., 1999).

6. Know the proper amount (i.e., type, frequency, duration, and intensity) of physical activity that is required to successfully achieve participants' goals.

   - Use a brief telephone call to talk with participants about the benefits of exercise and to make recommendations about walking frequency, intensity, and duration, and send participants mailings related to physical activity (Chen et al., 1998).

   - Provide participants with exercise fact sheets and information about stretching techniques, exercise safety, and assessment of fitness levels (Owen et al., 1987) and handouts (e.g., *Age Pages*) that complement participants' physical activity goals (Mayer et al., 1994).

   - Use an exercise video and resistance bands to provide participants with a home-based resistance exercise training program (Jette et al., 1999) to increase muscle strength and endurance.

7. Assess participants' skill level and, if necessary, practice and learn the skills they need to increase self-efficacy and achieve their goals. These may include *mastery experiences* to increase confidence by practicing successful involvement in physical activity, *vicarious experiences* to observe peer role models who reinforce personal steps toward skill development and confidence in one's own abilities, *verbal encouragement or persuasion* to counsel and guide participants and to enhance self-efficacy by helping them make incremental steps toward achieving their physical activity goals, and *emotional support* to help people stay positive and combat self-defeating thoughts.

   - *Mastery experiences*: Use a trained exercise leader to provide initial exercise instruction and exercise supervision to participants for 3 weeks (Dunn et al., 1999), or even during a single walk (Coleman et al., 1999). Provide instruction on how to monitor pulse rates (King et al., 1991) or use the Borg scale to monitor exercise intensity (Coleman et al., 1999). Collaborate with a physical therapist (Jette et al. 1999) or other physical activity leader (King et al. 1991) to work with older adults to develop home-based physical activity programs.

   - *Vicarious experiences*: Provide participants with a motivational video of physical activity role models (Jette et al., 1999; McAuley et al., 1994).

   - *Verbal encouragement or persuasion*: Have an activity counselor call participants periodically to promote physical activity self-efficacy and to encourage and enhance positive self-talk about walking (Chen et al., 1998).

   - *Emotional support*: Provide cognitive restructuring (to combat self-devastating thoughts) (Jette et al., 1999).

8. Identify and obtain positive social support for being physically active.

   - Use an activity counselor to call participants periodically throughout the physical activity intervention to provide social support and to help people come up with their own plan to increase their social support (Chen et al., 1998).

   - Form buddy groups of two or three people to provide each other with social support and encouragement to be active, and periodically give program participants a booster sheet to encourage them to support their buddies (McAuley et al., 1994).

   - Use an interactive computer-based telecommunication system to provide weekly computer-generated telephone counseling support to increase physical activity (Jarvis et al., 1997).

- Incorporate significant others into the activity plan for support and reinforcement of behaviors (Chen et al., 1998).

9. Monitor participants' progress and performance and make steady incremental progress toward a physical activity goal that cannot be immediately reached. Tools such as pedometers or accelerometers can help people track their progress toward physical activity goals.

- Use gradual progression or increases in exercise duration as part of a program (McAuley et al., 1994).
- Have participants use physical activity or exercise logs or attendance logs to monitor their progress (Coleman et al., 1999; Jette et al., 1999; King et al., 1991; McAuley et al., 1994).
- Monitor participants' progress, answer questions, and provide support and feedback by making telephone calls (Chen et al., 1998; Jette et al., 1999; King et al., 1991; McAuley et al., 1994) to counsel participants.
- Hold periodic meetings to provide participants with progress reports (McAuley et al., 1994), and provide participants with feedback forms to help them monitor their progress (Owen et al., 1987) or provide participants with booster sheets to help them document their performance improvements, mastery of program requirements, and goals (McAuley et al., 1994).
- Provide encouraging feedback or assess performance improvements by conducting monthly timed walks (McAuley et al., 1994) or by tracking different color and thickness of elastic resistance bands used by participants (Jette et al., 1999).

10. Resolve problems if incremental or overall goals are not being achieved. It may be necessary to revise goals, especially if they are set too high or incremental improvements are too ambitious because of skill level or the inability to be physically active due to seasonal conditions or other factors.

- Use a telephone counselor to help participants identify and overcome barriers to walking (Chen et al., 1998). Reinforce discussions with tip sheets about how to overcome barriers (Chen et al., 1998).
- During weekly meetings, have an activity counselor help participants overcome obstacles that are keeping them from reaching their walking goals (Coleman et al., 1999).
- Include home assignments as part of a lifestyle physical activity intervention to enhance behavioral skills to problem solve (Dunn et al., 1999).

11. Obtain positive reinforcement or incentives for progressing successfully.

- Provide participants with praise (Coleman et al., 1999) and verbal reinforcement (Dunn et al., 1999).
- Use modest incentives (stickers or $1 bill for turning in exercise logs) (Jette et al., 1999), or use monetary contracts to motivate participants to complete physical activity measures (Coleman et al., 1999).
- Have participants identify rewards they will give themselves when they attain their goals (Coleman et al., 1999).

12. Anticipate and plan for relapse or periods when regular physical activity is difficult or impossible to obtain. Booster sessions may be needed to help people re-engage or jump start their physical activity after a relapse.

- Use telephone counseling to help participants develop physical activity relapse prevention skills (Chen et al., 1998).
- Provide participants with worksheets to anticipate problems they may encounter in maintaining walking after an intervention ends (Coleman et al., 1999), or with mailings that include instructions on how to prevent exercise relapse (Owen et al., 1987).

The following study, which was referenced in the *Community Guide,* is described to illustrate how the preceding strategies can be combined to increase physical activity.

Example of a Successful Intervention

A 16-week walking program was conducted for the faculty and staff at the University of Buffalo to help them meet the 1995 Centers for Disease Control and Prevention and American College of Sports Medicine recommendation for physical activity (at least 30 minutes a day of moderate-intensity physical activity on most days of the week) (Coleman et al., 1999). The intervention was also intended to help study participants integrate their newly adopted physical activity into their lifestyle for long-term maintenance. The study was designed to evaluate the extent to which continuous or accumulated bouts of 30 minutes of walking changed aerobic fitness, body composition, and blood pressure measures. This walking program was directed toward faculty and staff who did not engage in moderate-intensity exercise for 30 minutes a day, 5 days a week, or who were not vigorously active for 20 minutes a day three times a week.

To determine what program would effectively increase walking, three groups were formed:

- Those who walked for 30 minutes continuously on 6 days per week
- Those who did 10-minute walking bouts three times a day, on 6 days per week
- Those who accumulated 30 minutes of walking with structured times of their choice by using bouts lasting a minimum of 5 minutes throughout the day on 6 days per week

Self-Monitoring and Reinforcement

- Participants were taught goal setting and self-management techniques.
- Participants were responsible for writing a personal contract.
- Participants were instructed to read and complete weekly lessons that were part of an exercise manual they received at the beginning of their program.
- An individual incentive was provided in the form of a monetary deposit. Participants deposited $50 into an account and portions were refunded back to them as they progressed through the program and completed activity and physiological assessments with the potential of a full refund.

Personal Feedback

- Weekly one-on-one discussions were conducted between the participants and a counselor.
- Participants completed a self-report daily diary regarding their levels of activity along with a description.
- The counselor reviewed assignments (including quizzes each week covering reading material from the participants' exercise manual) and walking logs

and provided assistance to participants on the status of reaching their goals, and determining solutions to obstacles.

- The counselor provided encouragement and feedback to participants on their progress and self- determined personal rewards.

Program Characteristics Participants Said Worked for Them Include:

- Making my walks part of my lifestyle
- Setting reasonable goals
- Support of my family and friends
- Walking instead of doing sedentary things
- Having a structured walking route
- Having several alternative walking routes

Lessons Learned

- Walking programs totaling 30 minutes per day, 6 days per week, resulted in significant changes in health. At the 16-week point there was a decrease in systolic blood pressure and increase in aerobic fitness; at a 32-week follow-up point significant changes at week 16 were maintained, and there was also a significant decrease in diastolic blood pressure and percent body fat.
- Most participants built on their walking foundation by increasing time spent walking as well as intensity of walking activities.
- Work environments may be especially useful for promoting habitual activity.

Translation Research Example

The Strong for Life program (Jette et al., 1999) was cited by the *Community Guide* as one example of an evidenced-based program to increase physical activity in sedentary older adults. The program consisted of a 35-minute videotaped session of 11 exercises performed by a trained leader. Participants use color-coded elastic bands of varying resistance. Those in the program received two home visits by a physical therapist who reviewed behavioral techniques to maintain program adherence and exercise progression and self-management strategies such as goal setting, rewards, behavioral contracts, and self-monitoring. This program resulted in significant improvements (compared with a control group) in isometric strength for hip extension, hip abduction, shoulder abduction, and knee extension in addition to a significant reduction (18 percent) in overall disability.

Community dissemination of Strong for Life was later attempted with a Robert Wood Johnson–sponsored collaboration between Faith in Action (Etkin et al., 2006) (which included more than 1,000 coalitions of all faiths and other community organizations) and the developers of Strong for Life. The home-based exercise program was provided to frail, homebound older adults in 10 sites selected from the Faith in Action network. Coordinators from these sites enrolled volunteer trainers who were trained by physical therapists to work with the study participants as part of a train-the-trainer program. The physical strength outcome measures performed by therapists as part of the original study (Jette et al., 1999) were not assessed by the volunteer educators; however, the coordinators at each site or the volunteers assessed the participants' satisfaction with the program, their program adherence, and health and functioning outcomes as measured by a Short-Form Health Survey. Participants significantly improved their social functioning at the 4-month follow-up, and 53 percent of the participants exercised at least two times per week. Findings also showed that 98.6 percent of the older adult participants and 100 percent of the volunteer trainers rated the Strong for Life program positively at 4-month follow-up. This study concluded that Strong for Life could be safely and successfully disseminated to a wide community group of frail older persons through the use of trained volunteers, a feasible public health intervention.

Conclusion

Good news! People can successfully overcome barriers and become more physically active, and behavior change theories and models have been successfully used to increase physical activity among diverse groups of the U.S. population. Because of their effectiveness, as recognized in the *Community Guide,* a Cochrane review, and an expanding literature on interventions using mediated approaches, individually-adapted health behavior change interventions can play an important role in community-based and public health efforts to promote physical activity. However, these interventions alone have not led to large-scale increases in population levels of physical activity. From a public health perspective, physical activity interventions that focus on individual behavior change have been undersupported. That is, initial increases in physical activity brought about by these interventions typically are not supported within the broader context of an ecological model that makes the healthy choice the easy choice in terms of helping sustain the physical activity behavior changes. Environmental and policy approaches are designed to provide opportunities, support, and cues to help people develop healthier behaviors, including physical activity behaviors, and serve as an important complement to individual-level programs (Brownson et al., 2006). Physical activity–friendly organizational and community-based policies (e.g., at schools, work sites, and health care settings) and social and physical environments that are accessible to all are needed to support and reinforce the initiation and maintenance of physical activity among the broad and diverse segments of the U.S. population.

Suggested Reading

To learn more about behavioral theory– or model-based physical activity interventions, read the following:

Blissmer B, McAuley E. 2002. Testing the requirements of stages of physical activity among adults: the comparative effectiveness of stage-matched, mismatched, standard care, and control interventions. *Annals of Behavioral Medicine* 24(3):181-189.

Buckworth J, Dishman RK. 2002. *Exercise Psychology.* Champaign, IL: Human Kinetics, 191-253.

Hallam, J. 2004. The long-term impact of a four-session work-site intervention on selected social cognitive theory variables linked to adult exercise adherence. *Health Education & Behavior* 31(1): 88-100.

Kim C-J, Hwang AR, Yoo JS. 2004. The impact of a stage-matched intervention to promote exercise behavior in participants with type 2 diabetes. *International Journal of Nursing Studies* 41:833-841.

Marcus BH, Forsyth LH. 2009. *Motivating People to be Physically Active.* Champaign, IL: Human Kinetics.

Marshall A, Bauman A, Owen N, et al. 2003. Population-based randomized controlled trial of a stage-targeted physical activity intervention. *Annals of Behavioral Medicine* 25(3):194-202.

Sallis J, Owen N. 1998. *Physical Activity and Behavioral Medicine.* Thousand Oaks, CA: Sage.

Woods C, Mutrie N, Scott M. 2002. Physical activity intervention: a transtheoretical model-based intervention designed to help sedentary young adults become active. *Health Education Research* 17(4):451-460.

For additional background on behavioral theories, see the following:

Bandura A. 1986. *Social Foundations of Thought and Action: A Social-Cognitive Theory.* Englewood Cliffs, NJ: Prentice Hall.

Glanz K, Rimer B. 2005. *Theory at a Glance: A Guide for Health Promotion Practice.* Bethesda, MD: National Cancer Institute.

Marcus BH, Banspach SW, Lefebvre RC, et al. 1992. Using the stages of change model to increase the adoption of physical activity among community participants. *American Journal of Health Promotion* 6(6):424-429.

Prochaska JO, di Clemente CC. 1984. *The Transtheoretical Approach: Crossing Traditional Boundaries of Change.* Homewood, IL: Dorsey Press.

Prochaska JO, DiClemente CC, Norcross JC. 1992. In search of how people change. *American Psychologist* 47:1102-1114.

Rosenstock IM. 1990. The health belief model: explaining health behavior through expectancies. *Health Behavior and Health Education: Theory, Research, and Practice.* San Francisco: Jossey-Bass.

Rosenstock IM, Strecher VJ, Becker MH. 1988. Social learning theory and the health belief model. *Health Education Quarterly* 15:175-183.

For information on adherence, see these publications:

Dishman RK, Washburn RA, Heath GW (Eds.). 2004. *Physical Activity Epidemiology.* Champaign, IL: Human Kinetics, 391-437.

Morgan WP, Dishman RK. (Eds.). 2001. The academy papers: Adherence to exercise and physical activity. *Quest* 53(3):277-398.

Sherwood N, Jeffery R. 2000. The behavioral determinants of exercise: implications for physical activity interventions. *Annual Review of Nutrition* 20:21-24.

Social Support Interventions in Community Settings

Social support interventions in community settings (Kahn et al., 2002; Zaza et al., 2005) focus on changing physical activity behavior through developing social networks that support behavior change. You can help increase physical activity by assisting people to create new social networks or by working within preexisting networks in a social setting outside the family, such as the workplace (Kahn et al., 2002; Zaza et al., 2005). These interventions influence the social environment. Studies have used social support physical activity interventions in community settings to encourage physical activity behavior in various ways. Social support interventions in community settings often focus on exercise groups by providing companionship and support to help group members achieve their physical activity and fitness goals. In many studies, participants received phone calls from other participants or from study staff to monitor their progress and encourage them to continue being physically active (Kahn et al., 2002). Several interventions included discussion groups where participants could talk about barriers to exercise and negative feelings about exercise. These interventions may also involve setting up a buddy system, contracting with others to achieve specified levels of physical activity, or organizing walking groups or other groups to provide friendship and support (Kahn et al., 2002; Zaza et al., 2005). Figure 4.1 provides examples of social support interventions across a logic model. Keep in mind that even low levels of social support can help people to increase the time they are physically active, but the more social support people have, the more likely they are to be active.

Inputs	Activities	Outputs	Outcomes		

Health coalition
 	
Health department
 	
Community sites:
 	
  Church site
 	
  Work site
 	
  University settings
	Create a buddy system
	
	Create social contracts
	
	Create an exercise (e.g., walking) group
		Pair participants with someone who provides encouragement and positive support
		
		Reflect on social contracts
		
		Information on how to find exercise (walking) partners
		
		Identify a leader to organize and facilitate exercise (walking) groups
		
		Identify times and routes for walking groups
			Short-term
			
			Increase knowledge of physical activity benefits
			
			Increase physical activity self-efficacy
			
			Identify and increase access to places where people can be physically active
			
			Better mood
				Intermediate
				
				Increase number of days per week person is active
				
				Increase duration of physical activity per day
				
				Increase intensity of physical activity over time (e.g., light- to moderate-intensity physical activity)
				
				Increase daily energy expenditure
				
				Increase aerobic capacity and cardiorespiratory fitness
					Long-term
					
					Prevent chronic diseases and disabilities
					
					Improve quality of life by making daily physical activity a part of routine behaviors

Figure 4.1 Logic model: Sample inputs, activities, outputs, and outcomes for changing physical activity behavior: Using social support interventions in community settings.

Task Force Recommendation on Social Support Interventions in Community Settings

The *Community Guide* identified nine interventions that used social support interventions in community settings to promote physical activity behavior (Avila and Hovell, 1994; Gill et al., 1984; Jason et al., 1991; King, 1988; King and Frederiksen, 1984; Kriska et al., 1986; Lombard et al., 1995; Simmons et al., 1998; Wankel et al., 1985). These nine studies were selected because they had suitable study designs and were well executed, following established decision rules (Briss et al., 2000; Briss et al., 2004). Several studies looked only at sedentary people, and the intervention was designed to get that group active.

Studies took place in the United States, Canada, and Australia, in community settings that included churches, community centers, universities, and work sites. The studies included men and women aged 18 years and older. According to the *Community Guide* (Kahn et al., 2002; Zaza et al., 2005), social support interventions in community settings should apply to diverse settings and populations, provided that the interventions are tailored to the target populations.

Interventions measured various outcomes to demonstrate changes in behaviors or fitness and health status. Outcome measures in social support community-based interventions included the number of times per day or week a person exercised, the length of time participants spent exercising, and increases in fitness as evidenced by measuring aerobic capacity. Changes in physical activity behaviors varied across studies. However, on average, number of times spent exercising increased 20 percent, time spent in physical activity increased by approximately 45 percent, and fitness—as measured by aerobic capacity—increased by 5 percent (Kahn et al., 2002; Zaza et al., 2005). Additional benefits of community-based social support interventions included decreases in body mass index and waist-to-hip ratio, a decrease in percent body fat of approximately 7 percent, increases in knowledge about exercise, increased confidence to be physically active (also known as self-efficacy), and increased numbers of social contacts. Based on the *Community Guide* rules of evidence, there is strong scientific evidence that social support interventions in community settings effectively increase levels of physical activity and energy expenditure and decrease body weight and fat (Kahn et al., 2002; Zaza et al., 2005). Two reviews published after the *Community Guide* provide additional evidence that social support interventions are effective (Hillsdon et al., 2005; Williams et al., 2008).

Practical Applications and Special Considerations

As you now know, social support community-based interventions are recommended to increase physical activity behaviors. These interventions can lead to benefits in addition to those described previously that are indicative of healthy communities, such as increased social cohesion, better-developed social networks, and an overall increase in social capital (Baker et al., 2000). Social support interventions can be used in any community, but there are some important things to keep in mind when implementing them in your community. This section addresses the broader macro community. There are also many micro communities (e.g., work sites) for which the same principles apply.

- Know your community. It is unique and its population's needs are often different than those in other communities. Talk to community leaders and look at census data. Use background information about activity levels, health outcomes, and community dynamics as you plan your intervention. Find out what the social networks are in your community (Heaney and Israel, 2002). How can you use those networks to provide intentional support to the community?

- To qualify as social support, an interpersonal relationship must provide some sort of assistance (Heaney and Israel, 2002). Social networks can provide support by affective (emotional), tangible, informational, and appraisal (sense of belonging) aspects of connections among and between individuals and more formal agencies and institutions (Baker et al., 2000). Decide what your intervention is working to change: knowledge, attitudes, or behavior. What specific support will be given in your intervention? Will it be emotional support (expressions of empathy, trust, and caring), instrumental support (tangible aid and services), informational support (advice, suggestions, and information), appraisal support (information for self-evaluation), or a combination of the four (Heaney and Israel, 2002)?

- Social support interventions should also take into account the following key considerations that guide other types of physical activity community interventions. Determine objectives of the interventions, its content, the format it will be delivered in, and who will deliver it. Behavioral theories are an excellent guide for intervention development, and some excellent theory-based interventions like those reviewed in the *Community Guide* can be adapted to fit your community. Part of planning is to create community buy-in for the intervention. Talk to community leaders and community groups and involve them in design and implementation. Produce written information that is at the appropriate reading level for your population and is culturally relevant. Include pictures of people from the community or pictures of people who look like people in the community as role models in the intervention materials. Suggest venues for activity that are available and accessible to the people in your community.

■ Measure the behaviors you plan to change. Include preintervention (pretest) measures in planning so that you know where your community is and where you want to go. It is also useful to know the rates of change in a similar community so you know that the change you have measured is actual change—this is called a control group. By measuring (posttest) outcomes, you can show how effective your program is.

■ Implement your intervention. Decide when social support in the community setting will be given—include community members in making these decisions. Contact media outlets and get free coverage for your program. Keep lines of communication open between community members and program staff. Try to adhere to your planned intervention but be flexible if it needs to be changed.

■ Share your results. Let the community (especially program participants) know how the program went—newsletters, newspaper articles, and a spot on the evening news are great ways to share results. Consider presenting your results at a scientific conference or writing a journal article to share your findings with other people who want to implement a similar program. Share both good and bad results as well as lessons learned; all the information is valuable.

Translational Research Examples

A successful social support study included in the *Community Guide* addressed physical activity training for weight loss in a group of overweight Latino women (Avila, 1994). This support group consisted of a 1-hour session per week, for 8 weeks, and included behavioral contacts, self-monitoring using diaries, exercise, and assistance from an assigned buddy. Women were taught problem-solving skills such as identifying weight-related or exercise-related problems, generating a plan for solving the problem, implementing the plan, evaluating the outcome, and reevaluating the plan and revising it if not successful. Compared with control subjects, women participating in the study intervention showed significant reductions in body mass index, waist-to-hip ratio, waist circumference, hip circumference, aerobic fitness level, and frequency of walking for exercise.

A physical activity intervention by Petersen and colleagues (2005) is an example of how social support interventions to enhance fitness among women have been used in another community setting. The Heart and Soul Physical Activity Program (HSPAP) (Petersen, et al., 2005), a church-based social support intervention that lasted 12 weeks, focused on increasing physical activity, energy expenditure, and cardiovascular fitness in rural women aged 35 to 65. This study compared the effects of an information-only intervention with a social support intervention. Components of the social support intervention included the following:

■ Social support: Group members established walking partners and developed a sense of belonging to the group. The group met weekly to share physical activity goals, challenges, and successes; receive helpful information to promote physical activity; and participate in a variety of 15-minute group activity sessions.

■ Tangible support: Group members helped one another achieve goals, including finding places to be physically active. Group members received an individualized physical activity plan, a personal copy of a walking video and an audiotape, and a pedometer.

Promoting Healthy Lifestyles: Alternative Models Effects (PHLAME)

Promoting Healthy Lifestyles: Alternative Models Effects (PHLAME) (Elliot et al., 2004) is a program initiated to investigate strategies to achieve and maintain healthy lifestyles among firefighters. The study compares the effects of two work-site health-promotion strategies: a team-based peer-taught curriculum and one-on-one meetings with a trained health counselor; a third group acted as a control. The program was implemented among professional firefighters, with each representing a team unit. Results from team-based health-promotion studies indicate that a team environment can powerfully affect members' attitudes and behaviors. The program created three teams of four firefighters, with one member trained as a group leader.

The team-based intervention contained the following elements:

▶ A team leader received a 60-minute orientation and a team guide.

▶ Team members received a workbook with activities for each meeting.

▶ There were 10 meetings; 5 weekly meetings the first 5 weeks and the other 5 spaced out over the remaining 4-1/2 months.

▶ Participants received physical activity information, training, and workout information.

▶ Nutrition information was provided, including serving sizes, nutritional content, and food analysis.

▶ Within-group team-building activities were conducted.

▶ Between-group competitions were held.

▶ Participants received visual and group reminders on weeks when the group did not meet.

Firefighters who participated in the intervention group had significantly reduced low-density lipoprotein cholesterol compared with the other two groups as well as increased personal exercise habits compared with the control group. Work shift group cohesion was increased in the team intervention.

■ Self-esteem: Group members were encouraged by having their successes rewarded, by being provided with positive feedback, and by having their goals monitored.

■ Journal keeping: Each woman received an HSPAP booklet that provided a place to describe her thoughts and feelings in a journal as well as track her goals, successes, and challenges.

Women in the intervention group increased their overall activity based on 7-day recall (i.e., time spent in recreational, transport, occupational, and household activities) to greater than 150 minutes per week. The intervention group increased energy expenditure from 1,219 to 2,677 kilocalories per week (including all forms of physical activity). Finally, women in the intervention group increased their fitness levels by 75 percent, as measured by maximal oxygen concentration (from 16.5 to 28.9 milliliters per kilogram of body weight per minute).

See the sidebar on page 90 for another example of a successful social support intervention.

Conclusion

Community-level social support interventions to promote physical activity show strong evidence of effectiveness. These interventions can be tailored to and applied in various settings. They are likely to be effective across a wide range of populations and settings and may be particularly useful in combination with other intervention strategies (e.g., enhancing access to places for physical activity) (Heath et al., 2006; Kahn et al., 2002). Individuals working in community settings should follow established methods of program planning, implementation, and evaluation (see chapter 7) when putting these interventions into practice.

Suggested Reading

Social Support Measurement and Intervention: A Guide for Health and Social Scientists. 2002. New York: Oxford University Press.

Heaney CA, Israel BA. 1999. Social networks and social support. In: Glanz K, Rimer B (Eds), *Health Behavior and Health Education: Theory, Research and Practice*. San Francisco: Jossey-Bass; pp. 179-205.

Polanyi M, Frank J, et al. *The Workplace as a Setting for Health Promotion*. 2000. Thousand Oaks, CA: Sage.

CHAPTER 5

Environmental and Policy Approaches to Promoting Physical Activity

James F. Sallis, Gregory W. Heath, Thomas L. Schmid, and Candace Rutt

Creation of or Enhanced Access to Places for Physical Activity Combined With Informational Outreach Activities

Interventions designed to create or provide access to places where people can be physically active often involve the efforts of employers, schools, coalitions, government agencies, and community members. These interventions commonly include providing access to weight and aerobic fitness equipment in fitness centers or community centers, creating walking trails, and providing access to school grounds. Many of these interventions incorporate components such as supervision of equipment use, health behavior education, and risk factor screening leading to physical activity counseling and referrals to health services. Interventions to create or enhance opportunities for people to be physically active have been accompanied by promotion of facility use or access to these opportunities.

People can be active almost anywhere, including places not primarily designed for physical activity. One can do calisthenics in a hotel room, walk down a gravel road, or play Wiffle ball on a street with low traffic volume. Thus, interventions to increase access to physical activity in places not primarily designed for physical activity are of interest. However, research studies that form the evidence base for the access recommendation generally focus on increasing access to places with a major purpose of providing settings for physical activity, such as gyms, playgrounds, and walking trails. The informational outreach part of the recommendation reinforces that the focus is on places specifically designed for physical activity. For example, health professionals would not normally conduct outreach activities to promote walking down a gravel street, because probably few people would do so. However, informational outreach is desirable when one builds a walking trail, because a large number of community residents will potentially use the trail, but not until they are aware of its existence.

Recommendations on Creating or Enhancing Access to Places for Physical Activity

The Task Force on Community Preventive Services identified 10 studies that addressed creating or enhancing access to places for physical activity combined with informational outreach activities (Kahn et al., 2002; Zaza et al., 2005) that met the inclusion criteria published in the *Guide to Community Preventive Services: What Works to Promote Health?* All of the studies reviewed were conducted in the United States (Blair et al., 1986; Brownson et al., 1996; Cady et al., 1985; Eddy et al., 1990; Heirich et al., 1993; Henritze et al., 1992; King et al., 1988; Larsen and Simons, 1993; Lewis et al., 1993; Linenger et al., 1991). Studies were conducted at work sites; in low-income communities; in urban, suburban, and rural areas; and among selected racial and ethnic populations. The task force indicated that given the variety of settings and populations included in this body of evidence, the results should be applicable to diverse settings and populations provided appropriate attention is paid to adapting the intervention to the target population (Kahn et al., 2002; Zaza et al., 2005).

Numerous and varied physical activity measures were obtained in the 10 studies representing this intervention area. Measures included changes in aerobic capacity (median increase of 5.1 percent; interquartile range, 2.8 percent to 9.6 percent), energy expenditure (median increase of 8.2 percent; interquartile range, –2.0 to 24.6 percent), reports of leisure-time physical activity (median increase of 2.9 percent; interquartile range, –6.0 to 8.5 percent), a measured exercise score (median increase of 13.7 percent; interquartile range, –1.8 to 69.6 percent), and reports of three or more exercise sessions per week or frequency of physical activity sessions per week (median increase of 48.4 percent; interquartile range, 21.0 to 83.8 percent). These different measures could not be combined to make a single quantitative summary score. Notably, the overall results of the various measures indicate that this type of intervention is effective in increasing physical activity. According to *Community Guide* rules, strong evidence shows that creating or enhancing access to places for physical activity combined with informational outreach activities is effective in increasing levels of physical activity, as measured by an increase in the percentage of people engaging in physical activity (Kahn et al., 2002; Zaza et al., 2005).

Practical Application and Special Considerations

In this chapter numerous examples are provided from a variety of settings that illustrate the effectiveness of creating or enhancing places to be physically active. These include schools, work sites, public recreation facilities, and other community organizations. These examples may be replicated or adapted for use in your specific setting, or they may serve as a catalyst to stimulate your thinking about developing and implementing other novel interventions related to access and outreach.

Schools

As discussed in chapter 4 (in the subsection titled Enhanced School-Based Physical Education), school physical education and health education curricula are often studied as methods of promoting youth physical activity, and these strategies can be effective. School buildings and grounds are widely available public resources for physical activity, and the access to well-designed facilities may affect physical activity among students and the community. A study of 24 middle schools evaluated the relationship between the school social and physical environment with students' physical activity (Sallis et al., 2001). Observers coded environmental characteristics including the entire size of the accessible play areas; improvements such as basketball hoops, soccer goals, and playground markings; and the presence of play equipment, supervision, and organized activities. Students' physical activity was observed during periods when they could choose to be active: before school, after lunch, and after school. Although student activity levels generally were low, they were strongly related to the social and physical environments at school. For example, about 10 times as many students chose to be active when supervision and improvements were high than when those supports were absent. Interesting differences between boys and girls were reported, with boys being most active on outdoor courts and girls being most active in indoor facilities.

Some schools may have policies to restrict students' and community members' access to school grounds outside of school hours. If so, these abundant public resources are underused, and these policies may have the most negative impact on low-income communities that lack other resources. Among the groups seeking solutions, the Denver Learning Landscapes Alliance (http://thunder1.cudenver.edu/cye/lla/home.html) is transforming school grounds into community parks, concentrating on low-income communities. Instead of remaining underdeveloped fields surrounded by fences, school grounds become community parks with play equipment, areas of natural vegetation, gardens, and welcoming gates. The impact of these school ground renovations on children's physical activity and social capital is being evaluated to determine whether this community-based strategy increases residents' physical activity. The Denver Learning Landscapes Alliance intervention should best be viewed as a promising practice until effectiveness data are available; however, the research by Sallis and colleagues (2001) suggests that such environmental modifications will have a positive effect on physical activity behaviors.

Walking and cycling to and from school provide physical activity for youth. The California Department of Transportation provided $66 million in funding over 3 years for Safe Routes to Schools grants to 270 schools (Boarnet et al., 2005). Funding was used to make physical improvements such as sidewalk and bike lane construction or enhancements. Some schools added promotional and educational programs to encourage people to use the improved streets. In Marin County, walking to school increased 64 percent and biking increased 114 percent after a combined intervention was put in place (Staunton et al., 2003). A statewide evaluation of 10 schools found that students who passed by the improved areas on their way to school increased walking and biking by 15 percent compared with 4 percent for students who did not pass by the improved areas (Boarnet et al., 2005). The California funding also supported traffic calming and street crossing improvements around some schools. These environmental interventions include examples of community-scale and street-scale urban design policies and practices to promote physical activity, which are discussed in more detail later in the chapter.

Work Sites

The relative impact of three different approaches to physical fitness at the work site on cardiovascular risk reduction was examined, based on before-and-after health screening of employees and

People can be active almost anywhere, including places not primarily designed for physical activity.

employees' reports of participation in physical activities (Heirich et al., 1993). In three automobile plants of similar size, three approaches to promoting physical activity for cardiovascular risk reduction were tested: in site 1, access to a physical fitness facility with certified exercised leaders; in site 2, individualized behavior change involving one-to-one counseling with at-risk employees that included counseling to increase exercise; and in site 3, a combination of one-to-one counseling with employees plus organized opportunities to exercise with colleagues (i.e., buddy systems and teams) using a 1-mile walking route established within the plant. A fourth site served as a control site. The program at site 1 had little measurable impact on cardiovascular risks and showed results similar to those at the control site. The programs that included counseling outreach only (site 2) or a combination of counseling outreach and access to opportunities to exercise within the plant (site 3) were more effective and led to better health outcomes than did the program without outreach (site 1) or the control site (site 4). Participants in programs with counseling outreach reported a greater frequency of exercise and reduced cardiovascular disease risk related to blood pressure control (among people with hypertension), weight loss (among the overweight), or smoking cessation. Site 3, which offered counseling plus exercise, showed the greatest improvements on outcome measures. These results provide evidence that systematic, ongoing counseling outreach to increase exercise among employees is more effective than the presence of fitness facilities without such outreach. Moreover, significant increases in the frequency of exercise can be sustained without a substantial investment in facilities.

Residential Public Housing

Lewis and colleagues (1993), who researched the effect of enhanced facilities plus outreach on increasing physical activity in a public housing community, reported

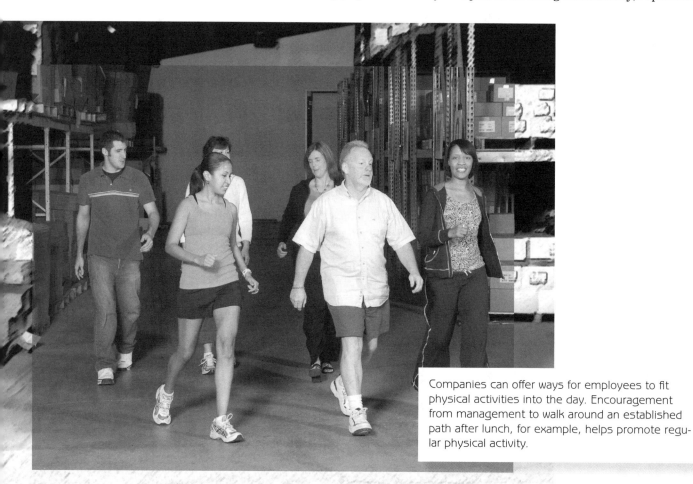

Companies can offer ways for employees to fit physical activities into the day. Encouragement from management to walk around an established path after lunch, for example, helps promote regular physical activity.

that outreach alone may not always be sufficient to motivate people to use enhanced facilities. The investigators found that outreach effectiveness can be influences by program staff who provide the counseling or outreach. The Physical Activity for Risk Reduction Project (PARR) (Lewis et al., 1993) sought to increase physical activity among low-income African American residents living in 1 of 13 public housing communities in Birmingham, Alabama, in part by enhancing existing physical activity facilities that were available in the communities. A unique aspect of this project was that lay exercise leaders were selected from among community residents representing each housing community and were an integral part of PARR's effort to encourage residents to be more active. PARR outreach efforts included recruiting residents for physical activity primarily through direct involvement with resident councils of the housing communities.

Two surveys conducted 1 year apart targeted about 80 households within each community. The first year's survey included questions on physical activity determinants, barriers, and preferences. Focus groups were formed, so both quantitative and qualitative data were available to shape and plan the interventions. The data confirmed the highly sedentary nature of the targeted population: less than 25 percent of the residents reported engaging in any kind of physical activity two or more times a week, and 31 percent said they got virtually no exercise.

Most of the public housing communities had facilities that could be used for physical activity, including playgrounds, open spaces, exercise equipment, and rooms that could be used for exercise programs. These facilities were enhanced by the community interventions. For example, each participating community received weightlifting equipment, provisions for aerobics programs (including audiotapes and portable tape players), and tools for screening participants (scales, stethoscopes, blood pressure monitors). As requested by the community residents, PARR staff incorporated activities such as games for children of both sexes, including indoor soccer; weightlifting for young adults of both sexes; aerobics and dance for women; basketball for men, and low-impact aerobics and walking for older adults regardless of sex. Although PARR staff encouraged people to form walking groups, several residents indicated that they were concerned about their safety while walking. PARR staff requested help from the local police to ensure that walking routes would remain safe.

PARR staff recruited and extensively trained individuals from each community, whom they paid as part-time leaders for the activity sessions. High turnover among the part-time lay activity leaders was an impediment to increasing physical activity among residents in some communities. Conversely, the single most important influence on participation in communities that were successful in increasing physical activity among their residents was the existence of strong lay leaders who remained in place during the intervention. These findings indicate that when addressing health and environmental disparities due to socioeconomic status or racial, ethnic, or cultural differences, outreach activities that accompany new or enhanced places for physical activity may need to go beyond merely informing people that these opportunities are available.

Public Recreation Facilities

Public parks and recreation facilities are widely used in the United States, with about 80 percent of the population using municipal facilities to some extent and a smaller but substantial percentage using park programs and services (Godbey et al., 2005). Various studies have shown that 30 to 65 percent of park users were engaged in physical activities or sports (Godbey et al., 2005). The contribution of public recreation facilities and programs to physical activity could be enhanced by optimizing the design of the facilities to support physical activity of various population groups, such as older adults and persons with disabilities, and promoting use of the facilities. The potential impact of improved park design was indicated by an Australian study reporting that adults with access to large and attractive public open spaces were 50 percent more likely walk for exercise regularly than those without such access (Giles-Corti et al., 2005).

The National Recreation and Park Association has partnered with the National Heart, Lung, and Blood Institute on the Hearts N' Parks Program, whose goal is to promote physical activity in parks to reduce the occurrence of chronic diseases. Interested recreation agencies became Hearts N' Parks magnet centers because of their interest in contributing to public health improvement and their ability to serve high-risk population groups. Youth efforts emphasized after-school and summer camp programs. Adult target populations were senior center attendees, city employees, and the general population of adult park users. A recent evaluation of magnet centers that developed multiple physical activity promotion programs found that 50 Hearts N' Parks magnet centers were operating in 11 states. Participants in programs were found to improved knowledge, attitudes, and physical activity behavior based on standardized survey procedures (www.nhlbi.nih.gov/health/prof/heart/obesity/hrt_n_pk/index.htm). The Hearts N' Parks magnet center program was conducted for 3 years with coordination but no funding from the national partners. This appears to be a valuable national effort that needs to be more widely disseminated.

There is some evidence that park and recreation professionals are enthusiastic about participating in more physical activity promotion. A survey of 44 recreation center directors in San Diego County found that most center directors wanted to provide more physical activity programs to youth, 75 percent were willing to partner with health professionals to train staff in physical activity leadership, and 59 percent wanted to improve the marketing of their programs. The most frequently cited barriers to offering more physical activity programs for youth were inadequate staff and training, departmental support, and funding (Moody et al., 2004). There is a need for increased collaboration between public health and recreation professionals to maximize the use of public recreation facilities for physical activity.

Promoting the Use of Facilities

According to Behavioral Risk Factor Surveillance System data in 1997, 60 percent of the population in the state of Missouri were overweight, and 65 percent were not sufficiently active to meet public health recommendations. To address this health problem, the Missouri Department of Health and Senior Services, with the assistance of community heart health coalitions throughout parts of rural Missouri, conducted activities to modify risk factors for cardiovascular disease, including physical inactivity. Community-wide events targeting physical inactivity included establishing aerobic exercise classes and walking clubs and developing walking trails (Brownson et al., 1996).

The Missouri Department of Health and Senior Services, with the assistance of a community heart health coalition, helped to fund the construction of walking trails in two communities through the Missouri Department of Transportation. Although a formal evaluation was not conducted, Department of Transportation staff had heard that trails were underused because of safety concerns and lack of amenities such as playground equipment and well-maintained restrooms. Because other communities were requesting funds to build trails, the state needed to know whether the investment would be worthwhile. To promote use of the existing trails, the state funded the health department to conduct an awareness campaign and trail enhancement activities in one of the communities with a 1-year-old trail. If community members were not more physically active after having both access to a walking trail and information about the trail and the benefits of regular physical activity, then the state probably would not fund additional trails.

The health department and a heart health coalition conducted the resulting Take Our Trail campaign for 3 months. Components of the Take Our Trail campaign are described through a composite of several articles (Brownson et al., 2005; Brownson et al., 2000; Eyler et al. 1999; Wiggs et al. 2006). The Take Our Trail campaign kicked off with a 3-mile Family Fun Walk and provided T-shirts and refreshments donated by local businesses. Throughout the campaign, signs were placed throughout the community to raise awareness of the trail. A simple brochure was sent to all programs in the local health department, as well as to clinics, church leaders, and the heart health coalition. The brochure contained information about the importance of physical activity, tips to increase walking, safety information, information about the trail, and names of people to contact for walking club information. The local television station created a public service announcement during the evening news to promote the trail and the importance of regular physical activity. The public transportation system placed signs inside buses. The heart health coalition helped develop walking clubs at work sites, churches, and social organizations. Local law enforcement officials agreed to patrol the walking trail periodically. The coalition worked with local business, city government, and churches to raise money to enhance the trail, adding amenities to the trails such as lights, benches, mile markers, painted lanes, and a water fountain.

The primary purposes of the evaluation were to determine whether a promotional campaign would increase the use of existing trails and increase the number of individuals who met recommended levels of physical activity. The Take Our Trail community had a 35 percent increase in trail use between 1 month before and 1 month after the springtime campaign compared with a 10 percent increase in the community without the campaign. Data from the walking trail counter indicated that trail usage was very high during Take Our Trail events. Use increased more with the formation of walking clubs in both communities (note: in the control community, several walking clubs formed naturally and were recorded in the event log system), but the increase in the Take Our Trail community was significantly higher. In addition, Sunday afternoon and Wednesday evening use increased with the creation of the church-based walking clubs (Brownson et al., 2005).

Interviews with stakeholders revealed that individuals in the campaign community felt safer while walking than did people in the community with a trail and no campaign, because of walking with partners (e.g., walking clubs), trail lights, and police patrols. More than 60 percent of trail users in both communities indicated an increase in their walking since the trail had existed.

All types of people used the trail, but especially women, older adults, athletes recovering from injuries, and people with medical conditions that required a low-impact activity. These included many of the groups who were targeted for use, especially older adults and people with low incomes. When asked how they became aware of the trail, most of the respondents indicated that they lived or worked near the trail or had heard about it at church or work, from their physicians, or from friends or family.

There is a need for increased collaboration between public health and recreation professionals to maximize the use of public recreation facilities for physical activity.

Evaluation of the Take Our Trail program suggested that the construction of walking trails increased physical activity and the implementation of a campaign to promote trail use further increased physical activity. These findings were shared with the Department of Transportation with a recommendation to build additional walking trails and support campaigns aimed at increasing trail usage. The report to the Department of Transportation also suggested that the focus of these campaigns include community-wide involvement in promoting the trail per se, promoting walking, and in making future trail enhancements.

Enhancing Physical Activity Through Community Organizations

Many community organizations provide physical activity facilities or programs, or they could do so. In the private sector, health clubs, dance studios, martial arts organizations, swimming clubs, and sports leagues are familiar examples. Nonprofit organizations, such as YMCAs, YWCAs, Boys and Girls Clubs, and sports leagues are great potential community partners. Faith-based organizations often have physical activity facilities and programs for their members, which could be made available to others in the community. Private and public housing developments have recreational and fitness facilities, as do many senior centers and residential settings for older adults. Thus, many resources throughout the nation can be used for recreational physical activity, and with improved promotion they can become better used. However, there do not appear to be any systematic studies of how the facilities and programs of these community organizations contribute to physical activity in their surrounding communities. Although there are undoubtedly many exemplary programs in these organizations, evaluation results related to outreach, access, or the programs themselves are lacking. The public health impact of these facilities and programs can be maximized by increasing the number of participants, increasing the frequency and duration of activity sessions, and sponsoring year-round programs, such as those offered by sports organizations, that include opportunities for participation by a variety of age groups and skill levels. Making resources available and accessible to the general community, including persons with disabilities, and offering reduced fees for low-income participants could also help reduce disparities in physical activity.

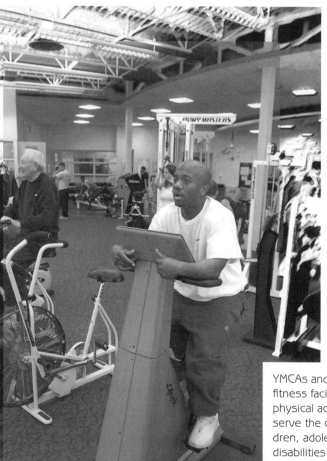

YMCAs and YWCAs and other local health and fitness facilities offer the general public access to physical activity opportunities. Increasingly, many serve the community with programming for children, adolescents, older adults, and persons with disabilities.

Costs, Benefits, and Funding

Two studies discussed in the *Community Guide* evaluated the costs and benefits of interventions to create or enhance access to places for physical activity. One 4-year study conducted at a fitness facility in Houston, Texas, for employees of an insurance company analyzed the costs and benefits of a structured physical fitness program (Bowne et al., 1984). Based on the quality assessment criteria used in the *Community Guide,* this study was classified as good (Carande-Kulis et al., 2000; *Guide to Community Preventive Services,* 2001). The program included regularly scheduled classes in aerobic dancing, calisthenics, and jogging as well as seminars on obesity, smoking, alcohol abuse, and stress reduction. Program benefits included savings in major medical costs, reduction in average number of disability days, and reduction in direct disability dollar costs. Program costs included personnel, nonsalary operating expenses, and medical claims. The adjusted estimates for benefits and costs for 1 year of the program per person were $1,106 and $451, respectively.

A second work site–based study was carried out for 5 years among 36,000 employees and retirees of an insurance company (Golaszewski et al., 1992), where a cost–benefit analysis of the company's health and fitness program was carried out by investigators. On the basis of the quality assessment criteria used in the *Community Guide,* this study was classified as good (Carande-Kulis et al., 2000; *Guide to Community Preventive Services,* 2001). The work site program included onsite health promotion centers, newsletters, medical reference texts, videotapes, and quarterly media campaigns. The cost analysis revealed cost savings from reduced health claims, a reduction in absenteeism, reduced death rate, and increased productivity. The costs of the program included personnel, indirect costs, capital equipment, materials, and rent. Adjusted estimates for benefits and costs were $139 million and $43 million, respectively.

A study conducted after the release of the *Community Guide* physical activity chapter by Wang and colleagues (2004) examined the cost of trail development and the number of users of four trails in Lincoln, Nebraska. The first year of trail development cost $289,035, of which 73 percent was construction cost. Of the 3,986 trail users, 88 percent indicated that they were physically active during their leisure time at least 3 days a week, including any activity on the trail. The average annual cost for people becoming more physically active was $98; for people who became active for general health improvement, it was $142; and for those who became active for weight loss, $884. The study provides a set of basic cost-effectiveness measures by compiling actual cost items of trail development, estimating the number and type of trail users, and identifying several physical activity-related outcomes.

Conclusion

This subsection of the chapter has provided several useful strategies for promoting physical activity through community outreach and increased access. These interventions are applicable in schools, work sites, recreation facilities, and other locations in the community. The concepts of access and outreach are complementary because it is necessary for people to have places for physical activity that are convenient, safe, and attractive, yet access to suitable places does not ensure high levels of use. Promotions and programs can inform and encourage people to take advantage of opportunities, but promotional strategies should not be expected to have much effect unless there are suitable places for activity. Undertaking these interventions requires collaborations among experts in physical design and promotional strategies, such as recreation, landscape architecture, marketing, social marketing, and community organization professionals. In designing facilities and promotional strategies, these professionals must consider the needs of diverse population groups, give high priority to groups with limited resources, and continually obtain community input so local needs can be met. The most effective strategies involve partnering with community groups from the very beginning, which can ensure the relevance of the interventions, build community capacity to continue the intervention, and enhance the chances for long-term influence on physical activity.

<u>Resources: Selected Access-Related Organizations and Web Sites</u>

CDC Physical Activity for Everyone—Trails for Health: www.cdc.gov/nccd-php/dnpa/physical/trails.htm

National Park Service Rivers, Trails and Conservation Assistance Program: www.nps.gov/rtca/

Bicycle and Pedestrian Programs: www.fhwa.dot.gov/environment/bikeped/bipedlnk.htm

Recreational Trails Program: www.fhwa.dot.gov/environment/rectrails/links.htm and www.fhwa.dot.gov/environment/rectrails/overview.htm

Federal Highway Administration (FHWA) Bicycle and Pedestrian Program: www.fhwa.dot.gov/environment/bikeped

FHWA Recreational Trails Program: www.fhwa.dot.gov/environment/rectrails

International Mountain Bicycling Association: www.imba.com/resources/grants/index.html

Bikes Belong Coalition: www.bikesbelong.org

CDC's KidsWalk-to-School: www.cdc.gov/nccdphp/dnpa/kidswalk/index.htm

National Center for Safe Routes to School: www.saferoutesinfo.org/

International Walk to School in the USA: www.bikewalk.org/saferoutestoschool.php

National Center for Walking and Bicycling www.activelivingresources.org/saferoutestoschool.php

Active and Safe Routes to School www.saferoutestoschool.ca/

www.saferoutestoschool.ca

Safe Routes to School: Practice and Promise: www.nhtsa.dot.gov/people/injury/pedbimot/bike/Safe-Routes-2004/

Community-Scale and Street-Scale Urban Design and Land Use Policies and Practices to Promote Physical Activity

Environmental and policy interventions related to urban design and land use can change the physical activity behavior of a large number of people in a geographic area, generating outreach well beyond what may be accomplished by individual or small-group interventions. Environmental and policy interventions can be used in conjunction with other interventions described in this book as informational, behavioral and social, and environmental and policy (e.g., enhanced access to places for physical activity with combined outreach activities) approaches. It is partly for these reasons that much research is currently being conducted evaluating environmental and policy interventions to increase physical activity.

Community-scale urban design and land use policies and practices support physical activity in geographic areas, generally several square kilometers or larger in area (Heath et al., 2006). Examples of community-scale interventions are zoning regulations; building codes; roadway design standards; policies that promote proximate placement of residential, commercial, and school properties; improved connectivity of streets and sidewalks; and increased population density while preserving green spaces.

Street-scale urban design is defined as design and land use policies that support physical activity in small geographic areas, generally limited to a few blocks. Examples include improved lighting, ease and safety of street crossing, sidewalk continuity, presence of traffic-calming structures, and aesthetic enhancements.

Transportation policy includes policies and practices that encourage and facilitate walking and bicycling for transportation, such as roadway design standards, expanding public transportation services, subsidizing public transportation, providing bicycle lanes and racks, and increasing the cost of parking (Heath et al., 2006).

This section explores the relationships between physical activity and transportation, community-scale, and street-scale urban designs, policies, and practices.

Recommendations for Using the Built Environment to Increase Physical Activity

In the United States, two expert panels, the Transportation Research Board/Institute of Medicine (TRB/IOM) and the Task Force on Community Preventive Services, have reviewed the evidence relating to how the built environment influences physical activity. The TRB/IOM report (Transportation Research Board and Institute of Medicine, 2005) concluded that the body of evidence linking the built environment to physical activity is at an early stage of development but that certain land use policies—higher population density, higher percentage of streets with a grid pattern, higher number of sidewalks, and higher employment density—are positively associated with greater walking. Accessibility (living or working closer to opportunities to be physically active) was also correlated with physical activity, as were design features and aesthetics, although these had weaker correlations.

The Task Force on Community Preventive Services also examined the literature with specific respect to community-scale urban design, street-scale urban design, and transportation policies and practices. Of 300 studies published between 1993 and 2003, 12 studies met inclusion criteria for evaluating the effectiveness of community-scale urban design and land use policies to increase physical activity. In these studies, physical activity outcomes included "change in pedestrians per hour per 1000 residents, percent change in pedestrians per 1000 housing units, percent trips, and distance and duration of the trip" (Heath et al., 2006, p. s60). A summary physical activity score across the diverse studies and outcome measures reviewed by the Task Force on Community Preventive Services was not calculated, but conclusions made based on a narrative review of findings indicate that community-scale urban design and land use policies are associated with higher levels of physical activity.

More than 100 studies published between 1987 and 2003 were identified that evaluated the effects of street-scale urban design and land use policies on physical activity. Of these, six studies using quasi-experimental, pre–post, or cross-sectional designs met the inclusion criteria for review by the task force. Outcome measures in these studies included "change or difference in the percentage of people walking, change or difference in the number of people active, and change or difference in the number of walkers, path users, or cyclists" (Heath et al., 2006, p. s62). There was an overall 35 percent (interquartile range, 16-62 percent) median increase in physical activity across study measures.

The task force concluded that there is sufficient evidence that community-scale and street-scale urban designs and land use policies are effective in increasing physical activity. Because only four studies met the *Community Guide* review criteria for transportation policy and practices, the task force described this area as having "'insufficient evidence" to make a recommendation. However, a large body of practice-based research and other research has been conducted since the initial *Community Guide* review. These new studies provide important information that helps inform practitioners about effective intervention strategies. A 2006 review by the National Institute for Health and Clinical Excellence (NICE) in the United Kingdom used a review process similar to the *Community Guide* to examine evidence for the effectiveness of transport interventions to increase physical activity. Twenty-six studies were reviewed across six main areas. In each case the preponderance of evidence was that slight to modest increases in walking and cycling (and outdoor play) were associated with these interventions. Categories of interventions included traffic calming, introduction or expansion of multiuse trails, closing or restricting use of roads, road user fees (tolls), improved cycling infrastructure, and programs that promote safe routes to school (NICE, 2006). Community-level, street-scale, and transportation-based interventions are often interrelated, and as the TRB/IOM and the *Community Guide* panels indicate, it was difficult to separate the effects of different environmental characteristics on physical activity behavior because many of the environmental variables are found together and are highly correlated. For instance, dense communities tend to have other characteristics associated with decreased automobile use and increased walking, such as higher parking costs, more mixed land use, lower automobile ownership rates, higher connectivity, and more mass transit options (Cervero and Radisch, 1996). The TRB/IOM, *Community Guide,* and NICE panels concluded that additional research is needed to disentangle the many interrelated and complex relationships characteristic of this research area.

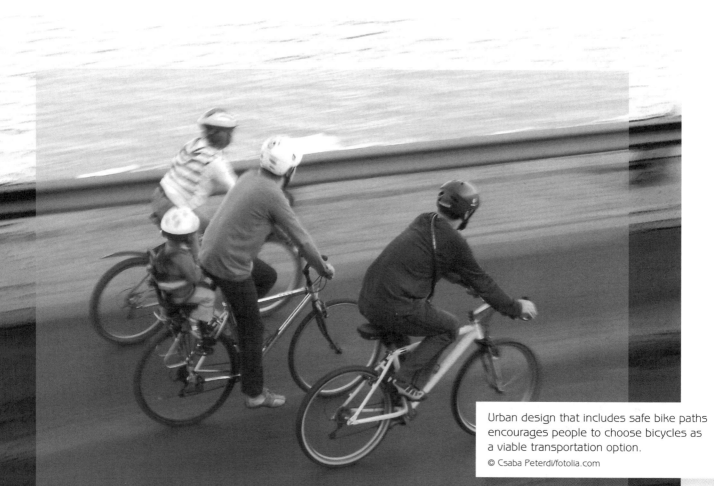

Urban design that includes safe bike paths encourages people to choose bicycles as a viable transportation option.
© Csaba Peterdi/fotolia.com

Practical Application and Special Considerations

Numerous examples illustrate the effectiveness of community-scale and street-scale urban design and land use policies and practices to promote physical activity. Similar to the interventions designed to increase access to physical activity that were discussed earlier in this chapter, community-scale and street-scale urban design interventions have been used in a variety of settings, including schools, work sites, and other community interventions.

Schools

Over the past half decade, public health advocates, transportation professionals, government officials, and parents have expressed increasing interest in encouraging children to walk and bike to school (CDC, 2004). Walk-to-school and safe routes to school programs are seen as an integral part of broader efforts to increase physical activity and active lifestyles in the population. The proportion of children walking or biking to school has declined by 60 percent over the past 25 years (CDC, 2004). Currently, few young people walk or bike to school, and most rely on nonactive forms of transportation, primarily automobiles and buses. Nationwide, only 10 percent of the trips to and from school are by nonmotorized means (CDC, 2004). Even among trips to and from school of 1 mile or less, only 28 percent are made by walking and only 1 percent are made by biking (CDC, 2004).

Schools are useful models for both environmental and policy interventions because the schools allow practitioners to use intuitive, logical, and data-based strategies. For instance, there is an increasing interest in where schools are located within a community because this has been found to affect many outcomes, including the ability of children to walk or bike to school. As noted previously, programs that promote safe routes to school can increase the percentage of students who commute to school by walking or bicycling (Boarnet et al., 2005; Staunton et al., 2003). Evidence also suggests that children who walk to school are more active during the rest of the day (Cooper et al., 2003; Tudor-Locke et al., 2003). The growing walk-to-school movement includes considerations about walkability, community access, and the school's contribution to the overall fabric of the community to the decision-making process. Local, urban-type schools (urban schools are those within the inner city as opposed to schools that are sited in the suburbs) can be conducive to students walking or cycling to school. Such schools are also good locations for the greater community to congregate for leisure activity and can serve as anchors to community structure. These schools can help define a community in comparison to big-box schools that tend to be more isolated or located on the fringes of a community.

Community partners who wish to promote physical activity through school placement, design, and access will need technical, practical, and political skills. They will also need tools to measure walkability to or around schools and theoretical and empirical approaches to guide the selection of community features to audit. These resources can be found on a variety of Web sites. These include the Active Living Research Web site (www.activelivingresearch.org), which provides synopses of recent research and links to measurement tools and related bibliographies. Advocacy groups such as walkinginfo.org also provide useful information. Policy-based guidance including tips on working with elected and appointed officials and examples of model codes, regulations, and design are provided through groups such as the National Governors Association (NGA), National Association of County and City Health Officials (NACCHO), and Surface Transportation Policy Project (STPP). For examples of practice-based experience, the Active Living by Design Web site provides related links, bibliographies, and case studies of community interventions. See table 5.1 for valuable Web resources related to environmental and policy interventions to promote physical activity in communities.

Table 5.1 Environmental and Policy Interventions to Promote Physical Activity

Organization	Web site	Summary
Research		
Active Living Research	www.activelivingresearch.org	Summaries of research findings, survey, assessment, and audit tools and extensive bibliography
National Institutes for Health and Clinical Excellence (UK) (NICE)	www.nice.org.uk	Systematic reviews and policy guidance
Practice		
Active Living by Design	www.activelivingbydesign.org/	Case studies, bibliography, and presentations
Pedestrian and Bicycle Information Center	www.walkinginfo.org	Practical material on developing and maintaining programs for safe routes to school, simple walkability checklists, and advocacy strategies
SUSTRANS (The sustainable transport charity)	www.sustrans.org.uk	UK-based pedestrian and cycling advocacy organization, resource library, case studies, and data on cycling and walking
CDC: KidsWalk-to-School	www.cdc.gov/nccdphp/dnpa/kidswalk/	Practical guidance, downloadable manual and presentations on implementing and evaluating walking to school programs
Regional Plan Association, Health Communities Initiative	www.rpa.org	Illustrative case studies on improving walkability through transit, school siting, and regional planning
PennSCAPEs	www.pennscapes.psu.edu	Policy and education tool (Web based) focusing on healthy and sustainable (walkable) community design
Policy and advocacy		
National Governor's Association	www.nga.org/portal/site/nga	Health communities initiatives; policy statement, and best-practices documents
National Association of County and City Health Officials and the American Planning Association	www.naccho.org	Nutrition and physical activity model policy, land use and health toolbox, PowerPoint presentations Includes "Land Use Planning 101"
Surface Transportation Policy Partnership	www.transact.org	Advocacy, policy, case studies, brief reports

Work Sites

Work sites have successfully used transportation and urban design policies and practices to increase walking and bicycling to work. One study of suburban workplaces listed "reducing motorized travel" as an advantage to pursuing **mixed-use developments** and suggested zoning and tax-incentive strategies to promote mixed use around workplaces. The report also found an association between the percentage of work trips by walking or bicycling and the share of commercial floor space devoted to retail around the workplace. Research showed that bringing additional land uses (e.g., places to shop, eat, or play) to a suburban workplace increases the number of non-work-related trips that can be taken on foot or bike and accessed directly from the work site without needing a motor vehicle (Cervero, 1988).

Another study examined how neighborhood environment is related to walking to work and found a significant relationship between a composite environmental score (aesthetics, traffic, destination) and walking to work (Craig et al., 2003). Mutrie and colleagues (2002) found that a simple intervention that provided information on behavior change, routes to work, and safety information significantly increased walking to work; however, the intervention did not affect cycling to work. This study was done in an urban area of the United Kingdom that had marked cycle routes, well-developed pedestrian amenities, and good access to transit. It is unclear whether such an intervention would be as effective in most U.S. cities, because they generally do not do not have well-developed pedestrian and bicycling infrastructures. The study by Mutrie and colleagues is also a good example of creating access to physical activity opportunities and enhancing their use by adding outreach activities, such as described earlier in the chapter. Similarly, the Nottingham Cycle-Friendly Employers project was designed to increase the number of employees who bicycle to work and for official work trips such as site visits (Cleary and McClintock, 2000). Incentives to increase physical activity included establishing secure bicycle parking at workplaces in addition to a variety of other environmental and policy changes:

- Provision of workplace showering and changing facilities
- Bicycle mileage allowances for short journeys on official business
- Interest-free loans for the purchase of bikes and equipment
- Purchase of company "pool" bicycles
- Publicity and information material
- Promotional events
- Establishment of bicycle user groups

The project's biggest success was in terms of encouraging existing cyclists to commute, but a 19.5 percent increase in cyclists using the UK cycling network was also found. Another study reported that a major benefit of successful walk- or cycle-to-work programs is that they promote lifestyle physical activity (habits that may endure) and improve aerobic fitness, decrease cardiovascular strain, increase use of fats as an energy source during physical activity, and lead to favorable changes in blood high-density lipoprotein cholesterol (Oja et al., 1998). A statistical modeling exercise explored factors that influence the choice to travel to work by bicycle or other means. The authors found that in the United Kingdom, a monetary incentive of 3 British pounds (about 5 dollars) per day would result in about a 55 percent increase in cycling to work. Incentives plus improved cycle routes, bicycle storage facilities, and showers at work would be the best way to increase cycling and reduce car commuting (Wardman et al., 2007).

Community Design and Physical Activity

As evident from the preceding discussion, transportation and urban design policies and practices can increase physical activity associated with specific community settings such as schools and work sites. Urban design on a broader community-wide scale can also influence physical activity behaviors, as the following studies illustrate.

Ewing and colleagues (2003) combined two national data sets, one that rated a community's level of sprawl and another generated by the Behavioral Risk Factor Survey, a nationwide survey that includes self-reported assessments of health and behavior. More than 200,000 people were included in the study. The sprawl index was based on a number of urban form features such as residential density (e.g., persons per square mile) and street accessibility (e.g., average block size, number of intersections). Scores ranged from 352 for compact Manhattan to 63 for sprawling Geauga County near Cleveland, Ohio. Results support the hypothesis that community design is associated with health and behavior (see sidebar). Even after statistically controlling for factors such as income, age, education, smoking, and race and ethnicity, the investigators found that people who lived in more sprawling communities were more likely to report less leisure-time walking, to be overweight, to eat fewer fruits and vegetables, and to have been told they have hypertension. Although the investigators did not report causal evidence, a variety of explanations for these findings implicate the automobile. People living in sprawling communities tend to spend more time in the car commuting, and this loss of free time may mean they have less leisure time during which to walk (Amarasinghe, 2006; Frank et al., 2004; Wen et al., 2006). It is also known that commuters are more likely to eat convenience foods and such foods are generally high in calories and sodium. Few drive-through windows feature fresh fruits and vegetables.

Frank and colleagues (2003, 2004, 2006) built on traditional automobile travel survey methods to compare a wide range of built environment variables such as land use mix (types of uses such as commercial, industrial, residential, and recreational) in a particular area, connectivity (how easy it is and how many ways there are to get from one place to another), density (number of people who live or work in an area), and recreational opportunities (green spaces, parks, gyms, and trails) with self-reported and objectively measured levels of physical activity. This study, called SMARTRAQ, included more than 8,000 households in the Atlanta metropolitan region. All respondents provided information on their travel habits and general level of physical activity. A subsample of respondents provided additional and more detailed information on their level and type of physical activity; some also provided objectively measured activity by wearing accelerometers. Both

---

Every 50-point increase in sprawl was associated with

- 14 minutes less walking per month,
- a 0.17 increase in body mass index (~1 pound or .45 kg per person), and
- a 10 percent increase in the odds of being obese.

From Ewing et al. 2003.

self-reported and objectively measured levels of physical activity were found to be significantly related to community design and, as Ewing and colleagues (2003) found, these results are significant at both a statistical and a practical level: Even in low-density Atlanta, for instance, as shown in figure 5.1, those living in less densely populated areas had a higher mean body mass index (BMI) than those in more densely populated areas. Figure 5.2 illustrates the differences in travel required to visit a neighbor in a traditional grid-style community as opposed to a typical suburban "lollypop" configuration. Although the air distances ("as the crow flies") are the same, the distances traveled on the ground are quite different. Significant associations were also found for land use mix and connectivity: Increases in these factors were associated with more physical activity and lower BMIs. In contrast, as illustrated by figure 5.3, more time spent in a car was associated with greater BMIs. (See sidebar for relationships between community design characteristics and walking and bicycling behaviors.)

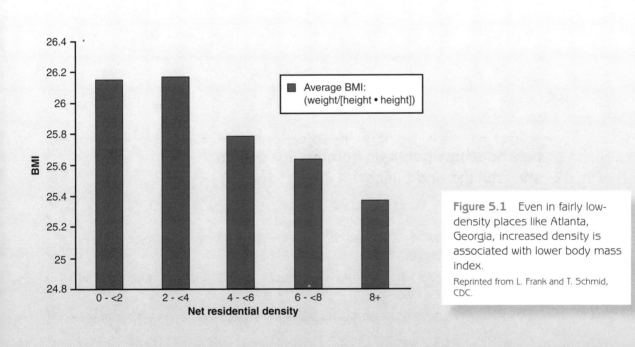

Figure 5.1 Even in fairly low-density places like Atlanta, Georgia, increased density is associated with lower body mass index.

Reprinted from L. Frank and T. Schmid, CDC.

Figure 5.2 Some neighborhood designs require people to travel much farther to go the same distance. Visiting a friend in the right panel requires more walking than visiting a friend who lives the same air distance in the left panel.

From *Health and Community Design* by Lawrence D. Frank, Peter O. Engelke, and Thomas L. Schmid. Copyright © 2003 Lawrence D. Frank and Peter O. Engelke. Reproduced by permission of Island Press, Washington, DC.

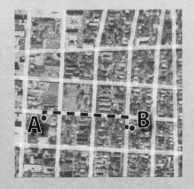
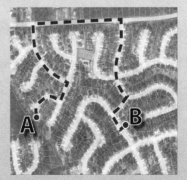

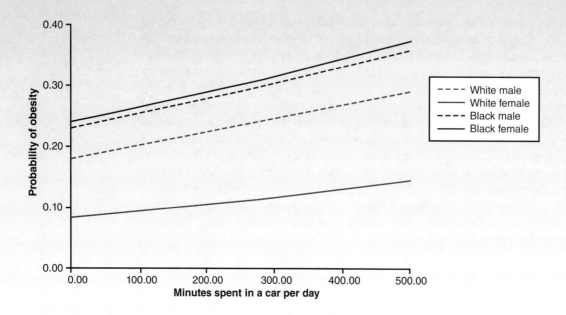

Figure 5.3 Each minute spent in a car is associated with an increase in the chance of being obese.

Reprinted from *Journal of Preventive Medicine*, Vol. 27 (4), L. Frank, M. Andresen, and T. Schmid, "Obesity relationships with community design, physical activity, and time spent in cars," pg. 87-96. Copyright 2004, with permission from Elsevier.

Relationships between community design and walking and biking

▸ Street network characteristics: Greater connectivity increases walking and biking.

▸ Street design: Traffic-calming pedestrian and bike amenities are associated with walking.

▸ Street design: Bike and walk facilities separated from traffic increase safety.

▸ Density: Walking and cycling increase with increased density (of household, work, retail).

▸ Land use mix: Greater mix is associated with increased walking and cycling.

▸ Site design: "New Urbanist" design with building closer to the street and pedestrian-oriented site design may be related to increased walking.

From *Health and Community Design* by Lawrence D. Frank, Peter O. Engelke, and Thomas L. Schmid. Copyright © 2003 by Lawrence D. Frank and Peter O. Engelke. Reproduced by permission of Island Press, Washington, DC.

Adding to the research of Ewing and colleagues (2003) and Frank and colleagues (2003, 2004, 2006), Moudon and colleagues (2006) evaluated relationships between those who walk enough to meet health recommendations and specific places in the environment that might serve as destinations. As shown in figure 5.4, people in Seattle who meet physical activity recommendations are more likely to live near destinations such as grocery stores, libraries, day care centers, and neighborhood centers. Another study based in Seattle used a walkability scale similar to that used in the Atlanta SMARTRAQ study and found similar results. For adults in the Seattle area, a 5 percent increase in walkability was associated with a 32.1 percent increase in time spent in active transport (e.g., walking, cycling), a .23 decrease in BMI, fewer miles traveled by vehicle, and less auto-based pollution (Frank et al., 2006).

Other countries, for example, Germany, the United Kingdom, and Colombia, have adopted design policies and practices that effectively promote and increase physical activity. From 1972 to 1995, the mode share of urban bicycling trips increased by 50 percent in Germany. This large increase is thought to be due to several policy changes that increased the safety, speed, and convenience of bicycling. The policies included giving cyclists right of way over cars, designating streets that are one way for cars and two way for cyclists, providing direct routes for cyclists but circuitous routes for cars, giving permission for cyclists but not cars to make left and right turns, providing advanced green lights for cyclists, providing bicycle safety training for children, holding bicycling festivals, increasing bike racks at transit stations, providing bike rental facilities, and creating an integrated well-marked system for cyclists. Other policies were focused on making automobile

Figure 5.4 People in Seattle who walk enough to meet recommendations (i.e., sufficient walkers) tend to live closer to restaurants, libraries, grocery stores, and neighborhood centers (NC, which are combinations of destinations) than people who do not walk enough (i.e., nonwalkers)

Reprinted, by permission, from A Mouden et al., 2006, "Operational definitions of walkable neighborhood: Theoretical and Empirical Insights," *Journal of Physical Activity and Health* 3(S1): S99-S117.

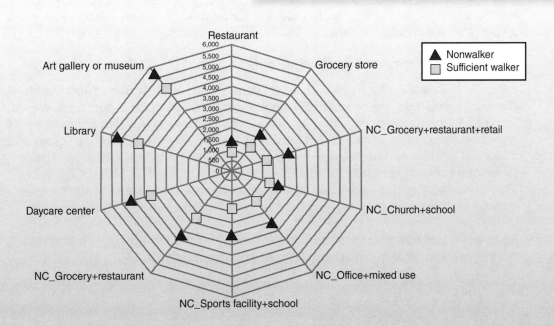

use more expensive and difficult (overall costs for automobile use are three times as much in Germany as in the United States). These policies included traffic calming, reducing speed limits, eliminating free parking, and decreasing the number of parking spaces (Pucher, 1997). An important element of a rational community mobility plan includes mass transit. Recent research in New York found that adding a commuter rail stop attracted new riders who used to drive, and many of the new riders reported meaningful increases in their level of activity; they reported increasing their total amount of activity per week, in many cases enough to move them from the "insufficient" to "meeting recommendations" categories of physical activity (Greenberg et al., 2005). Americans who use transit average 19 minutes of daily walking going to and from transit (Besser and Dannenberg, 2005). Werner and Evens (2007) also found increased walking by transit users. Train commuters were four times more likely to walk 10,000 steps per day and walked an average of 30 percent more steps per day than car commuters (Werner and Evens, 2007).

The United Kingdom has made substantial investments (~£210 million) in its bicycling network. In the year 2000 there were about 4,800 miles of bicycling network. By 2008 this had increased to over 12,000 miles. Data from 7,300 bicycle users were collected in 2000 and 2001; 43 percent used the trail for transportation and 53 percent used it for recreation; 42 percent said the trail network had helped them increase their physical activity by a large amount; 28 percent said the trail network had helped them increase their physical activity by a small amount; and 30 percent said the network did not change their total amount of physical activity (Lawlor et al., 2003).

In Bogotá, Colombia, a culture and environment very different from much of the United States, a recent study of the relationships between built form and transportation infrastructure found that even in this high-density, highly connected, highly mixed, and transport-friendly environment, the amounts of transportation-related and leisure-time physical activity are influenced by the environment in which people live. For instance, road facility designs and designations like street density, connectivity, and proximity to ciclovia (bicycle routes) lanes are associated with nonmotorized travel for utilitarian purposes, whereas density of parks and green space is associated with meeting physical activity recommendations through leisure time (Gomez et al., 2006). Country levels of active transport are also related to levels of obesity. An ecological study in Europe, North America, and Australia found a strong and significant correlation ($r = .86$, $p < .001$) between levels of active transportation and levels of obesity (Bassett et al., 2008).

The Built Environment and Diverse Subgroups of the U.S. Population

Earlier in this chapter (pp. 103-104), select conclusions made by the expert panels that developed the *Community Guide* review and TRB/IOM joint report were summarized. In the *Community Guide,* an additional conclusion was that community-scale and street-scale urban design interventions are likely to generalize across a variety of settings and population groups "provided appropriate attention is paid to adapting the intervention to the target population" (Heath et al., 2006, p. S61). This caveat to pay close attention to the target population is true for any type of community-based physical activity intervention, as demonstrated by the research in this area. The evidence indicates that nuances in how men and women, different age groups, and different racial and ethnic groups interact uniquely with the built environment need to be considered; these are discussed next.

General Relationships

Although general relationships between design and levels of physical activity generally hold, they are not universal. Just as the individual determinants of physical activity vary by gender, the importance of environmental factors in determining physical activity also varies by gender. Suminski and colleagues (2005) found that safety and destinations predicted whether women walked for exercise but did not predict whether men walked for exercise. In

> *The relationships between urban form and physical activity may differ not only by gender and age but also by race and ethnicity.*

another study, increases in men's vigorous-intensity physical activity were related to neighborhood environment, convenience of exercise facilities, and presence of exercise equipment in the home. For women, the absence of any kind of facilities was related to lower levels of physical activity (Sallis et al., 1992; Shaw et al., 1991).

There may also be differences in how the built environment encourages or discourages physical activity by age group. For instance, the immediate environment around the home may be more important for children, adolescents younger than 16 years of age, and elderly people who cannot drive because they have more limited mobility. New analyses suggest that the overall relationships between community form and patterns of activity also hold for young people in the SMARTRAQ study. In these analyses, Kerr and colleagues (2007) found that youth through young adults (5-20 years of age) reported significantly greater walking if they lived in places with either greater mix, connectivity, residential density, or recreational open space. In the Netherlands, the number of days in which youth 6 to 11 years of age met physical activity recommendations increased with increased access to sports facilities and to green space and residential areas with limited access to traffic. Parking spaces, intersections, and heavy bus and truck traffic were associated with less physical activity (de Vries et al., 2007). A small study in Seattle found significant relationships between community form (density) and level of activity among seniors (Frank et al., 2003), and similar results were found in Missouri (Fuzhong et al., 2005).

The relationships between **urban form** and physical activity may differ not only by gender and age but also by race and ethnicity. Evidence of these racial and ethnic differences may inform some of the differences found in levels of physical activity between the majority population and minorities. For instance, in contrast to previous research, Rutt and Coleman (2005b) found that in a predominantly Hispanic population along the U.S. and Mexico border, regular walkers were more likely to walk in places that had fewer physical activity facilities. In addition, greater land use mix was associated with higher BMIs (Rutt and Coleman, 2005a). These disparate findings may be due to subtle environmental differences that mediate the relationship between the built environment and health. For instance, in the Rutt and Coleman (2005a) study, land-use mix was measured as the total number of nonresidential buildings divided by the total number of buildings, and thus the type of use was not determined. As suggested by Moudon and colleagues (2006) and illustrated in figure 5.4, the type of use may prove to be important in future research with some types being correlated with increased physical activity (post office, corner store) and other uses linked with increased BMI (fast food outlets, restaurants). In a national study of adolescents, Gordon-Larsen (2006) found that those living in neighborhoods of low socioeconomic status (SES) had significantly less access to attractive recreation areas; these neighborhoods may have had the same number of facilities compared with other areas in the community but these facilities were rated as much less attractive, safe, and accessible). In a similar vein, Lee and Moudon (2006) found that although the number of facilities (parks, green space, gyms, community centers) were roughly equal between communities, physical activity resources near public housing had much greater number of "incivilities;" that is, more litter, graffiti, unattended dogs, and unsafe traffic conditions, all of which are reported to discourage physical activity. Thus, in addition to measuring access to facilities, researchers and practitioners should examine the type and quality of facilities because they may act as important equity and social justice mediators of physical activity behavior and health outcomes.

Self-Selection Bias

The higher rates of pedestrian travel found in traditional communities may not be entirely explained by their urban form or by the interaction of urban form with gender, age, race and ethnicity, or SES characteristics. Other factors, such as the types of individuals who choose to live in those communities and the web of interrelations between those people, may influence travel behavior (McNally and Kulkarni, 1996; Shriver, 1997). Factors such as personality, attitudes, and values may in part determine the type of community or neighborhood in which people choose to reside. Although we need to learn more about such factors, the data suggest that both self-selection and environmental design have an independent influence on levels of physical activity. Handy and colleagues (2006) report that an analysis of two California-based studies found that the built environment affects walking behavior even after other important variables are considered, such as SES, race, income, attitudes, and preferences. In a national survey in the United States (Librett et al., 2007), level of activity and preference for type of community—urban, suburban, or rural—had only a marginal significance in predicting level of physical activity. The authors concluded that self-selection may play a role in explaining some of the difference in levels of physical activity between communities, but community design also makes a significant contribution to these differences. An analysis of a substudy on housing preferences in the SMARTRAQ data provides similar findings: There is significant unmet demand for housing in urban walkable communities. The authors concluded that "both neighborhood preferences and the built environment explain walking frequency and vehicle travel . . . thus the built environment appears to be both an enabler and disabler of physical activity" (Frank at al., 2006, p. 1900).

Conclusions and Future Research

A growing body of evidence supports the hypothesis that how we build our communities matters. Decisions about community design and investment in transportation infrastructure can have a measurable and meaningful influence on the type and amount of physical activity that individuals engage in as well as health and quality of life. This is not an indictment of any particular form of community development but rather is an effort to place physical activity and public health considerations into planning, transportation, and related community design decisions. All community types have features that can encourage or discourage healthful levels of physical activity. It is the role of public health practitioners and their allies to promote community design that encourages physical activity while eliminating those features that discourage physical activity. This role is not limited to traditional public

Place physical activity and public health considerations into planning, transportation, and related decisions.

health venues but extends to all areas in which such decisions are made, including planning and transportation boards, departments of education and recreation, and work site health committees.

Future research must establish more effective measures of both the built environment and the type and amount of physical activity assessed and must better specify and control mediators, moderators, and confounders of the environment and physical activity. Although true experimental designs, which would involve randomly assigning individuals to neighborhoods and then following them over time, are not practical, it is possible to take advantage of natural experiments in communities where environmental changes are planned. For instance, baseline measures of activity could be compared with level of activity after the environment is changed, or individuals could be followed as they move from one neighborhood to another in order to determine whether they are more or less active after they moved. The redevelopment of communities after disasters, such as New Orleans and the Gulf Coast after Hurricane Katrina, may provide other opportunities to evaluate the relationship between the *re*built environment and physical activity and health. Practice-based research should be integrated into the literature and the decision-making process. Further refinement of predictive models is needed so that practical guidance can be provided. For instance, how much environmental and policy change, and in what combination, is required before meaningful changes in behavior can be expected? Are efforts below this threshold a waste of resources?

Resources

Demers M. 2006. Walk for Your Life: Restoring Neighborhood Walkways to Enhance Community Life, Improve Street Safety and Reduce Obesity. Ridgefield, CT: Vital Health.

Frank LD, Engelke PO, Schmid TL. 2003. Health and Community Design: The Impact of the Built Environment on Physical Activity. Washington, DC: Island Press.

Garreau J. 1992. Edge Cities: Life on the New Frontier. New York: Random House.

Heath GW, Brownson RC, Kruger J, Miles R, Powell KE, Ramsey LT; Task Force on Community Preventive Services. 2006. The effectiveness of environmental and policy interventions to increase physical activity: a systematic review. Journal of Physical Activity and Health 3(suppl. 1):S55-S76.

Jacobs J. 1961. The Death and Life of Great American Cities. New York: Random House, USA Vintage Books.

Leyden K. 2003. Social capital and the built environment: the importance of walkable neighborhoods. American Journal of Public Health 93:1546-1551.

Putnam R. 2001. Bowling Alone: The Collapse and Revival of American Community. New York: Simon & Schuster.

Schwanen T, Mokhtarian PL. 2004. The extent and determinants of dissonance between actual and preferred residential neighborhood type. Environment and Planning B: Planning and Design 31:759-784.

Schwanen T, Mokhtarian PL. 2005. What if you live in the wrong neighborhood? The impact of residential neighborhood type dissonance on distance traveled. Transportation Research Part D 10:127-151.

Transportation Research Board and Institute of Medicine. 2005. Does the Built Environment Influence Physical Activity? Examining the Evidence. Washington, DC: National Academies Press.

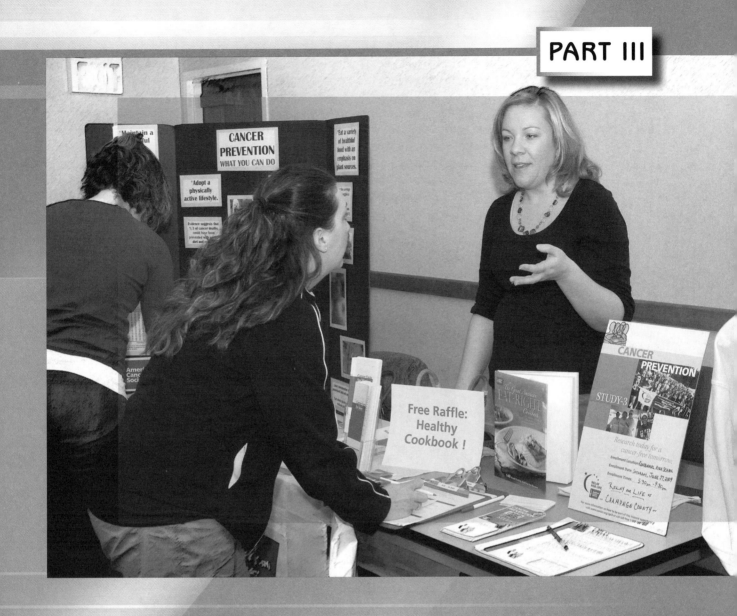

PART III

Planning, Implementing, and Evaluating Your Intervention or Program

You learned in Part I what you need to know—about why to promote physical activity and how much physical activity to promote for general health. You learned in Part II about three approaches and eight effective and recommended intervention categories to increase physical activity. It is time to get to work!

In this section, you will learn the basics of effective partnering and the nuts and bolts of planning and evaluation. Chapter 6 covers the art of partnering in a way that leads to action—more effective action than could be taken on by any one person or organization. You will also be led to think about various sectors with whom to partner depending on your situation. Some may come as a surprise to you.

Chapter 7 covers planning, that is, planning for the implementation of your physical activity promotion efforts, interventions, or programs and planning for the evaluation of such efforts. Program evaluation is the key to continuous quality improvement. Your interventions and programs can only be improved by knowing what is working and what is not. In Chapter 7, you will see how closely program planning and evaluation are intertwined.

CHAPTER **6**

Partnerships

Tamara Vehige Calise, Refilwe Moeti,
and Jacqueline N. Epping

The most effective approach to promoting physical activity may require working in partnership with individuals and organizations in your community. Public health leaders recognize the importance of partnerships. As Dr. David Satcher, former Surgeon General of the United States, stated, "Success in public health work requires partnerships" (Satcher, 1996, p.1707). Comprehensive physical activity programs may require participation and commitment from different segments of your community, many of which may not have worked together previously or may have little background in physical activity and public health. One mechanism to garner support for and involvement in promoting physical activity is to form a partnership.

The *American Heritage Dictionary* (2006) defines a partnership as "a relationship between individuals or groups that is characterized by mutual cooperation and responsibility, as for the achievement of a specified goal." Partnerships can take many forms. Three commonly used forms are cooperation, coordination, and collaboration. Cooperative partnerships are informal relationships without a commonly defined mission, structure, or planning effort. Coordination requires more formal relationships and an understanding of the compatibility of each partner's mission. Collaborative partnerships combine previously separate organizations or individuals into a new and separate structure, and partners are fully committed to a common mission. Collaborative partnerships involve considerable planning and communication at multiple levels, and resources are pooled or acquired by the partnership, rather than the individual partners (Mattessich et al., 2001).

The kind of partnership to use depends on your goal; a partnership may at various times include elements of all three of the partnerships just described. Most of the discussion of partnerships in this chapter focuses on effectively promoting physical activity by joining together personnel and resources, that is, a collaborative partnership.

Although partners may not have worked together previously and may not even have a public health background or experience, their interest in promoting physical activity allows them to

- share a vision or mission (see sidebar Healthy Maine Walks);
- share common goals or objectives;
- share their diverse history of experiences that could provide valuable lessons to the partnership;
- facilitate efforts or serve as effective channels for reaching the target audience; and
- provide access to staff, volunteers, facilities, equipment, materials, funding, or other resources that will assist in promoting the partnership.

Key Steps to an Effective Partnership

The following steps can increase the chance of a successful partnership. Each step is discussed in detail subsequently.

Healthy Maine Walks: A Shared Vision

The Healthy Maine Walks Coalition was established in late 2002. The coalition consists of a group of state-level organizations with a shared interest in trails and health. With financial support of the Maine Center for Disease Control and Prevention's Physical Activity and Nutrition Program, the coalition maintains a Web site (www.healthymainewalks.org) that promotes walking opportunities throughout the state. The coalition has about a dozen member organizations representing a variety of community sectors. These include the East Coast Greenway Alliance, Governor's Council on Physical Activity, GrowSmart Maine, Maine Department of Conservation, Maine Department of Transportation, Maine Nutrition Network, Maine Physical Activity and Nutrition Program, Maine Recreation and Park Association, National Park Service River & Trails Program, Rails-to-Trails Conservancy, and the Southern Maine Volkssport Association. These partners recognized the need for some longer-range thinking regarding the coalition and Web site. The partners initially addressed how the Web site could most effectively be used, whether there was a reason for the coalition to continue to meet, and, if so, what activities the coalition could address next. The coalition partners agreed to continue to meet, and to develop a strategic plan. One coalition member from the Department of Transportation offered to provide a professional facilitator to assist with the development of a 3-year strategic plan. Ultimately the entire coalition was involved in the planning discussions to develop the plan's goals and objectives. The partners agreed to work on two of the three goals during the first year, and these serve as the basis for periodic meeting agendas. The coalition operates within an informal structure, with no bylaws or formal processes in place for decision making or allocating staff and resources to activities.

Personal communication with Rebecca Drewette-Card, Physical Activity Coordinator, Maine Center for Disease Control and Prevention, Physical Activity and Nutrition Program, 12/15/08.

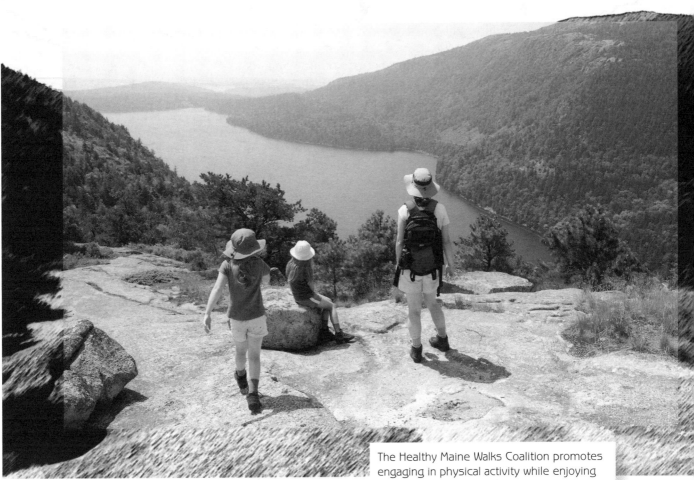

The Healthy Maine Walks Coalition promotes engaging in physical activity while enjoying Maine's beautiful natural resources.
©Richard Freeda/Aurora Photos/Getty Images

- Step 1: Determine whether a partnership is necessary to accomplish your physical activity goals and objectives.
- Step 2: Determine whether potential partners have the capacity to support the physical activity partnership and its proposed actions.
- Step 3: Recruit partners.
- Step 4: Establish leadership.
- Step 5: Determine one or more common goals.
- Step 6: Determine the partners' level of involvement and cooperation in the partnership.
- Step 7: Define the partnership's operational structure.
- Step 8: Keep the long-term goal in view.
- Step 9: Start with reasonable short-term objectives.
- Step 10: Evaluate the partnership.

Step 1: Determine Whether a Partnership Is Necessary

Although there are many benefits to forming a partnership, there are also challenges and drawbacks. Examples are presented in table 6.1

Before starting a partnership, you must determine whether it is an appropriate mechanism for accomplishing desired goals and objectives. Consider the pros and cons of a partnership, and remember that it is just one tool that can be used to promote physical activity. In some cases, you may determine that you and your organization best reach your goals and objectives independently. For example, the most appropriate strategy to address your goals and objectives may be to develop a Web page, write a newsletter, or otherwise act independently.

Answering the questions in table 6.2 might help you determine whether forming a partnership is the best approach for achieving what you would like to accomplish.

Table 6.1   Benefits and Challenges to Forming a Partnership

Benefits	Challenges
Forming a partnership broadens community support and strengthens the community's trust in your program.	Time and patience are needed to network, assess, and understand the target community and its needs and assets.
One or more partners can address a comprehensive range of factors related to physical activity, from personal knowledge and skills to environmental factors.	Bringing a diverse group of people and organizations together can be difficult.
Working in partnership eliminates duplication of effort.	It can be challenging to accommodate partner goals while accomplishing overarching community goals.
A partnership allows you to direct more resources (people and funding) toward promoting physical activity and helps bridge gaps.	Maintaining group interest and a collaborative process over time may not be easy.
A partnership shares the power of leaders and other influential people.	Forming a partnership can result in significant delays in achieving tangible outcomes.
A partnership achieves a bigger impact (i.e., reaches people within your target population in greater numbers and with greater effectiveness).	
Forming a partnership shares knowledge and expertise (e.g., training capability) and enhances credibility.	

Table 6.2 Questions to Help You Decide Whether
to Form a Partnership

	Yes	No
Will your goals and objectives for promoting physical activity be better reached by involving more individuals or organizations than by working alone?		
Would a partnership help potential partners achieve goals they could not achieve alone?		
▶ Will strengths emerge when a group of different people come together?		
▶ Will perspectives, resources, and skills of a broad array of community partners be available?		
▶ Will people be encouraged to use their expertise to address new areas and feel free to challenge accepted opinions or knowledge?		
Do key community leaders or decision makers show interest in and support for a partnership to promote physical activity? If not . . .		
▶ Do you know what information these key leaders need to realize the full advantage of the partnership?		
▶ Do you know how to provide them with that information?		
Are there gaps in the following resources that potential partners might be able to provide?		
▶ Expertise in physical activity and public health		
▶ Expertise in evaluation		
▶ Leadership and oversight of the partnership		
▶ Other personnel or staff support		
▶ Finances		
▶ Office space, equipment, or supplies		
▶ Access to places and opportunities to be physically active (e.g., recreational space, facilities, or programs)		
Are there specific advantages to a partnership, such as reaching a population group, influencing decision makers, or leveraging resources?		

Step 2: Determine Whether Potential Partners Have the Capacity and Interest to Support the Partnership

Identifying partners takes time and careful planning but is an important step in determining the size and type of partnership that is formed. Before you develop your list of potential partners, inventory your organization's strengths and weaknesses. Answer questions such as the following:

- What does my organization have to offer in accomplishing our physical activity goals or objectives?
- What resources, personnel, funding, programmatic expertise, visibility, or credibility does my organization have? (You may not need to partner if you have all the prerequisites.)

Once you have identified your organization's strengths and weaknesses, identify partners who might complement your strengths as well those who might fill gaps. For example, if you find physical activity–related disparities among certain subgroups of the community and you lack access to these groups, identify potential partners who already have a relationship with and access to these groups.

Physical activity promotion needs to occur within various community sectors to be effective, so potential partners should include organizations from many different community sectors (also see the sidebar):

- Government
- Health
- Education
- Transportation
- Business
- Media
- Recreation
- Urban planners and developers

Examples of Potential Partners to Promote Physical Activity

Government sector

National, state, and local elected officials

Representatives of federal, state, county, or city government

Regional or local planning commissions

State or county department of health or mental health

State or county cooperative extension service

State or county department of education

State or county department of transportation (SAFETEA program); bicycle and pedestrian coordinators; Safe Routes to School coordinators

State or county department of parks and recreation

Governor's or mayor's council on physical fitness and sports

Local council on physical fitness and sports or wellness

State department of natural resources

State department of tourism

Public utility companies

Area agencies on aging

Law enforcement agencies

State, county, or local crime prevention task forces

Emergency rescue agencies (e.g., medical and fire)

Libraries

Public housing communities

State or county zoning board

Health sector

Wellness councils or coalitions

State and local health departments (chronic disease divisions)

State and local health and fitness coalitions

Hospitals and clinics

Private practicing physicians

Physical and occupational therapists

Cardiovascular rehabilitation centers

Professional medical associations and auxiliaries

Emergency medical teams

Mental health centers or crisis intervention centers

Insurance companies and health maintenance organizations

Health and fitness organizations, such as local chapters of the

- ▶ American College of Sports Medicine;
- ▶ National Association of Sport and Physical Education; and
- ▶ American Association of Health, Physical Education, Recreation and Dance

National and state health education associations, such as the

- ▶ American Association for Health Education,
- ▶ Society of Public Health Educators,
- ▶ National Society of Physical Activity Practitioners in Public Health, and
- ▶ American Public Health Association, Health Education Section

National and state nursing and medical associations, such as the

- ▶ American Nurses' Association,
- ▶ American Association of Occupational Health Nurses,
- ▶ American Medical Association,
- ▶ National Medical Association,
- ▶ American Academy of Family Physicians,
- ▶ American College of Occupational Medicine, and
- ▶ American College of Preventive Medicine

Education sector

State and local departments of education

Universities and colleges

Technical schools

Public elementary, middle, and high schools

Private elementary, middle, and high schools

School boards

Day care centers, preschool programs, and after-school programs

Special education programs

Parent–teacher associations

School wellness captains

State and local chapters of professional teachers and administrators associations, such as the

- ▶ National Education Association,
- ▶ American Federation of Teachers,
- ▶ National Association of Elementary School Principals,
- ▶ National Association of Secondary School Principals, and
- ▶ American Association of School Administrators

Transportation and environmental development sector

Environmental Protection Agency (EPA)

State and local department of transportation officials; bicycle and pedestrian coordinators; Safe Routes to School coordinators

National and state highway traffic and safety officials

City and regional planning commissions; urban planners

Colleges and institutes of city and regional or urban planning and research

Colleges and schools of architecture, civil engineering, landscape design, and social ecology

Colleges and schools of law and criminal justice

Professional associations and environmental advocacy groups, such as the

- ▶ American Planning Association,
- ▶ American Institute of Architects,
- ▶ Urban Land Institute,
- ▶ Congress for the New Urbanism,
- ▶ Citizen Planner Institute,
- ▶ Institute of Transportation Engineers,

(continued)

▶ Partnership for a Walkable America,

▶ Bicycle Federation of America,

▶ Rails-to-Trails Conservancy,

▶ Insurance Institute for Highway Safety,

▶ Surface Transportation Policy Project,

▶ International Federation of Pedestrians,

▶ Pedestrian Federation of America, and

▶ National Coalition for Promoting Physical Activity

Healthy Communities project staff

Sierra Club; private walking, hiking, bicycling, and other sporting organizations

Private nature, garden, and other outdoor conservation organizations

County commissioners regulating zoning laws

Business sector

Chamber of commerce

Business coalitions and labor organizations

Large and small businesses and industries

Real estate agencies

Work site wellness coordinators

Shopping mall managers

Fitness clubs and health spas

Athletic or sporting goods industries

Professional sports teams

Media and communication sector

Television stations (cable and public)

Radio station managers

Newspaper editors (daily and weekly; state and local), especially health section editors

Newsletter editors

Electronic mail and Internet consultants

Professional journal editors

Health and fitness publication editors

Public relations and marketing professionals or consultants

Recreation sector

National Park Service

National, state, or local parks

Local park and recreation departments

YMCA and YWCA

Senior centers

Community centers

Walking, hiking, or running clubs

Community team sports clubs (e.g., softball, soccer, basketball, volleyball, football, and ice hockey) for youth, adults, or special populations

Outdoor sporting clubs of any kind, such as hiking, walking, bicycling, skiing, tennis, golf, orienteering, and sailing

Special Olympics or Wheelchair Sports, Inc.

Sports governing bodies and state athletic associations

State Games associations (e.g., Senior Games and Corporate Games)

Faith sector

Clergy and ministerial associations or councils

Churches, synagogues, and other places of worship

Women's groups and men's groups

Youth groups

Faith-based recreation facilities, camps

Voluntary or service organization sector

American Heart Association

American Red Cross

National Arthritis Foundation

American Lung Association

American Diabetes Association

Special public or private foundations

Neighborhood or homeowner associations

Girl Scouts of America, Boy Scouts of America, Boys and Girls Clubs of America, 4-H clubs, and other youth organizations

AARP, elder hostels, seniors' organizations, National Council on Aging, and American Society on Aging

Rotary, Lions, Kiwanis, Jaycees, and other service organizations

League of Women Voters, Junior League, and other predominantly women's organizations

Graduate students in schools of public health, medical students, physical therapy students, and education students (particularly physical education or health education)

College fraternities and sororities

Local physicians, sports figures, and celebrities

Taken from U.S. Department of Health & Human Services, 1999, p. 169.

- Faith-based organizations
- Voluntary or service organizations
- Organizations that focus on specific populations, such as older adults, people with disabilities, women, or people from specific racial and ethnic groups, socioeconomic groups, or types of community (rural vs. urban)

MOVE Missoula (see sidebar) is an example of a partnership that includes a variety of partners who represent various community sectors.

Assess the Capacity of Potential Partners

Once partners have been identified, you must assess their capacity to provide resources that complement those of your organization. Questions to consider when determining whether specific partners have the capacity to become involved in a partnership include the following:

- Does the potential partner have an interest or investment in the intended activities or outcomes?
- Does the potential partner have financial resources?
- Does the potential partner have available time and trained physical activity personnel?
- Does the potential partner have knowledge, expertise, or skills that will be beneficial to the partnership (e.g., evaluation)?
- Does the potential partner have an infrastructure that can help support and sustain the partnership (e.g., providing a meeting place, typing minutes, servicing sites for physical activity programs)?
- Does the potential partner have credibility in the community?

Every partner may not be able to contribute or provide resources in all of these areas but should be able to complement or add to the overall strength of the partnership.

MOVE Missoula Community Partnership Promotes Physical Activity

Eat Smart Move More is Missoula, Montana's, version of a multilevel community initiative to increase physical activity and healthy eating. The partnership consists of representatives from the University of Montana, schools, health care industry, businesses, media, and other community organizations. This partnership has made several key accomplishments, resulting in positive impacts on the Missoula community. For example, through schools that are part of the nation-wide Coordinated Approach to Child Health (CATCH) program, city parks and St. Patrick Hospital in Missoula work together to promote physical activity and healthy eating in children through curriculum, policy change, and parent outreach. Other partnerships include Safe Routes to School efforts including Walking School Bus programs and active after-school programs.

A recent project was a pilot Missoula Worksite Health Promotion Campaign. The campaign work group surveyed staff at the participating work sites about their interest in nutrition and physical activity programs. Using the results, employers adopted several environmental and policy changes, including allowing time for activity during work, providing on-site exercise facilities, and encouraging active transportation to and from work. Additionally, the work group initiated a break-time walking program and campaign, awarding employees with incentives for participating in the program. Media partners documented the success of the efforts in the local newspaper and shared information with the community and other work sites.

Other community-wide events have included the Be a User Campaign, which distributes CD-ROM walking maps as well as bookmarks that encourage dog walking, and a Healthy Built Environment campaign. As a result of committed individuals and organizations with a common goal, these Eat Smart Move More partnerships continue to evolve and make a positive impact on their community and the people who live, work, and play in Missoula.

Personal communication with Greg Oliver, Health Promotion Director, Missoula City-County Health Department, Missoula, MT, and Catherine Costakis, Physical Activity Coordinator, Montana Nutrition and Physical Activity Program, Montana State University, Bozeman, MT, 12/15/2008.

Step 3: Recruit Partners

Selecting the right individuals and representatives of organizations for your partnership is important. Recruit not only institutional representatives but also community members who will be served or affected by the activities or outcomes of the partnership, that is, stakeholders. Partnerships are more likely to be effective and long-lasting when individuals, community-based organizations, and institutions that will be affected by the effort are involved.

In the recruiting process, think about the benefits and costs of participation from the standpoint of the potential partner. Likely partners will assess whether the benefits of joining and participating in the partnership exceed the costs (e.g., time and resources). Advantages of joining a partnership may include the following:

- Ability to identify key strategic approaches to reaching an organization's physical activity goals by getting input from a diverse group of partners.
- Access to a network with people who have similar interests and have the potential to pool knowledge and resources (see sidebar about New York's Walkable Communities Conference).
- Opportunity to build on strengths and combined resources, avoid redundancy, and maximize impact.

There may also be reasons why potential partners will not want to join a partnership or invest the time to be an active contributing member. Barriers may include the following (adapted from U.S. Department of Health & Human Services, 1999, p. 165):

- Negative prior experiences
- An institutional culture that discourages partnering
- Competition for scarce resources
- Poor leadership and no clear direction
- Control of the partnership by one organization or individual
- Inadequate participation by key partners
- Vague delineation of partners' roles, responsibilities, resources, or time commitments
- Differences among partners regarding values, vision, goals, or actions
- Unwillingness to negotiate or compromise on important issues

New York's Walkable Communities Conference Attracts Nontraditional Partners and Meeting Participants

Several New York state agencies (e.g., health, transportation, state, and motor vehicles) and state-level nonprofit organizations (e.g., parks and trails, bicycling, state physical activity coalition) sponsored three conferences on walkable communities starting in 2001. The group convened after participants recognized, while working on smaller collaborations, that they shared common goals. They realized that pooling resources would allow them to hold a larger conference, bring in more prominent speakers, attract a more diverse audience, and ultimately increase collaboration among a variety of disciplines. The attendance at the conferences has ranged from 100 to 160 participants. The disciplines represented include bicycle and pedestrian advocacy, local government, public health, traffic safety, law enforcement, transportation, planning, and architecture. The group plans to sponsor a conference every 2 years. Each agency has one or two staff members who work on the conference, and at least four agencies contribute financially to the event.

Personal communication with Amy Jesaitis, Healthy Heart Program, New York State Health Department, 12/18/08.

Working with other organizations can be challenging. Try to understand these barriers and address them in advance. As partners are recruited, they will need to explore their motivations for joining as well as the barriers and the potential benefits of participating.

Recommended Additional Reading

For additional examples of partners that represent many different sectors see U.S. Department of Health and Human Services, Public Health Service, Centers for Disease Control and Prevention, National Center for Chronic Disease Prevention and Health Promotion, Division of Nutrition and Physical Activity. Promoting Physical Activity: A Guide for Community Action. Champaign, IL: Human Kinetics, 1999, pp. 163-179.

Step 4: Establish Leadership

Successful partnerships require effective leadership to ensure a clear decision-making process, agreed-upon rules, well-planned activities and meetings, and effective communication. It is important to have a collaborative leader who is able to empower the partners and advance the collaborative process. A collaborative leader will be able to inspire commitment and action, help partners to reach agreement and solve problems, and ensure and sustain participation from all partners to accomplish short- and long-term goals (Chrislip and Larson, 1995).

Step 5: Determine One or More Common Goals

A common challenge to collaborating with people and organizations is resolving differences and finding ways to meet a variety of needs while making progress toward a shared vision (see sidebar about Maine's Active Community Environments Workgroup). It is important from the outset that all partners know and agree on the partnership's vision, mission, goals and objectives. Expect, invite, and be prepared to address the differences in the individual collaboration methods of various partners. The partnership needs to transcend these differences to achieve a common purpose and a common goal.

It is important to address differing goals and objectives of partners, for your vision may be related but in some respects different. For example, your organization may want to increase physical activity, whereas an environmental justice organization may want to reduce air pollution. These goals are quite different but both can be met, for example, by increasing the number of people who walk and bike for transportation and reducing their reliance on car use.

Two features that are critical to finding common ground among partners are communication and developing trust.

Maine's Active Community Environments Workgroup Faces the Challenge of a Common Language and Mission

The Maine Centers for Disease Control and Prevention (CDC), Physical Activity and Nutrition Program (PANP), and colleagues from Maine CDC's Community Health Promotion Program, the Department of Transportation, and the State Planning Office formed a workgroup to explore whether these agencies could work together on issues surrounding the built environment. Because the partners come from different agencies that have diverse missions, the workgroup will need to overcome their unique perspectives, develop a common language or acquire an understanding of the language used in the different agencies, and identify objectives and goals that all can agree upon and support. The group developed a common definition of *active community environments*. The group is building relationships by emphasizing an understanding of each agency's work and mission. This will help lay the groundwork for any future collaboration. Despite challenges, representatives from the different agencies continue to participate in the workgroup and the Department of Conservation recently joined the group. One outcome of this group was a Built Environment and Physical Activity conference in May 2008. In an Active Community Environments Workgroup meeting, representatives of PANP and the Department of Transportation realized they were planning similar training conferences, so they decided to combine resources and provide a joint training conference. Workgroup members from the State Planning Office assisted with various aspects of the day. The 2009 Active Communities Conference was held in May 2009. There are many challenges to overcome when partners who do not traditionally work together attempt to collaborate (e.g., different terminology, perceived importance of different outcomes related to physical activity). However, many of the contemporary problems that communities face, including environmental and policy issues, may ultimately be best addressed by such collaborative efforts.

Personal communication with Rebecca Drewette-Card, Physical Activity Coordinator, Maine Center for Disease Control and Prevention, 12/15/08.

Communication is the sharing of ideas and opinions. Partners must work consciously to increase their level of communication by being open and willing to listen to each other. Effective communication includes the following:

- Ability to empathize and identify with people with whom you are communicating
- Appropriate use and understanding of verbal and nonverbal communication methods (can different partners speak the same language?)
- Use of different dynamics of communication (tones, content, and structure) by which messages are delivered

Open, regular communication will help foster trust and credibility among partners. Developing trust is a reciprocal process that takes time. Building trust is essential for a functional partnership and requires that all partners understand and honor their roles, responsibilities, and rights, in addition to everyone else's.

Step 6: Determine the Partner's Level of Involvement and Cooperation in the Partnership

As discussed earlier, levels of involvement and cooperation may vary among partnerships, ranging from minimal involvement to more detailed mutual sharing, and may include the following (Mattessich et al., 2001):

- Cooperation: Partners exchange information, schedule or alter activities to be mutually beneficial, and each uses their resources, expertise, people, time, influence, access, funds, or physical property to achieve a common purpose.

- Coordination: While maintaining their autonomy, partners exchange information, schedule or alter activities to be mutually beneficial, and work together to achieve a common purpose. Resources may be shared. The partnership adds strength to activities and may avoid duplication in effort. It involves a certain degree of trust and overlap in responsibilities.

- Collaboration: Partners work together from the beginning to the end, sharing information, altering schedules and activities, and sharing the risks, responsibilities, and rewards. Resources are pooled or jointly acquired; partners help each other become better at what they do best. Partners at multiple levels of each of the organizations or settings meet regularly to plan and carry out specific activities to meet their objectives. Although in a collaboration you may lose your autonomy, you may gain a great deal more from what the collaborative partnership can achieve than what you might have been able to achieve alone.

Step 7: Define the Partnership's Operational Structure

For a well-functioning partnership to achieve its goals and objectives, all partners must consider and agree on level of formality, type of partnership, roles and responsibilities of each partner, and resources.

Formality

A variety of partnership structures can be adopted by partners, ranging from a formal arrangement (e.g., a written agreement or contract) to a more loosely structured, informal model (e.g., operate with a common understanding or consensus among partners). The precise operational structure and level of formality should be selected by partners and should reflect the needs of the participants and the community as well as the goals and objectives of the partnership. The range of operational structures and levels of formality is quite wide. For example, in noncontractual partnerships, partners sometimes sign a formal agreement called a Memorandum of Understanding, which allows them to contribute funding or in-kind support to a specified project; see sidebar Memorandum of Understanding (MOU): A National-Level Partnership.

Memorandum of Understanding (MOU): A National-Level Partnership

The Centers for Disease Control and Prevention (CDC), Division of Nutrition, Physical Activity and Obesity, partners with federal agencies and other recreation organizations through a MOU-based interagency workgroup to promote the development and use of parks and recreation facilities by providing technical assistance to stakeholder organizations. As of 2008, the partnership included collaboration among the Department of Health and Human Services (CDC, Indian Health Service, and Office of Public Health and Science), Department of Agriculture (Forest Service and Center for Nutrition Policy and Promotion), Department of the Interior (Bureau of Indian Affairs, Bureau of Land Management, Bureau of Reclamation, Fish and Wildlife Service, and National Park Service), and the Department of the Army (Army Corps of Engineers). The purpose of the MOU is for the collaborating agencies "to work together to promote uses and benefits of the Nation's public lands and water resources to enhance the physical and psychological health and well-being of the American people . . . and to help promote healthy lifestyles through sound nutrition, physical activity, and recreation in America's great outdoors" (Centers for Disease Control and Prevention, 2009). Although this MOU is an example of federal agencies working together to promote public health through outdoor recreation, it is possible that a similar MOU could be formed among community-based public health and parks and recreation agencies.

Another type of formal agreement is a cooperative agreement. In this case, one organization funds another organization to carry out the activities that both organizations agree on. For example, the CDC has a cooperative agreement with 25 state health agencies to fund state programs in nutrition, physical activity, and obesity. Partnerships can be structured a number of ways, including the following (taken from U.S. Department of Health & Human Services, 1999, p. 166):

■ Advisory council: A group of individuals selected to provide suggestions and guidance to organizations or programs.

■ Alliance: Semiofficial grouping of organizations connected by a common cause.

■ Coalition: Varied partners united around common interests or problems, addressing their goals through cooperation, advocacy, capacity building, social change, and community action. Although member organizations are autonomous, free to enter or leave the group, commitment among those who assume leadership is necessary to achieve a coalition's success.

■ Collaborative: The most organized and structured form of partnership: a new entity formed by a group of partners working in collaboration to accomplish a shared vision, mission, goals, and objectives.

- Network: Spontaneous and often loosely knit communication links between individuals or organizations as a means of maintaining contact or keeping informed. Network structures are less formal and hierarchical than most other forms of partnerships

  - Consortium: A formal relationship among professional individuals or organizations linked by similarities in the services they provide or in the audiences they reach. The relationships among consortium members are generally more structured than in a network or alliance but less so than in a coalition or collaborative.

  - Task force: A group of individuals who want to accomplish a specific, predetermined series of activities, most often at the request of an overseeing body.

Roles and Responsibilities

Identifying roles and responsibilities plays an important part in the success of a partnership. Partners should discuss and agree on their roles and responsibilities and how they will contribute to the goals and objectives of the partnership. When partners discuss and agree upon roles and responsibilities early in the process, they ensure alignment of their needs, interests, and resources, helping the partnership to succeed in the long run. These are a few examples of roles and responsibilities:

- Providing funding
- Providing oversight
- Providing training
- Contributing products or services
- Providing transportation
- Planning and organizing meetings
- Printing and disseminating reports or other materials

Resources

As a group, partners must discuss and agree on the resources that are present and those that are needed. The type and level of resources needed by a partnership depend on the physical activity projects and activities planned.

Step 8: Keep the Long-Term Goal in View

Short-term goals should be small steps toward the long-term goal. To achieve short-term and long-term goals, partners need to be dedicated to participating in meetings, implementing relevant activities, and sharing progress and reports with the community and funders. During this process, obstacles may arise. Partners must be patient and persistent in achieving short-term objectives while keeping the long-term goal in sight.

Step 9: Start With Reasonable Short-Term Objectives

It is best to start with realistic short-term objectives, that is, objectives that are achievable. Achieving short-term objectives early in the partnership provides momentum and helps partners build the stamina that will be needed during challenging tasks and difficult times. Early tasks should be significant enough to be both challenging and achievable, neither trivial nor too difficult. It is best to start small and work your way up to bigger and more complex tasks as the partnership matures and shows results. Developing objectives to guide your partnership activities is discussed more in chapter 7, Program Planning and Evaluation.

Step 10: Evaluate the Partnership

To be effective, the partnership needs to be evaluated and necessary adjustments made. Evaluation of the partnership is an ongoing process that begins very early (e.g., evaluating whether you have the necessary partners) and continues over the course of the partnership. It's important to evaluate how well the partnership is functioning (level of partner participation, appropriate pace, appropriate partners, clear roles and responsibilities) as well as external factors that might influence the partnership's direction (e.g., changes in the political and social climate, changes in available resources).

Keep track of progress toward the desired objectives (both short and long term) and use indicators to determine whether results have been achieved. For example, indicators of whether a program implemented or supported by the partnership is using community resources as intended include the number of volunteers, the types of volunteer activities that are occurring, and the amount of time volunteers are working. It's also important to note unintended consequences of the partnership and its activities. For example, an unintended positive consequence might be that individual partners without a history of working in physical activity develop new ways of looking at their own agendas, to include or assess physical activity.

If results are not achieved or some aspect of the partnership is not working, you should adjust the partnership agreement, contract, work plan, or implementation activities to address the problem. All partners must consider and agree to any modifications or changes that are made.

If the evaluation indicates that the partnership is not meeting its goals or objectives, you may need to consider disbanding the partnership. If this is necessary, it is important to end the partnership in a way that is respectful to all partners.

Conclusion

Forming partnerships can be the catalyst to planning, implementing, and evaluating successful public health interventions, including physical activity interventions. Many physical activity interventions, particularly community-wide and policy- and environmental-level interventions, need to rest on a solid partnership foundation if they are to be effective.

Recommended Readings

Braithwaite R, Taylor S, Austin J. 2000. *Building Health Coalitions in the Black Community*. Thousand Oaks, CA: Sage.

Brown C. 1984. *The Art of Coalition Building: A Guide for Community Leaders*. New York: American Jewish Committee.

Butterfoss FD. 2004. The coalition technical assistance and training framework: helping community coalitions help themselves. *Health Promotion Practice* 5(2):118-126.

Butterfoss FD, Goodman RM, Wandersman A. 1993. Community coalitions for health promotion and disease prevention. *Health Education Research: Theory and Practice* 8(3):315-330.

Butterfoss FD, Goodman RM, Wandersman A. 1996. Community coalitions for prevention and health promotion: factors predicting satisfaction, participation and planning. *Health Education Quarterly* 23(1):65-79.

Butterfoss FD, Kegler MK. 2002. Toward a comprehensive understanding of community coalitions: moving from practice to theory. In: DiClemente RJ, Crosby RA, Kegler MC (Eds.), *Emerging Theories in Health Promotion Practice and Research: Strategies for Improving Public Health*. San Francisco: Jossey-Bass; pp. 157-193.

Center for the Advancement of Collaborative Strategies in Health, New York Academy of Medicine. Partnership Self-Assessment Tool. Available at www.partnershiptool.net.

Centers for Disease Control and Prevention. 2004. *Principles of Community Engagement.* Atlanta: U.S. Department of Health and Human Services; 2004. Available at http://www.cdc.gov/phppo/pce.

Florin P, Mitchell R, Stevenson J. 1993. Identifying training and technical assistance needs in community coalitions: a developmental approach. *Health Education Research: Theory and Practice* 8(3):417-432.

Francisco VT, Paine AL, Fawcett SB. 1993. A methodology for monitoring and evaluating community health coalitions. *Health Education Research* 8(3):403-416.

Goldstein SM. 1997. Community coalitions: A self-assessment tool. *American Journal of Health Promotion* 11(6):430-435.

Goodman RM. 1998. Principles and tools for evaluating community-based prevention and health promotion programs. *Journal of Public Health Management and Practice* 4(2):37-47.

Goodman RM, Wandersman A, Chinman M, et al. 1996. An ecological assessment of community based interventions for prevention and health promotion: approaches to measuring community coalitions. *American Journal of Community Psychology* 24(1):33-36.

Hanson P. 1989-1990. Citizen involvement in community health promotion: a role application of CDC's PATCH model. *International Quarterly of Community Health Education* 9(3):177-186.

Kaye G, Wolff T (Eds). 1997. *From the Ground Up! A Workbook on Coalition Building and Community Development*. Amherst, MA: AHEC Community Partners.

Kreuter MW, Lezin NA, Young LA. 2000. Evaluating community-based collaborative mechanisms: implications for practitioners. *Health Promotion Practice* 1(1):49-63.

Mattessich PW, Monsey BR. 1992. *Collaboration: What Makes It Work? A Review of Research Literature on Factors Influencing Successful Collaboration*. St. Paul, MN: Amherst H. Wilder Foundation.

McLeroy KR, Kegler MC, Steckler AB, et al. 1994. Community coalitions for health promotion: summary and further reflections [editorial]. *Health Education Research* 9(1):1-11.

Sofaer S. 2004. *Working Together, Moving Ahead: A Manual to Support Effective Community Health Coalitions*. New York: Baruch College, School of Public Affairs.

US Department of Health and Human Services. 2002. Physical Activity Evaluation Handbook. Atlanta, GA: US Department of Health and Human Services, Centers for Disease Control and Prevention.

Wandersman A, Florin P, Friedmann R, et al. 1987. Who participates, who does not, and why? An analysis of voluntary neighborhood organizations in the United States and Israel. *Sociological Forum* 2(3):534-555.

Wandersman A, Valois R, Ochs L, et al. 1996. Toward a social ecology of community coalitions. *American Journal of Health Promotion* 10(4):299-307.

CHAPTER 7

Program Planning and Evaluation

Sarah Levin Martin and Lauren M. Workman

You probably have heard it before, but it cannot be said enough: Planning and evaluation go hand in hand. More specifically, planning for implementation and planning for evaluation should go hand in hand. When developing physical activity promotion program and activities, consider how you will promote increased physical activity as well as how you will monitor the program's execution, impacts, and outcomes.

> Program planning is more than a to-do list, and evaluation planning is more than administering before-and-after questionnaires. Evaluation involves asking meaningful questions, gathering information, summarizing responses, reporting information, and using your findings to fine-tune your delivery of messages and services. If you carefully select and track appropriate progress indicators from the very start of your program, you will have the information you need to measure the program's success (U.S. Department of Health & Human Services [DHHS], 1999, p 146).

This chapter outlines the principles of program planning and those of program evaluation and describes how the two are interrelated.

Program Planning

As you are planning, create an approach that will account for who is going to do what, when, where, and how (and for how much money). Following are questions to consider as you plan your program (see sidebar). These questions will help you conceptualize your program, foresee barriers, and keep your overall goals in mind.

Carefully conducted program planning begins much before a work plan can be developed—it begins with an assessment of current conditions. This is referred to as a formative assessment. Formative assessment is a process designed to enhance understanding of the target audience's characteristics, attitudes, beliefs, values,

Questions to Consider as You Determine Your Expectations

▸ What is your goal or vision? What do you hope to accomplish?

▸ Who is your target population? How would you portray their characteristics and lifestyle?

▸ What does your target population need and want?

▸ What current target population attitudes or behaviors are you trying to change?

▸ What action do you want your target population to take as a direct result of your intervention?

▸ When and where are members of your target population most open to your message or call to action? What channels might reach your population effectively?

▸ Which components of behavior change will your intervention address (i.e., awareness, knowledge, motivation, readiness, self-efficacy, social support, or environmental support)?

▸ What specifically do you propose to do? What are your objectives?

▸ When will the proposed activities take place? What is your timetable?

▸ Who needs to be involved in carrying out the plan? What resources are required? With whom can you partner?

▸ What resistance might you encounter? From whom? How can you involve potential resisters in planning and implementation?

▸ To what extent do stakeholders, gatekeepers, and intermediaries support your plans?

▸ How will you know if you have achieved your objectives? What will "success" look like?

▸ What would be the consequences of doing nothing at all?

From USDHHS, 1999, p. 147

behaviors, determinants, benefits, and barriers to behavior change to inform a strategy for interventions and programs. It is the "precede" of the precede–proceed model, that is, the diagnosis of social, epidemiological, behavioral, environmental, educational, organizational, and administrative and policy factors (Green & Krueter, 1992), similar to the market research involved in social marketing (Andreasen, 1995).

At a minimum, the formative assessment will include a look at needs and resources in a community. In gathering these data, consider questioning several people and using a variety of methods (DHHS, 2002):

- People
  - Organizational and agency staff
  - Physical activity program staff
  - Community leaders

- Funding officials
- General public

There are various ways to collect data:

- From surveys
  - Face-to-face
  - Telephone
  - E-mail
  - Postal mail
- From interviews (structured or unstructured)
  - Face to face
  - Telephone
  - Public forums
  - Focus groups
- From documents
  - Grant proposals
  - Newsletters
  - Press releases
  - Administrative records
  - Current or previous intervention attendance lists
- From existing data
  - Behavioral Risk Factor Surveillance System (BRFSS)
  - Youth Risk Behavioral System (YRBS)
  - National Health and Nutrition Examination Survey (NHANES)
  - National Health Interview Survey (NHIS)
  - Crime reports
  - Other public domain research-based surveys
  - Directories
- From observations
  - Direct observations of behavior or a physical environment
  - Indirect observations (e.g., video camera or infrared light counters)

Based on the findings of the formative assessment, you are ready to begin thinking about your program. It is best to work with a group of people who are interested in the issue to plan the program and its evaluation. These are referred to as **stakeholders,** and they fall into four main categories (DHHS, 2002):

1. Implementers: those who implement, manage operations, and evaluate the program
2. Partners: those who support overall program goals and efforts to implement and evaluate the program
3. Participants: those who will be affected by the program
4. Decision makers: those with decision-making power over the program

It's important to begin by working with stakeholders to determine a vision and mission, which will help articulate a foundation and direction for your program and its evaluation.

Vision and Mission

As commonly defined in strategic planning, a vision is a guiding image of success or an ideal condition; for example, "Our vision is people of all ages being active in an activity-friendly community." A mission is a statement of general purpose; it communicates your essence: "Our coalition's mission is to promote physical activity to all levels of the community."

Next, you can work with stakeholders to determine the goals and objectives. These should be consistent with the vision and the mission. Take some time to carefully consider and construct objectives because these will be the keys to conducting the evaluation.

Goals and Objectives

A goal is a broad statement of purpose. For example, "Our goal is to increase the physical activity level of community members by making more physical activity opportunities accessible to all."

An objective describes results expected to be reached. Objectives are most useful when they are SMART: specific, measurable, achievable, relevant, and time-bound (DHHS, 2002).

- Specific: who (target population) and what (action or activity)
- Measurable: how much change is expected
- Achievable: realistic given current resources and constraints
- Relevant: within the scope of the program purposes
- Time-bound: when the objective will be met

For example, "One of our objectives is to expand the physical activity offerings of the Parks and Recreation Department by 50% by December 2011." Evaluation planning can actually precede program planning. In other words, you may know, or want to know, what questions to answer before you know what program or intervention will be implemented.

Once the vision, mission, goals, and objectives are established, it is time to start thinking about strategies to reach your goals and objectives. In conjunction with considering the activities that will be conducted, consider what is needed to make the activities happen—these are the inputs.

Inputs

Inputs are the staff, partners, and financial and other resources that make it possible to implement activities. Examples of diverse inputs include these:

- Your own staff time and expertise
- A partner's donation of gymnasium time
- The city chamber of commerce's donation of financial resources
- The public support of the mayor
- An existing trail

Activities

When you plan physical activity interventions, consider evidence-based interventions, that is, interventions that have been shown to work. *The Guide to Community Preventive Services: What Works to Promote Health? (Community Guide)* (Heath et al., 2006; Kahn et al., 2002; Zaza et al., 2005) includes eight recommended physical activity intervention categories within three broad approaches and are described more fully in Part II. Selecting one or more of these interventions and tailoring them based on a formative assessment will increase the chances of having an effective intervention.

Writing a work plan and developing a logic model that specifies the details of your activities can be very helpful. The work plan should include a time line with a detailed description of tasks and an identified person who agrees to do them, as described in table 7.1.

Table 7.1 Work Plan for Beginning a New Volleyball League

Who	What	Where	When	How
Mark J. of the city parks department	Run a new adult volleyball league	At the city park gymnasium	Tuesday nights from 7 to 9 p.m.	Advertise the new league in the newspaper; identify volunteer captains to recruit teams; hire referees

A logic model shows the logical relationships or connections between activities and outcomes; it should illustrate something like "if this happens, the result will be this." A fully developed logic model should include the inputs (i.e., the resources that will be put into implementing the program), the activities that will occur, and the outcomes of those activities. It can be useful to sequence the outcomes as short term, intermediate, and long term.

An innovative physical activity program called Walk a Hound, Lose a Pound (WAHLAP) is used here as an example of how to operationalize or put into practice a logic model. WAHLAP promotes walking to enhance health and fitness among both dog walkers and dogs and helps homeless dogs socialize and receive visibility to increase their chances of finding a home (see sidebar for program description).

Once a logic model was developed to serve as a roadmap to guide planning and evaluation of WAHLAP (see logic model, figure 7.1), the relevant process and outcome measures could be determined. Process measures included recording the number and type of organizations and individuals who provided resources, that is, what inputs were provided for the program and when those inputs were applied. (The program, initiated in 2003, is currently ongoing, and as the program has grown the number and type of inputs and activities have expanded beyond those in the original logic model.) Likewise, program activities have been measured and tracked over time, not only to determine whether and to what extent the original proposed activities occurred but to record and evaluate new activities. For example, the program originally took

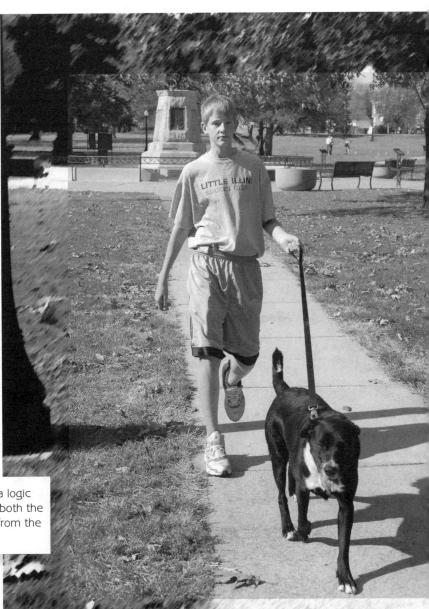

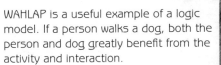
WAHLAP is a useful example of a logic model. If a person walks a dog, both the person and dog greatly benefit from the activity and interaction.

The Indianapolis, Indiana, Walk a Hound, Lose a Pound (WAHLAP) Program

This unique collaboration brings together partners with diverse individual goals and objectives. These differing goals and objectives are being addressed through a common mission, motto, and overall goal for the dog walking program. Partners and stakeholders include organizations and individuals with primary goals related to the following:

1. Improving animal welfare
   - City of Indianapolis Animal Care and Control
   - Humane Society of Indianapolis
   - Local Foster Groups (Alliance for Responsible Pet Ownership)
   - Friends of Indianapolis Dogs Outside (FIDO)
   - Indiana Paw
   - Doggone Connection
2. Increasing physical fitness and reducing obesity and other chronic diseases
   - The National Institute for Fitness and Sport (NIFS)
   - FitCity, Indy Parks
3. Promoting use of local parks
   - Indianapolis Parks and Recreation Department
   - White River State Park and Greenway
4. Promoting community service
   - Program volunteers
5. Participating in enjoyable and purposeful physical activity
   - Individual and family program participants

WAHLAP is a community program that involves community participants who volunteer to walk shelter and other homeless dogs in local parks. The collaborative program's motto is "More than just a walk in the park!" The mission is "improving the lives of people and homeless animals through fitness and physical activity." The major goals are to affect the growing rate of obesity by increasing physical activity through a creative and fun approach to physical fitness, to address the plight of homeless animals and increase their adoptability through provision of exercise and socialization, and to increase community awareness of issues related to animal welfare. Although some of the stakeholders differ greatly in terms of their goals and objectives, the motto, mission, goals, and program activities address individual goals and objectives and create the common ground needed for an effective partnership.

WAHLAP website: www.walkahound.org. Accessed 01/02/09.

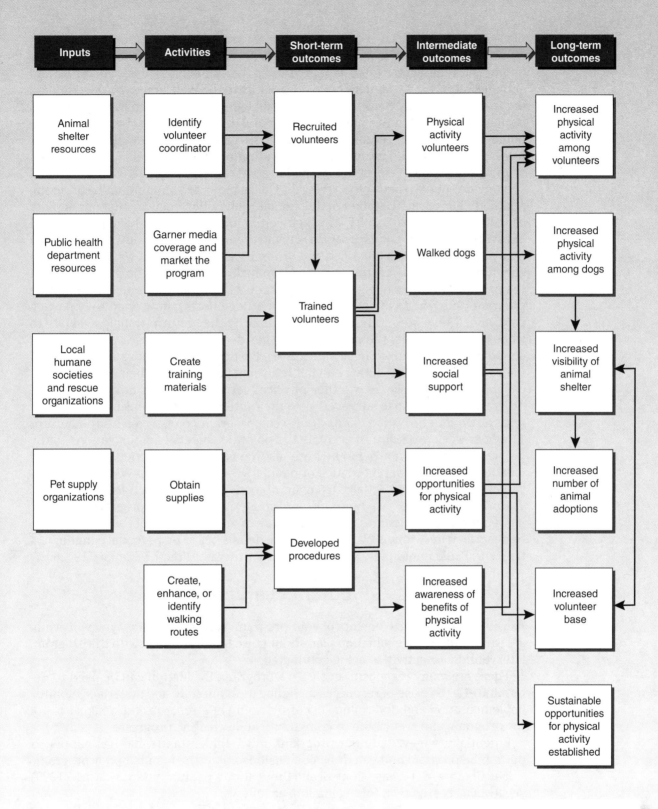

Figure 7.1 Walk a Hound Lose a Pound logic model.

place in one location. Over time, as a result of partnerships with local park and recreation programs, the program expanded to multiple locations. This increased the number and characteristics of volunteers and the number and type of materials and supplies required. The number and type of hits to the Web site, www.walkahound. org, can help evaluate response to and participation in the program. Indicators for many of the outcomes have been clear and easy to measure. For example, the number of volunteers recruited and trained to walk dogs, the number of dogs that have been walked, and the number of dog adoptions are easily tallied from records such as sign-in sheets, program administrative records, and participating animal shelter and animal rescue group records. One unexpected outcome of the program, related to increasing visibility of the animal shelter, has been an offshoot activity called Habitat for Dogmanity, in which community volunteers have participated in events to build doghouses for dogs in need. Another related outcome has been that participants have identified the program as a meaningful way to engage in community service activities. Surveys, administered when participants sign in at the program events, collect information such as how participants learned of the program (to evaluate effectiveness of marketing efforts), how often they participate, and, if they are returning participants, why they return (to help evaluate to what extent the dogs, the program, or other determinants might provide social support for being more physically active). Participants are also surveyed about their baseline physical activity and, if returning participants, their current physical activity (to determine whether physical activity increases as a result of the program). They are also surveyed as to their interest in variations in the program (e.g., a regular structured 3-5 day per week program compared with the current 1 day per week program) to evaluate the potential effects of modifications to the program. The program personnel are also considering collecting demographic data to determine characteristics of people who participate in WAHLAP and assessing their physical activity using an objective measure such as pedometers. The program has kept yearly records and created a list of major program activities, innovations, and outcomes so that the growth and evolution of the program can be described over time. (WAHLAP program details based on personal communication with Paula Puntenney, RN, MA, WAHLAP Program Director, January 19, 2009.)

Program Evaluation

As you determine the elements of your program, keep in mind how you will evaluate each of them. An evaluation plan should be carefully aligned with the program, intervention, or activities being conducted.

There are many reasons to evaluate a program. Evaluation can be used to determine **effective** use of resources including funding, staff, and materials; monitor implementation and determine success; document strengths and weaknesses of the program; and contribute to community and scientific progress.

Essentially, we evaluate our programs so we understand what has happened during the program and can draw conclusions about the results of our program.

The Centers for Disease Control and Prevention's **evaluation framework** (1999) suggests a six-step plan for evaluation, as follows:

1. Engage stakeholders
2. Describe and plan the program
3. Focus on evaluation
4. Gather credible evidence
5. Justify conclusions
6. Ensure use

Engage Stakeholders

To develop an adequate understanding of different perspectives, interests, and program expectations, aim to engage a diverse group of stakeholders. The evaluation stakeholder group may be a subset of your main stakeholder group, depending on the size and scope of the program and the ways you intend to use your evaluation results. Engage those who have a vested interest in the outcomes of the program.

Describe and Plan the Program

As stated earlier in this chapter, it is ideal to begin thinking about evaluation as you develop your program. However, consider the stage of program development and plan your evaluation plan accordingly. For example, is this a new program, or are you refining an existing program? To answer to this question will have significant impact on your evaluation plans.

To focus your evaluation plan, review your mission, goals, objectives, strategies, and available resources. Reassessing your program will help to structure the evaluation plan around the proposed elements. A **logic model** can be helpful in conceptualizing the program elements. As discussed earlier in this chapter, a logic model is a visual representation of the hypothesized links between program elements. Logic models can facilitate evaluation of the linkages between chosen elements.

Focus on Evaluation

Once you have described your program, you can focus on the evaluation plan. Account for questions stakeholders may have, the intended uses and users of your evaluation results, and the overall purpose of your program (e.g., to gain insight, change practices, assess effects). Refining your evaluation plans will allow you to meet the expectations of your stakeholders and use your resources efficiently. This step will entail creating evaluation questions, choosing an evaluation design and developing a timeline.

Evaluation questions will help clarify what you hope to learn from your proposed program and should be related to your planned goals and objectives. These questions should be directly linked to inputs, activities, expected results or outcomes, and possibly contextual factors that may influence the program (such as the political climate, the environmental climate, other programs or activities).

Process and Outcome Evaluation

There are two primary phases, or types, of evaluation: process and outcome. As the name implies, process evaluation views the process of delivering the intervention and documents how your program was implemented. **Outcome evaluation** pertains to the results of having delivered the intervention and focuses on the expected findings (short-term, intermediate, and long-term outcomes) of your project. An outcome evaluation most often relies on a preintervention (i.e., baseline) measure that is compared with the same postintervention measure—so the first outcome measure will be collected before any process measures are available. For example, prior to the start of a proposed point-of-decision intervention (e.g., placing signs to encourage people to use the stairs), a baseline measure of stair and escalator use should be obtained. The implementation of program components and the process evaluation should start after the baseline measures are obtained. Process and outcome evaluations can be diagrammed (see figure 7.2).

Process evaluation relates to program inputs and activities, so as you plan activities and how they will be carried out (i.e., what inputs), think about process measures that will let you know whether the process is occurring as intended.

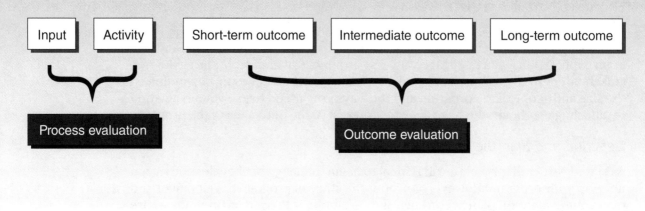

Figure 7.2   This simple diagram clearly illustrates how planning and evaluation are intertwined.

Objectives that are determined in the planning stage can easily be translated into outcomes that can be measured.

Some outcomes naturally precede other outcomes. Depending on the time frame of the program or intervention, you may be able to realistically reach only short-term outcomes. These might include improvements in knowledge and attitudes about being physically active, which may change faster than physical activity behavior, which in the long run will affect health status such as blood pressure or weight (see figure 7.3).

Evaluation Designs

An important consideration for program evaluation is that it is not intervention research; there are some important differences. In intervention research in its truest sense, you are testing an intervention compared with the absence of that intervention (control) or with an inert intervention (placebo) or directly comparing two interventions (comparative effectiveness). Thus, delivery of the intervention being tested must be unalterable (i.e., it cannot be changed once implementation begins). In program evaluation, you are examining the value or worth of a program at the same time that you are attempting to make it the best that it can be. Using process measures allows the program to be altered to make it better and improve the chances of success. In intervention research, it is important to have an objective evaluator (i.e., someone who is not involved in the intervention). In program evaluation, the evaluator should be someone intimately knowledgeable about the program because that person is best able to make appropriate improvements.

Differences aside, evaluation designs for program evaluation come from the research field. Many evaluation designs commonly rely on the following pre- or quasi-experimental research designs (Cook & Campbell, 1979; DHHS, 2002) (see figure 7.4).

Including a comparison group strengthens the evaluation design considerably because it controls for many potential threats to the validity of the findings. Drawing from classic research terms, consider the "threat" of history—was it just time passing that changed the outcome of interest or was it the intervention? Without a comparison group, we cannot say. The same is true for the use of assessment tools or instrumentation—was just measuring the participants what made them change or was it the intervention? Another threat that is difficult to control is selection

Outcome evaluation		
Short-term outcome	Intermediate outcome	Long-term outcome
Knowledge Attitude	Physical activity behavior	Blood pressure Weight

Figure 7.3 Outcome diagram.

Pre- and post- one-sample tests:	X_1 O X_2 (Where X is the measure and O is the intervention)
Pre- and post- two-sample tests:	X_1 O X_2 (intervention group) X_1 X_2 (comparison group)
Time-series design:	X_1 O X_2 X_3 X_4 X_5 (intervention group) X_1 X_2 X_3 X_4 X_5 (comparison group)

Figure 7.4 Experimental design.

bias. Unless participants are randomly assigned to groups (e.g., intervention or control), it is possible that some characteristics of the participants, or social or physical environmental influences other than the intervention, caused them to change. Controlling for threats to validity such as history, instrumentation, and selection bias are issues typically more related to experimental research than programmatic activities (Cook & Campbell, 1979). However, if resources allow you to control any of these threats to validity you should do so, because such efforts can strengthen program evaluation.

Gather Credible Evidence

After an evaluation plan is in place, data collection can begin. Consider how the information will be collected, who will collect it, and where the data will come from.

Indicators, Data Sources, and Performance Measures

For every evaluation question, there should be one or more **indicators.** An indicator is exactly that—it tells you whether what you are measuring has occurred. For example, if you want to know whether participants in a walking program increased their walking, then "number of steps walked" would be a great indicator. It is usually best to have more than one indicator, because it is difficult to measure some indicators precisely. For example, to use "number of steps walked" as one indicator, you would have to rely on the participants' being able to report their number of steps walked accurately. This will be difficult to do without using an objective measure of physical activity, such as a step counter or pedometer. You could also add a second indicator such as "minutes walked." This indicator might be easier for participants to recall, and by using more than one indicator you may obtain both additional information and the option to cross-validate your results.

For every indicator, there should be one or more data sources. A data source is the means by which to measure an indicator. In the previous example, the data source for number of steps walked could be a pedometer, and the data source for minutes walked would be a stopwatch. Findings from the data sources (e.g., logs, questionnaires, or interviews) can be recorded and subsequently conveyed to evaluation staff. Table 7.2 lists multiple indicators and data sources as examples of things to consider for process evaluation.

Thought should go into selecting indicators and data sources that ultimately help you achieve your performance measures. It takes careful planning to find a balance between what is feasible and what is accurate. Sometimes the most accurate measures are not feasible given time or resource limits. You should consider two things in this regard:

- Triangulation—Using multiple data sources allows for more than one perspective on indicators; select more than one indicator for every question, and select one or more data sources for every indicator.

- Mixing qualitative and quantitative data—Quantitative measures can provide part of the picture (e.g., the number of successful program completers); qualitative measures can provide additional information (e.g., interviews with program completers and noncompleters can give you the reasons behind the numbers).

Data Collection

During careful planning for evaluation you selected indicators and data sources, so collecting the data is then a matter of course. Someone, however, has to make sure it happens. Usually, there is a senior evaluator with oversight over data collectors. Data collectors work directly with participants to gather the data. The skills necessary to be a data collector depend on the data sources. For example, if interviews are being conducted, data collectors need qualitative skills and training to adhere to a standardized interview protocol. If objective measurement instru-

Table 7.2 Process Evaluation

Activity	Indicators	Data sources	Performance measure
Run a new adult volleyball league	Volleyball games	Observation	Tuesday night games from 7 to 9 p.m.
Advertise	Number of ads	Newspaper clippings	A month of weekend ads
Identify captains	Number of captains and teams	Registration forms	Eight captains and teams
Hire referees	Number of referees needed	Interviews with referees	Two referees per game

ments are being used such as accelerometers, which measure movement, someone with technological skills is needed to calibrate and maintain the accelerometers, instruct people in proper use, and obtain, analyze, and interpret the recorded data.

Justify Conclusions

After data collection, the next step is to analyze and interpret the data. A critical review of the evaluation data will allow program personnel to create and substantiate conclusions about the program. Moreover, findings will provide a basis for an action plan to improve or maintain the program or even replicate the program for the benefit of many more people.

Analyses

The most basic steps in quantitative data analysis are as follows (DHHS, 2002):

- Enter the data into a computer program, such as Access, Excel, SPSS, or SAS.
- Check for data entry errors (e.g., double entry).
- Tabulate the data (e.g., calculate the number of participants and their attendance or program adherence; percentage of participants meeting physical activity recommendations; percentage of participants who walked to school every day).
- Stratify data (i.e., analyze it by community, gender, age, race or ethnicity, income level, fitness level).
- Make comparisons (e.g., differences between pretests and posttests data or between a comparison and an intervention group or community).
- Present data in a clear and uncomplicated format.

The most basic steps in qualitative analyses are as follows (Warden and Wong, 2007):

- Review your data; transcribe interviews and information obtained from focus groups; review observation notes.
- Code data from interviews and other notes. Look for similar themes and organize data into meaningful categories. Alternatively, data can be entered into a qualitative analysis computer program, such as Nudist or Atlis Ti, for coding.
- Identify patterns (e.g., similar comments made by various program participants).
- Summarize findings appropriately for your intended audience.

Interpretation

What do the quotes, numbers, frequencies, averages, and statistical test results that emerge from data analyses say about your program? For this process, the senior evaluator should communicate with those who care about the evaluation findings (i.e., evaluation stakeholders).

- Are findings similar to what was expected? If not, why?
- Are there alternative explanations for the findings?
- How do the findings compare with those of similar programs?
- Was the program or intervention delivered as intended?
- What are the limitations of the evaluation? For example, are there potential biases? Do findings pertain to groups other than those evaluated?
- If multiple indicators were used to answer the same evaluation question, were similar or predicted findings obtained for each indicator?
- What insights do the qualitative data provide?

Ensure Use: Reporting Your Findings

The most important question to ask throughout the evaluation process is "will the evaluation results be used?" Do not collect data that won't be used. Do not analyze data in a way that is not useful. And, by all means, share findings so that they can be used! After the data have been analyzed and interpreted, ensure use of the findings by disseminating the information. When you are working with communities, it is of utmost importance to share the program evaluation findings with relevant stakeholders and to implement findings related to program changes.

There are some points to keep in mind to ensure that evaluation findings will be used. Of key importance is making action-oriented recommendations. Recommendations for continuing, expanding, redesigning, or abandoning a physical activity program may follow directly from the program evaluation findings. When making these decisions, remember the following tips:

■ Consider stakeholders' values and align recommendations when possible. For example, one stakeholder may be interested in reducing the incidence of chronic diseases and another stakeholder in reducing the reliance on cars for transportation in the same community. You must give stakeholders the data they need to support their separate positions (e.g., did the development of walking and bicycle trails increase physical activity among community members and, if yes, why? Did people claim they walked for health or transportation reasons?).

■ Share draft recommendations with stakeholders and solicit feedback.

■ Relate recommendations to the original purposes and uses of the evaluation.

■ Determine who should receive recommendations from the stakeholders in order to promote use of the evaluation findings and target them appropriately for each audience that will receive them. Ideally, this should be done as you focus your evaluation early in the process.

Next, consider how to effectively share this information. Your strategy should consider format and channels.

Format

An evaluation report will be necessary, and this will require that the audience be considered. Are the stakeholders scientists or community members? Reports summarizing the results of the evaluation should be easy for the intended audience to understand and appropriate for that audience. Moreover, different stakeholders may have different questions they will need answered. Thus, depending on the audiences, more than one report may need to be prepared. This will require that someone from the project staff, perhaps the project evaluator, be designated to create reports.

In the report,

■ summarize the evaluation plan and procedures,
■ list the strengths and weaknesses of the evaluation,
■ list the pros and cons of each recommendation,
■ present clear and succinct results in tables and graphs, and
■ summarize the stakeholders' roles and involvement in both the project and the follow-up plans.

Channels

Decide how to get the information to the intended audiences. You might use the following:

- Mailings
- Web sites
- Community forums
- Media (television, radio, newspaper) (Share findings with stakeholders first, so they are not surprised by the media reports.)
- Personal contacts (including telephone individual or conference calls)
- Listservs
- Organizations' newsletters

Follow-Up

Because of the effort required, reaching justified conclusions and making sound recommendations can seem like an end in itself; however, active follow-up is needed for several reasons:

- To remind stakeholders and the audience of the intended uses of the evaluation results
- To reflect on how the evaluation findings may change or improve your program in the future
- To prevent lessons learned from being lost or ignored in the process of making complex program or policy decisions
- To prevent misuse of results by ensuring that evidence is applied to the questions that were the evaluation's central focus and that the results are not taken out of context

Conclusion

This chapter emphasizes the importance of evaluating programs and physical activity initiatives. Previous chapters focusing on evidenced-based physical activity interventions, by their very nature, also point to the importance of evaluation. Given scarce resources and numerous public health problems, it will be very difficult to ask key policy makers and decision makers to support and fund physical activity programs and interventions that lack evidence that they are efficacious (i.e., that they work under ideal or controlled conditions) or effective (that they work in real-world field settings). Implementing physical activity interventions, programs, and other initiatives requires an understanding of how well they are implemented (process evaluation) and what impact or outcomes they have regarding changing behavior or health status (outcome evaluation). When these kinds of evaluations occur, then other people, organizations, and communities can more confidently consider adopting and translating the interventions and programs for use in their own unique settings. Without such assessments, it is appropriate to ask whether interventions, programs, or initiatives that are not evidenced based and have not been evaluated should take place. The money may be better spent on other interventions or public health issues that rest on a more solid foundation of evaluation and effectiveness. Knowing what we know about the risks of inactivity and benefits of physical activity, evaluating our efforts to increase physical activity using community- and population-based interventions and programs is of paramount importance. Planning for implementation and planning for evaluation should, indeed, go hand in hand.

Suggested Readings

Centers for Disease Control and Prevention. 1999. Framework for program evaluation in public health. *MMWR Recommendations and Reports* 48(RR-11):1-40. Available at www.cdc.gov/mmwr/preview/mmwrhtml/rr4811a1.htm

Mathison SA (Ed). 2004. *Encyclopedia of Evaluation*. Thousand Oaks, CA: Sage.

Patton MQ. 1996. *Utilization-Focused Evaluation,* 3rd edition. Thousand Oaks, CA: Sage.

Welk G (Ed). 2002. *Physical Activity Assessments for Health-Related Research*. Champaign, IL: Human Kinetics.

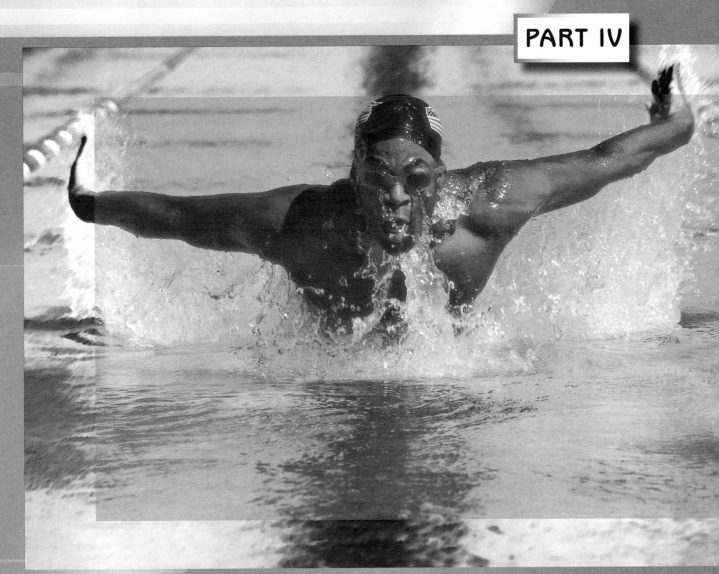
© Stockbyte

PART IV

Resources for Action

This section provides additional resources and information about select topics related to physical activity and public health. These materials may increase your knowledge about promoting physical activity in your community and assist your efforts to help people become active—and stay active.

Appendix A, Physical Activity and Disabilities, provides you with important information to help create interventions and available and accessible programs and opportunities that support the needs of people with disabilities. The National Center on Physical Activity and Disability (NCPAD) is discussed. Contact information is listed for a number of organizations and agencies that provide information about, and opportunities for, physical activity among persons with disabilities.

Appendix B, Physical Activity Surveillance, details concepts that are important in physical activity surveillance and describes surveillance systems that are utilized to conduct epidemiologic research, surveillance of physical activity prevalence estimates and physical activity trends over time, and monitoring of national objectives.

Appendix C, Physical Activity and Fitness (HP 2010 Progress Review), discusses the Healthy People 2010 physical activity objectives. This appendix provides information on programs, resources, and initiatives used to achieve the Healthy People 2010 objectives. These objectives may help support or clarify your own objectives for your initiative, program, or intervention. Monitor physical activity information on Web sites such as government health agencies and professional organizations for the soon to be released Healthy People 2020 objectives.

Appendix D, Physical Activity and Health: A Report of the Surgeon General is an executive summary of this important 1996 document that helped influence and advance the field of physical activity and public health.

Appendix E, Selected Organizations for Promoting Physical Activity, lists information about organizations and programs across the country that have a focus on physical activity. You're sure to find something in these resources that will help your efforts to promote physical activity in your community and to develop, implement, and evaluate physical activity programs and interventions.

Physical Activity and Disability

James H. Rimmer

The lack of participation in regular and beneficial physical activity is a serious public health concern for all Americans, but it is even more acute for the estimated 52 million Americans with disabilities who are demonstrably at much greater risk for developing the types of serious health problems associated with a sedentary lifestyle (Rimmer et al., 1996). Despite the enormous health benefits that can be derived from regular physical activity, people with disabilities are one of the most physically inactive groups in society. *Healthy People 2010* uses cross-sectional surveys to outline current levels of physical activity and exercise for various subpopulations in the United States and lists goals for the year 2010 (USHHS, 2000). This report states that people with disabilities are currently much less active than their nondisabled counterparts and participate in less regular moderate and vigorous physical activity. In addition, people with disabilities report a substantially high number of secondary conditions that are directly or indirectly associated with their disability but in most cases are considered preventable (e.g., fatigue, weight gain, pain).

Efforts to eliminate health disparities must address issues, needs, and barriers of people with disabilities for positive lifestyle change. The level of physical inactivity observed among people with disabilities has been linked to an increase in the severity of disability and erosion of involvement in community activities. These patterns of low physical activity reported among people with disabilities raise serious concern regarding their health and well-being, particularly as they enter their later years, when the effects of the natural aging process are compounded by years of sedentary living and severe deconditioning.

NCPAD: A Comprehensive Electronic and Interactive Information Center on Physical Activity and Disability

The National Center on Physical Activity and Disability (NCPAD) is an online health promotion resource whose mission is to reduce the incidence of secondary conditions and improve the overall quality of life for persons with disabilities through promotion of beneficial levels of physical activity and healthy, active lifestyles.

Developed as a cooperative agreement between the University of Illinois at Chicago (UIC) and the Division of Human Development and Disability at the National Center on Birth Defects and Developmental Disabilities, Centers for Disease Control and Prevention (CDC), NCPAD collects, organizes, synthesizes, and develops materials to inform consumers, guide practitioners, facilitate development of best practices, and foster future research.

NCPAD's Web site (www.ncpad.org) provides a wide array of resources on physical activity and disability:

- *NCPAD-News:* a monthly e-newsletter
- Video clips and video-enabled fact sheets on disability, chronic health conditions, and physical activity, including fitness, recreation, and sports
- Searchable national directories of accessible physical activity programs, adaptive equipment suppliers, organizations, accessible parks, and personal fitness trainers who work with individuals with disabilities and chronic health conditions
- Health promotion topics related to nutrition, wellness, disability, and programming
- Calendar of events on upcoming conferences and expositions in physical activity and disability
- Listings on jobs and grants in physical activity and disability

To access NCPAD's resources, go to www.ncpad.org, or contact NCPAD at 800-900-8086, ncpad@uic.edu, or 312-355-4058 (Fax).

Legislation and Guidelines

Legislation protecting the rights of people with disabilities is critical for ensuring equal access and opportunity for all Americans. Today, many legislators continue to support new bills and amendments to existing laws that advocate for the rights of people with disabilities. These laws have made it possible for people with disabilities to have a higher quality of life and live independently in the community.

The Americans with Disabilities Act Public Law 101-336

The Americans with Disabilities Act (ADA) is a civil rights law that prohibits the discrimination of people with disabilities and ensures that programs and services are equally accessible to individuals with and without disabilities. The ADA has implications for anyone planning and conducting physical activity programs. There are five titles within the ADA:

- Title I: Employment
- Title II: State & Local Governments
- Title III: Places of Public Accommodations
- Title IV: Telecommunications
- Title V: Miscellaneous Provisions (such as insurance coverage)

The ADA defines an *individual with a disability* as a person who

- has a physical or mental impairment that substantially limits one or more "major life activities" (i.e., caring for oneself, walking, seeing, hearing, speaking, learning, and working);
- has a record of such an impairment; or
- is regarded as having such an impairment.

Title II of the ADA, which covers state and local governments, may be of particular interest to professionals who are involved in or are developing accessible physical activity programs. Title II prohibits state and local governments and their departments from discriminating against people with disabilities in their programs, activities, and services. Programs and services must be provided in an integrated setting, unless separate or different measures are necessary to ensure equal opportunity.

For more information on the Americans with Disabilities Act, contact

U.S. Department of Justice
950 Pennsylvania Ave. NW
Civil Rights Division
Disability Rights Section—NYAV
Washington, DC 20530
Phone: 800-514-0301 (voice)
TTY: 800-514-0383
Fax: 202-307-1198
www.usdoj.gov/crt/ada/adahom1.htm

Americans with Disabilities Act Accessibility Guidelines (ADAAG) for Recreation Facilities

In 2002, the Architectural and Transportation Barriers Compliance Board (Access Board) issued final accessibility guidelines that will serve as the basis for standards to be adopted by the Department of Justice for new construction and alterations of recreation facilities covered by the ADA. The guidelines ensure that newly constructed and altered recreation facilities meet the requirements of the ADA and are readily accessible to and usable by individuals with disabilities. State and local governments that provide recreation facilities have a separate obligation under Title II of the ADA to provide program accessibility, which may require the removal of architectural barriers in existing facilities. Private entities who own, lease (or lease to), or operate recreation facilities have a separate obligation under Title III of the ADA to remove architectural barriers in existing facilities where such action is readily achievable (i.e., easily accomplishable and able to be carried out without much difficulty or expense). (From www.access-board.gov/recreation/final.htm)

The guidelines include scoping and technical provisions for the following:

- Amusement rides
- Boating facilities
- Fishing piers and platforms
- Golf courses
- Miniature golf
- Sports facilities
- Swimming pools and spas

Summaries of the *Accessibility Guidelines for Recreation Facilities* may be downloaded at www.access-board.gov/recreation/guides/index.htm.

The Individuals with Disabilities Education Improvement Act (IDEA of 2004)

The Individuals with Disabilities Education (IDEA) Improvement Act (PL 108-446 of 2004) ensures that school-aged children and youth who have a disability receive a free appropriate public education that emphasizes special education and related services. Special education is provided, at no cost to the parents, to meet the unique needs of a child with a disability, including:

- instruction conducted in the classroom, in the home, in hospitals and institutions, and in other settings; and
- instruction in physical education, which includes adapted physical education, movement education, and motor development.

Related services are transportation and other supportive services that will help students benefit from the special education program and prepare them for further education, employment, and independent living. These services may include speech and language pathology and audiology services, interpreting services, psychological services, physical and occupational therapy, recreation, including therapeutic recreation, and social work services.

IDEA Resources

- IDEA 2004 (PL 108-446) online: www.copyright.gov/legislation/pl108-446.pdf
- IDEA Partnership: www.ideapartnership.org
- IDEA: Guide to Frequently Asked Questions:
- http:// republicans.edlabor.house.gov/archive/issues/109th/education/idea/ideafaq.pdf
- U.S. Department of Education, IDEA 2004 Resources: www.ed.gov/policy/speced/guid/idea/idea2004.html
- Wrightslaw: www.wrightslaw.com/idea/

Additional resources are available:
Paciorek MJ, Jones JA. 2001. *Disability Sport and Recreation Resources*, 3rd edition. Traverse City, MI: Cooper.

National Disability Physical Activity & Recreation Related Organizations (General)

Adaptive Adventure
27888 Meadow Dr.
Evergreen, CO 80437
Phone: 877-679-2770
Fax: 303-670-8290
e-mail: Info@AdaptiveAdventures.org
www.adaptiveadventures.org

American Alliance for Health, Physical
    Education, Recreation and Dance
1900 Association Dr.
Reston, VA 20191-1598
Phone: 800-213-7193
www.aahperd.org

American Amputee Soccer Association
Seattle, WA
Phone: 302-529-0701
e-mail: rgh@ampsoccer.org
www.ampsoccer.org

American College of Sports Medicine
401 W. Michigan St.
Indianapolis, IN 46202
Phone: 317-637-9200
Fax: 317-634-7817
e-mail: publicinfo@acsm.org
www.acsm.org

American Association of Challenged Divers
P.O. Box 501405
San Diego, CA 92150-1405
Phone: 619-597-8978
e-mail: pinnacle@cts.com

American Hearing Impaired Hockey
   Association
1143 West Lake St.
Chicago, IL 60607
Phone: 312-226-5880
TTY: 773-767-3130
Fax: 312-829-2098
e-mail: info@ahiha.org
www.ahiha.org

American Therapeutic Recreation Association
1414 Prince St., Ste. 204
Alexandria, VA 22314
Phone: 703-683-9420
Fax: 703-683-9431
www.atra-online.com

American Wheelchair Bowling Association
P.O. Box 69
Clover, VA 24534-0069
Phone: 434-454-2269
Fax: 434-454-6276
e-mail: bowlawba@aol.com
www.awba.org

American Wheelchair Table Tennis
   Association
23 Parker St.
Port Chester, NY 10573
Phone: 914-937-3932
e-mail: johnsonjennifer@yahoo.com

Bankshot Sports
785 F Rockville Pike, Ste. 504
Rockville, MD 20852
Phone: 800-933-0140
Fax: 301-309-0263
e-mail: info@bankshot.com
www.Bankshot.com

BlazeSports
U.S. Disabled Athletes Fund, Inc.
280 Interstate North Circle
Atlanta, GA 30339
Phone: 770-850-8199
Fax: 770-850.8179
e-mail: blazesports@blazesports.com
www.blazesports.com

Cerebral Palsy International Sports and
   Recreation Association
P.O. Box 16
6666 ZG Heteren
The Netherlands
Phone: +31-26-47-22-593
Fax: +31-26-47-23-914
e-mail: contact@cpisra.org
www.cpisra.org

Disabled Sports USA
451 Hungerford Dr., Ste. 00
Rockville, MD 20850
Phone: 301-217-0960
Fax: 301-217-0968
e-mail: information@dsusa.org
www.dsusa.org

Dwarf Athletic Association of America
418 Willow Way
Lewisville, TX 75077
Phone: 972-317-8299
Fax: 972-966-0184
e-mail: daaa@flash.net
www.daaa.org

Fore Hope (therapeutic golf)
925 Darby Creek Dr.
Galloway, OH 43119
Phone: 614-870-7299
Fax: 614-870-7245
e-mail: info@forehope.org
www.forehope.org

Handicapped Scuba Association International
1104 El Prado
San Clemente, CA 92672-4637
Phone: 949-498-4540
Fax: 949-498-6128
e-mail: hsa@hsascuba.com
www.hsascuba.com

International Paralympic Committee
Adenauerallee 212-214
53113 Bonn
Germany
Phone: +49-228-2097-200
Fax: +49-228-2097-209
e-mail: info@paralympic.org
www.paralympic.org

International Paralympic Table Tennis
107 Jenne St.
Santa Cruz, CA 95060
Phone: 831-457-1713
e-mail: bizde@gotnet.com
www.ipttc.org

National Amputee Golf Association
11 Walnut Hill Rd.
Amherst, NH 03031
Phone: 800-633-6242
Fax: 603-672-2987
e-mail: info@nagagolf.org
www.nagagolf.org

National Beep Baseball Association
5568 Boulder Crest St.
Columbus, OH 43235
Phone: 785-234-2156
e-mail: info@nbba.org
www.nbba.org

National Center on Accessibility
501 North Morton St., Ste. 109
Bloomington, IN 47404
Voice: 812-856-4422
TTY: 812-856-4421
Fax: 812-856-4480
e-mail: nca@indiana.edu
www.indiana.edu/~nca/

National Disability Sports Alliance
  (affiliated with Blazesports)
25 West Independence Way
Kingston, RI 02881
Phone: 401-792-7130
e-mail: info@blazesports.org
www.blazesports.org

National Instructors Association for Divers
  with Disabilities
P.O. Box 798
Moss Landing, CA 95039
Phone: 831-633-3006
Fax: 831-633-2889
e-mail: stonley@pacbell.net
www.niadd.org

National Park Service
1849 C St. NW
Washington, DC 20240
Phone: 202-208-6843
e-mail: Kendra_Peel@nps.gov
www.nps.gov

National Recreation and Park Association
22377 Belmont Ridge Rd.
Ashburn, VA 20148-4501
Phone: 703-858-0784
Fax: 703-858-0794
e-mail: membership@nrpa.org
www.nrpa.org

National Senior Games Association
P.O. Box 82059
Baton Rouge, LA 70884-2059
Phone: 225-766-6800
Fax: 225-766-9115
e-mail: nsga@nsga.com
www.NSGA.com

National Wheelchair Basketball Association
6165 Lehman Dr., Ste. 101
Colorado Springs, CO 80918
Phone: 719-266-4082
Fax: 719-266-4876
e-mail: toddhatfield@nwba.org
www.nwba.org

National Wheelchair Softball Association
6000 W. Floyd Ave., #110
Denver, CO 80227
Phone: 303-936-5587
e-mail: paraathlete@comcast.net
www.wheelchairsoftball.org

North American Riding for the
  Handicapped Association
P.O. Box 33150
Denver, CO 80233
Phone: 800-369-7433
Fax: 303-252-4610
e-mail: NARHA@NARHA.ORG
www.narha.org

Physically Challenged Golf Association
34 Dale Road
Avon, CT 06001
Phone: 860-676-2035
No Web site available

SABAH: Skating Athletes Bold at Heart
2607 Niagara Street
Buffalo, NY 14207
Phone: 716-362-9600
fax: 716-362-9601
e-mail: sabah@sabhinc.org
www.sabahinc.org

Outdoors for All Foundation
2 Nickerson Street, Suite 101
Seattle, WA 98109-1652
www.outdoorsforall.org

Special Olympics
1133 19th St. NW
Washington, DC 20036-3604
Phone: 800-700-8585
Fax: 202-824-0200
e-mail: info@specialolympics.org
www.specialolympics.org

United States Adaptive Recreation Center
43101 Goldmine Dr.
Big Bear Lake, CA 92315-2897
Phone: 909-584-0269
TTY: 800-735-2929
Fax: 909-585-6805
e-mail: mail@usarc.org
www.usarc.org

United States Association of Blind Athletes
33 N. Institute St.
Colorado Springs, CO 80903
Phone: 719-630-0422
Fax: 719-630-0616
www.usaba.org

United States Deaf Ski and Snowboard
   Association
1772 Saddle Hill Dr.
Logan, UT 84321
Phone: 435-752-2702
Fax: 810-279-4063
e-mail: Secretary@usdssa.org
www.usdssa.org

United States Electric Wheelchair Hockey
   Association
7216 39th Ave. North
Minneapolis, MN 55427
Phone: 763-535-4736
e-mail: info@powerhockey.com
www.powerhockey.com

United States Flag Football for the Deaf
P.O. Box 230853
Centreville, VA 20120
e-mail: secretary@usffd.org
www.usffd.org

United States Handcycling
P.O. Box 3538
Evergreen, CO 80437
Phone: 303-679-2770
e-mail: info@ushf.org
www.ushf.org

United States Paralympics
One Olympic Plaza
Colorado Springs, CO 80909
Phone: 719-866-2030
Fax: 719-866-2029
e-mail: paralympicinfo@usoc.org
http://usparalympics.org/

US Sled Hockey Team
25 Club Valley Drive
East Falmouth, MA
02536 508-564-6740
e-mail: ksaint12@adelphia.net
www.usahockey.com//Template_Usahockey
   .aspx?NAV=TU_10&ID=194136

USA Deaf Sports Federation
102 North Krohn Pl.
Sioux Falls, SD 57103-1800
Phone: 605-367-5760
TTY: 605-367-5761
Fax: 605-977-6625
e-mail: HomeOffice@usdeafsports.org
www.usdeafsports.org

Wheelchair Sports, USA
1668 320th Way
Earlham, IA 50072
Phone: 515-833-2450
e-mail: wsusa@aol.com
www.wsusa.org

General Disability-Related Organizations

Alzheimer's Association
225 N. Michigan Ave., 17th Floor
Chicago, IL 60601
Phone: 800-272-3900
e-mail: info@alz.org
www.alz.org

American Association on Intellectual and
   Developmental Disabilities
444 North Capitol St. NW, Ste. 846
Washington, DC 20001-1512
Phone: 800-424-3688
Fax: 202-387-2193
www.aamr.org

American Cancer Society
1599 Clifton Rd. NE
Atlanta, GA 30329
Phone: 800-227-2345
TTY: 866-228-4327
www.cancer.org

American Diabetes Association
1701 North Beauregard St.
Alexandria, VA 22311
Phone: 800-342-2383
e-mail: AskADA@diabetes.org
www.diabetes.org

American Heart Association
7272 Greenville Ave.
Dallas, TX 75231
Phone: 800-242-8721
www.americanheart.org

American Lung Association
61 Broadway, 6th Floor
New York, NY 10006
Phone: 800-548-8252
www.lungusa.org

American Obesity Association
1250 24th St. NW, Ste. 300
Washington, DC 20037
Phone: 202-776-7711
Fax: 202-776-7712
e-mail: webmaster@obesity.org
www.obesity.org

American Paraplegia Society
75-20 Astoria Blvd.
Jackson Heights, NY 11370
Phone: 718-803-3782
Fax: 718-803-0414
e-mail: aps@unitedspinal.org
www.apssci.org

American Society of Hypertension
148 Madison Ave., 5th Floor
New York, NY 10016
Phone: 212-696-9099
Fax: 212-696-0711
e-mail: ash@ash-us.org
www.ash-us.org

American Spinal Injury Association
2020 Peachtree Rd., NW
Atlanta, GA 30309-1402
Phone: 404-355-9772
Fax: 404-355-1826
www.asia-spinalinjury.org

American Stroke Association
7272 Greenville Ave.
Dallas, TX 75231
Phone: 888-478-7653
www.strokeassociation.org

Amputee Coalition of America
900 East Hill Ave., Ste. 285
Knoxville, TN 37915-2568
Phone: 888-267-5669
TTY: 865-525-4512
Fax: 865-525-7917
www.amputee-coalition.org

Arc of the United States
1010 Wayne Ave., Ste. 650
Silver Spring, MD 20910
Phone: 301-565-3842
Fax: 301-565-3843
www.thearc.org

Arthritis Foundation
P.O. Box 7669
Atlanta, GA 30357-0669
Phone: 800-568-4045
www.arthritis.org

Autism Society of America
7910 Woodmont Ave., Ste. 300
Bethesda, MD 20814-3067
Phone: 800-328-8476
www.autism-society.org

Brain Injury Association of America
8201 Greensboro Dr., Ste. 611
McLean, VA 22102
Phone: 800-444-6443
www.biausa.org

British Columbia Fibromyalgia Society
PO Box 42504
105-1005 Columbia St.
New Westminster, British Columbia V3M
  6H5
Canada
Phone: 888-353-6322
Fax: 604-878-7707
e-mail: info@mefm.bc.ca
www.mefm.bc.ca/bcfm

Christopher and Dana Reeve Paralysis
  Resource Center
636 Morris Turnpike, Ste. 3A
Short Hills, NJ 07078
Phone: 800-539-7309
e-mail: info@ChristopherReeve.org
www.paralysis.org

Chronic Fatigue and Immune Dysfunction
  Syndrome Association of America
P.O. Box 220398
Charlotte, NC 28222-0398
Phone: 704-365-2343
www.cfids.org

Easter Seals
230 West Monroe St., Ste. 1800
Chicago, IL 60606
Phone: 800-221-6827
TTY: 312-726-4258
Fax: 312-726-1494
www.easterseals.com

Lupus Foundation of America
2000 L St. NW, Ste. 710
Washington, DC 20036
Phone: 800-558-0121
Fax: 202-349-1156
e-mail: info@lupus.org
www.lupus.org

Muscular Dystrophy Association—USA
National Headquarters
3300 E. Sunrise Dr.
Tucson, AZ 85718
Phone: 800-344-4863
e-mail: mda@mdausa.org
www.mdausa.org

National Breast Cancer Foundation
One Hanover Park
16633 North Dallas Parkway, Ste. 600
Addison, TX 75001
e-mail: info@nationalbreastcancer.org
www.nationalbreastcancer.org

National Ability Center
P.O. Box 682799
Park City, UT 84068
Phone: 435-649-3991
TTY: 435-649-3991
Fax: 435-658-3992
e-mail: info@nac1985.org
http://69.2.249.50/

National Center on Accessibility
501 North Morton St., Ste. 109
Bloomington, IN 47404-3732
Phone: 812-856-4422
TTY: 812-856-4421
Fax: 812-856-4480
e-mail: nca@indiana.edu
www.ncaonline.org

National Council on Disability
1331 F St. NW, Ste. 850
Washington, DC 20004
Phone: 202-272-2004
TTY: 202-272-2074
Fax: 202-272-2022
e-mail: ncd@ncd.gov
www.ncd.gov

National Down Syndrome Society
666 Broadway
New York, NY 10012
Phone: 800-221-4602
e-mail: info@ndss.org
www.ndss.org

National Fibromyalgia Association
2121 S. Towne Centre, Ste. 300
Anaheim, CA 92806
Phone: 714-921-0150
Fax: 714-921-6920
e-mail: nfanurse@comcast.net
www.fmaware.org

National Heart, Lung, and Blood Institute
P.O. Box 30105
Bethesda, MD 20824-0105
Phone: 301-592-8573
Fax: 240-629-3255
e-mail: nhlbiinfo@nhlbi.nih.gov
www.nhlbi.nih.gov

National Mental Health Association
2001 N. Beauregard St., 12th Floor
Alexandria, VA 22311
Phone: 800-969-6642
TTY: 800-433-5959
Fax: 703-684-5968
www.nmha.org

National Multiple Sclerosis Society
733 Third Ave.
New York, NY 10017
Phone: 800-344-4867
www.nmss.org

National Osteoporosis Foundation
1232 22nd St. NW
Washington, DC 20037-1292
Phone: 202-223-2226
www.nof.org

National Parkinson Foundation
1501 N.W. 9th Ave.
Bob Hope Rd.
Miami, FL 33136-1494
Phone: 800-327-4545
e-mail: Mailbox@npf.med.miami.edu
www.parkinson.org

Osteoporosis and Related Bone Diseases
    National Resource Center
2 AMS Circle
Bethesda, MD 20892-3676
Phone: 800-624-2663
TTY: 202-466-4315
Fax: 202-293-2356
e-mail: niamsboneinfro@mail.nih.gov
www.osteo.org

Paralyzed Veterans of America
801 Eighteenth St. NW
Washington, DC 20006-3517
Phone: 800-424-8200
TTY: 800-795-4327
e-mail: info@pva.org
www.pva.org

William Black Medical Building Columbia–
Presbyterian Medical Center
Parkinson's Disease Foundation
710 W. 168th St.
New York, NY 10032-9982
Phone: 800-457-6676
e-mail: info@pdf.org
www.pdf.org

Post-Polio Health International
4207 Lindell Blvd., #110
St. Louis, MO 63108-2915
Phone: 314-534-0475
Fax: 314-534-5070
e-mail: info@post-polio.org
www.post-polio.org

Rehabilitation Institute of Chicago (RIC)
Sports and Fitness Center
710 N. Lake Shore Dr., 3rd Floor
Chicago, IL 60611
Phone: 312-238-5002
Fax: 312-238-5017
www.richealthfit.org

Rehabilitation, Research and Training
Center on Aging with Developmental
Disabilities
1640 West Roosevelt Rd., M/C 626
Chicago, IL 60608-6904
Phone: 800-996-8845
TTY: 312-413-0453
Fax: 312-996-6942
www.rrtcadd.org/index.html

Spina Bifida Association of America
4590 MacArthur Blvd. NW, Ste. 250
Washington, DC 20007-4226
Phone: 800-621-3141
e-mail: sbaa@sbaa.org
www.sbaa.org

United Cerebral Palsy
1660 L St. NW, Ste. 700
Washington, DC 20036
Phone: 800-872-5827
TTY: 202-973-7197
Fax: 202-776-0414
e-mail: webmaster@ucp.org
www.ucp.org/

United States Access Board
1331 F St. NW, Ste. 1000
Washington, DC 20004-1111
Phone: 800-872-2253
TTY: 800-993-2822
Fax: 202-272-0081
e-mail: info@access-board.gov
www.access-board.gov

Physical Activity Surveillance

Sandra A. Ham

Physical activity surveillance tracks population levels of physical activity behaviors, programs, and policies in adults and youth. *Healthy People 2010* (2020 soon to be released) provides national public health objectives that guide most of the physical activity surveillance activities in the United States. This appendix begins with background on some concepts that are important in physical activity surveillance and then describes the surveillance systems that are part of *Healthy People 2010*.

Background

Physical activities are often classified into domains that reflect the purpose of the activity. A common four-category classification is as follows:

- Occupational (work-related)
- Domestic (housework, yard work, physically active care for children and adults, chores)
- Transportation (walking or bicycling for the purposes of going somewhere)
- Leisure time (discretionary or recreational time for hobbies, sports, and exercise)

Existing physical activity assessment questionnaires differ as to which domains are measured, and few assess multiple domains. Historically, strategies to promote physical activity have emphasized increases in leisure-time physical activity, and, consequently, many questionnaires focus on only this domain. More recently, strategies to promote physical activity have emphasized the health benefits of all kinds of physical activity. Consequently, more physical activity assessment questionnaires are being designed to measure more than one, if not all four, domains of activity.

Physical Activity Assessment

Physical activity can be assessed in three general ways: questionnaire, observation and direct measurement, and diary. Physical activity questionnaires measure activities by asking a respondent to recall and report recent or usual participation in activities or in sedentary behaviors, usually over a set period of time. Methods of observation and direct measurement include electronic devices (e.g., pedometers, motion detectors, heart rate monitors) designed to record an individual's movements or physiological responses to movement and direct observation (e.g., watching and recording playground use during school recess). Diary assessment of physical activity involves requiring an individual to record all activity for a defined period of time (usually a week or a day). Once data from each of these assessment methods are gathered, estimates or indicators of energy expenditure or indices of physical activity are obtained.

U.S. national health surveys that assess and track physical activity in individuals typically include short sets of questions as just one of many sets of health-related questions. No national surveys currently use a long, detailed physical activity questionnaire, such as those typically used in research studies. One national health survey has used direct measurement (National Health and Nutrition Examination Survey 2003-2004, available at www.cdc.gov/nchs/about/major/nhanes/nhanes2003-2004/nhanes03_04.htm), and no national physical activity or health surveys have yet used observational methods of physical activity assessment. In addition to asking about cardiovascular-related physical activities, some national health surveys query muscle-strengthening and flexibility activities. Travel and transportation surveys, designed to track individual transportation and movement habits, rely on diaries for information on daily walking and bicycling habits.

Physical Activity Questionnaire Scoring

Once assessment is completed, responses must be summarized for reporting and research purposes. Methods to create summary scores from physical activity questionnaires can result in either continuous scores (such as total kilocalories expended in physical activity over a given time period) or categorical scores (e.g., low, medium, or high levels of physical activity). A frequently used scoring algorithm in U.S. national surveys relies on an external standard (pre-established physical activity recommendations or guidelines such as those established by the Centers for Disease Control and Prevention and American College of Sports Medicine or the *2008 Physical Activity Guidelines for Americans*). Individual survey respondents are classified into three levels: active (meeting physical activity recommendations or guidelines), insufficiently active (some reported physical activity but not enough to meet existing recommendations or guidelines), and inactive (no reported physical activity). All public health indicators used for tracking progress toward meeting the *Healthy People* objectives, including measures of physical activity, are categorical summary measures (meets/does not meet the objective).

Surveillance Systems

Five national surveys provide information on physical activity levels of the U.S. population, and two surveys contain relevant data on policies and programs for physical activity promotion (table B.1). Each survey uses a different set of questions, because the purposes of each survey differ. Compiling and evaluating data from all sources provides a more complete picture of the physical activity levels and trends among Americans than can be obtained from evaluating results from a single surveillance system.

Results from these surveys paint a similar picture—most Americans are not physically active at recommended levels, and most schools and work sites can do more to improve physical activity levels. Each survey, however, shows slightly different results and this, taken collectively, has the potential for confusion. Each of the surveys is described next. To reduce confusion when citing results, you should include the name of the survey, the year of the results, and the domains of physical activity that were assessed.

Table B.1   U.S. Physical Activity Surveillance Data Sources

Survey	Mode of data collection	Target population	Frequency of data collection	Physical activity domains
General Health Surveys				
BRFSS	Telephone interview	Adults (>18 years of age) in U.S. states, territories, and District of Columbia ~430,00 respondents in 2007 www.cdc.gov/brfss/	Ongoing, annual	Leisure time Domestic Transportation
NHIS	Personal interview	Adults in U.S. states and District of Columbia ~22,000 adult respondents in 2008 www.cdc.gov/nchs/nhis.htm	Ongoing, annual	Leisure time
Specialized Surveys				
NHANES	Interview/ examination	Children and adults in U.S. ~10,000 respondents in 2005-2006 www.cdc.gov/nchs/nhanes.htm	Ongoing, annual	Leisure Time Domestic Transportation
YRBS	School-based survey	High school students in U.S. ~14,000 respondents in 2007 www.cdc.gov/HealthyYouth/yrbs/	Every 2 years	Leisure time Domestic Transportation
NHTS	Household survey	U.S. households 155,000 households in 2008 http://nhts.ornl.gov	Every 5-7 years	Transportation
Policy Surveys				
SHPPS	Mail survey	U.S. school districts, state education organizations, and classrooms www.cdc.gov/HealthyYouth/shpps/	Periodic	Physical activity policies and curricula
NWHPS	Employer survey	U.S. work sites Proprietary data/not in the public domain	Periodic	Physical activity and fitness programs

U.S. National Surveys for Physical Activity: General Health Surveys

The CDC conducts two surveys of general health conditions and behaviors in the U.S. population. These surveys collect data on general physical and mental health status, health conditions, health behaviors, other risk factors, and special topics of interest in a given year. Physical activity questions are on the core surveys every year or alternating years.

Behavioral Risk Factor Surveillance System (BRFSS)

Begun in 1984, the BRFSS is a telephone survey that provides ongoing statistics on major behavioral risk factors among American adults, with an emphasis on state- and local-level surveillance and comparisons across states. The BRFSS collects data from more than 400,000 people in 50 states, the District of Columbia, Puerto Rico, the U.S. Virgin Islands, and Guam. The main purpose of the physical activity portion of the BRFSS is to track the proportion of respondents who meet or exceed CDC recommendations for sufficient physical activity. Historically, two sets of physical activity questions have been addressed in the BRFSS. Between 1984 and 2000, the questions focused on measurement of only one domain of physical activity—specifically, leisure-time physical activity—using open-ended questions. Beginning in 2001, a different set of the BRFSS questions was implemented to capture data on three key physical activity domains: leisure time, domestic, and transportation. Occupational physical activity was also queried in the BRFSS survey but, because it did not measure frequency, intensity, and duration, did not contribute to a physical activity summary score. The main results from the survey are the proportions of American adults who are active, insufficiently active, and inactive.

National Health Interview Survey (NHIS)

The NHIS provides statistics about the health of Americans with a major emphasis on national-level estimates to track progress toward national health objectives (currently, *Healthy People 2010*). The NHIS is a large CDC survey (approximately 30,000 households and 75,000 respondents with approximately 30,000 eligible for the Sample Adult questionnaire) that relies on personal interviews for data collection. From 1997 through 2010, the main purpose of the physical activity questions on the NHIS was to provide information relative to progress to *Healthy People 2010* objectives 22-1 through 22-5. Between 1985 and 1996, the NHIS periodically assessed physical activity using closed-ended activity questions; in 1997, a revised set of questions, again using a closed-ended format, was implemented. Both versions of the NHIS physical activity questions query the leisure-time physical activity domain. Notably, the current NHIS physical activity questions include an assessment of light- to moderate-intensity physical activities, which is different from other questionnaires that focus only on moderate- and vigorous-intensity activities.

U.S. National Surveys for Physical Activity: Specialized Health Surveys

Because general health surveys are limited in the level of detail of data that can be collected for health indicators or population subgroups, specialized surveys provide supplementary data. These surveys are conducted by several federal agencies to serve multiple sectors of society that are related to physical activity behaviors and programs.

National Health and Nutrition Examination Survey (NHANES)

The NHANES provides statistics about the health of Americans through a combination of personal interview and direct physical examination. It is substantially smaller (approximately 10,000 persons in 1999-2000) than either the BRFSS or the NHIS, but it provides much more specialized information than can be collected in the other surveys. Although the NHANES collects information on children and adults on many aspects of health, it has traditionally emphasized relationships among dietary intake, nutrition, and health outcomes. The current physical activity questions in NHANES were first used in 1999. For adults, three domains (leisure time, domestic, and transportation) are measured by separate questions in closed-ended format in the survey. For children, leisure-time physical activity is assessed. Sedentary behaviors are also assessed for children and adults. Of note, through 2006, the NHANES physical examination included a cardiovascular fitness evaluation (submaximal treadmill test), a musculoskeletal fitness test (strength testing), and from 2003 to 2006, direct monitoring (motion sensors). These are the only national data available on physical fitness measures and direct monitoring in adults.

Youth Risk Behavior Survey (YRBS)

The YRBS is a national school-based survey of school students (grades 9-12). YRBS is a large CDC survey with more than 15,000 respondents. The purpose of the survey is to help determine national prevalence and age at initiation of key health-risk behaviors. Physical activity data from the YRBS are used to monitor progress toward *Healthy People 2010* objectives 22-6 through 22-11. Current YRBS physical activity questions use a closed-ended format and measure factors related to physical activity participation (including moderate intensity, vigorous intensity, and muscle strengthening and flexibility), physical education class attendance and availability, and television viewing habits. Three domains of activity (leisure time, transportation, and domestic) are measured in the YRBS. Occupational activity is not thought to be a major source of physical activity in this age group.

National Household Travel Survey (NHTS)

The NHTS is also formerly known as the Nationwide Personal Transportation Survey and the American Travel Survey. It is a U.S. Department of Transportation survey of travel modes, commuting habits, and long-distance trips. The NHTS provides national estimates of daily trip frequency, trip distance, means of transportation, and trip time for persons of all ages. The unit of analysis in this survey is the trip rather than the individual respondent. The NHTS provides information for the transportation-related physical activity domain. This survey is periodic (approximately every 5 years), with survey data available for 1969, 1977, 1983, 1990, 1995, 2001, and 2008. Estimates from this survey are used to track progress toward *Healthy People 2010* objectives 22-14 and 22-15 regarding walking and bicycling habits in general and to school in particular. Of note, the NHTS has dozens of regional counterparts that are conducted by regional transportation authorities, a federal requirement for those regions to receive federal highway funds. Unlike the BRFSS (with its state-based estimates), these regional surveys are not coordinated by a federal agency to ensure consistent implementation protocols and quality control. Comparisons of results among regions and with national estimates are therefore not advised.

U.S. National Surveys for Physical Activity: Policy Surveys

Healthy People 2010 used two policy surveys to collect data on school health policies and worksite health promotion policies. These surveys were conducted less often than the population health surveys. Nevertheless, they provide a valuable window to the trends in policies that influence physical activity behaviors.

School Health Policies and Programs Study (SHPPS)

The SHPPS is a periodic national mail survey designed to assess school health policies and programs at the state, district, and classroom level in elementary, middle, and high schools. State education agencies, district level representatives, and designated school staff classroom faculty provide the respondent base for this survey. Physical activity questions on the SHPPS assess physical education curriculum offerings, availability of recess and intramural sports programs, and state and district curricular requirements for physical education. Physical activity data from the SHPPS measure progress toward *Healthy People 2010* objectives 22-8 and 22-12.

National Worksite Health Promotion Survey (NWHPS)

The NWHPS is a periodic national survey of employers designed to assess work-site health policies and programs. The survey was conducted by the Association for Worksite Health Promotion in 1985, 1992, 1999, and 2004. Physical activity questions on the NWHPS assess work-site physical activity program offerings at the work site, through the health care plan, or both. Physical activity data from the NWHPS measured progress toward *Healthy People 2010* objective 22-13.

APPENDIX C

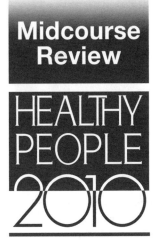

Midcourse Review

HEALTHY PEOPLE 2010

Physical Activity and Fitness **22**

Co-Lead Agencies:
Centers for Disease Control and Prevention
President's Council on Physical Fitness and Sports

Contents

Goal: Improve health, fitness, and quality of life through daily physical activity.

Introduction[*]

Recognition of physical inactivity as an important public health problem has evolved rapidly since moderate-intensity physical activity was first recommended for overall health benefits in 1996 by the landmark *Physical Activity and Health: A Report of the Surgeon General.*[1] Physical activity plays a key role in the Healthy People 2010 overarching goals of increasing quality and years of healthy life and eliminating health disparities. Physical activity is associated with decreased risk of cardiovascular disease, stroke, diabetes, colorectal and breast cancer, and osteoporosis.[1] Other benefits of active lifestyles include the following:

- Improved mood and feelings of well-being.
- Better control of body weight, blood glucose, blood pressure, and cholesterol.
- Enhanced independent living among older adults.
- Better health benefits for people who have chronic diseases or disabilities.
- Increased quality of life for all persons.[1]

The focus area for physical activity and fitness has 15 objectives related to participation in physical activities and access to physical activity and fitness programs and facilities at schools and worksites. Progress toward the targets occurred for several objectives; changes were similar in all populations. No progress was made in eliminating disparities in physical activity participation.

Modifications to Objectives and Subobjectives

The following discussion highlights the modifications, including changes, additions, and deletions, to this focus area's objectives and subobjectives as a result of the midcourse review.

Two objectives were modified following publication of *Healthy People 2010.* Earlier in the decade, the operational definition for increasing moderate-intensity physical activity in adults (22-2) was changed from moderate activity only to include activities of at least moderate intensity. Scientific evidence has demonstrated that persons who engage in vigorous-intensity physical activities at least 3 days per week for 20 minutes per occasion accrue overall health benefits.[1] Thus, adults who meet the objective for vigorous physical activity also meet the objective for moderate physical activity.

For clarity and consistency, the wording of moderate physical activity among adolescents (22-6) was revised to specify "moderate physical activity for at least 30 minutes per day 5 or more days per week," rather than "for at least 30 minutes on 5 or more of the previous 7 days per week."

---

[*] Unless otherwise noted, data referenced in this focus area come from Healthy People 2010 and can be located at http://wonder.cdc.gov/data2010. See the section on DATA2010 in the Technical Appendix for more information.

Physical activity at school facilities (22-12) became measurable, with a baseline of 35 percent and a target of 50 percent of public and private schools providing community access to school physical activity facilities for all persons outside of normal school hours (that is, before and after the school day, on weekends, and during summer and other vacations).

Progress Toward Healthy People 2010 Targets

The following discussion highlights objectives that met or exceeded their 2010 targets; moved toward the targets, demonstrated no change, or moved away from the targets; and those that lacked data to assess progress. Progress is illustrated in the Progress Quotient bar chart (see Figure 22-1), which displays the percent of targeted change achieved for objectives and subobjectives with sufficient data to assess progress.

Objectives that met or exceeded their targets. No physical activity and fitness objectives met their targets at the time of the midcourse review.

Objectives that moved toward their targets. Five physical activity and fitness objectives for adults and two for adolescents in grades 9 through 12 moved toward their targets. Reducing the proportion of adults who do not participate in some form of leisure-time physical activity (22-1) moved toward its target of 20 percent, achieving 15 percent of its targeted change. Compared with a baseline of 40 percent of the population being inactive in 1997, 37 percent reported no leisure-time physical activity in 2003. Regular moderate or vigorous physical activity (22-2) moved toward its target of 50 percent, achieving 6 percent of the targeted change. Regular vigorous physical activity (22-3) achieved 14 percent of the targeted change, moving toward its target of 30 percent. Muscular strength and endurance (22-4) and flexibility exercises among adults (22-5) also advanced toward their targets, achieving 17 percent and 8 percent of the targeted change, respectively.

Improvement in physical activity levels of Americans may relate to the steady increase in the visibility of physical inactivity as a health issue and to a growing number of initiatives that seek to promote physical activity. A public health initiative that identifies interventions to promote physical activity is the *Community Guide to Preventive Services.*[2] This resource for public health practitioners recommends evidence-based intervention strategies for modifying behavioral, environmental, and policy correlates of active lifestyles. In addition, many State health programs use national guidelines and recommendations to promote healthy behaviors to reduce the burden of cardiovascular disease, stroke, cancer, and obesity and to increase healthful behavior in youth.[3]

Gains were made among students in grades 9 through 12 for objectives addressing physical activity during physical education class (22-10) and television viewing time (22-11). The proportion of students in grades 9 through 12 who spent at least half of physical education class time being active reached 8 percent of its targeted change. The increased use of school-based programs may have contributed to the increase in active physical education time. For example, the Sports Play and Active Recreation for Kids (SPARK)[4] and the Coordinated Approach to Child Health (CATCH)[5] programs provide teachers with information and ideas on ways to increase activity time during physical education classes. The proportion of adolescents who limited television viewing to 2 or fewer hours a day increased from 57 percent in 1999 to 62 percent in 2003, achieving 28 percent of the targeted change and moving toward its target of 75 percent. An increase in time spent multitasking, such as playing video games, instant messaging, or doing homework while the television is on, might have influenced the change in television viewing.[6]

Objectives that demonstrated no change. None of the objectives for this focus area remained static since the launch of Healthy People 2010.

Objectives that moved away from their targets. The objective covering moderate physical activity among students in grades 9 through 12 (22-6) moved away from its target. From a baseline of 27 percent in 1999, the proportion of students who participated in such activity dropped to 25 percent in 2003, moving away from the target of 35 percent. Vigorous physical activity (22-7) and participation in daily physical education in schools (22-9) among students in grades 9 through 12 also moved away from their targets. Even though most States have mandates for physical education, decisions on curriculum content and specific requirements often fall to local school districts or individual schools, which leads to a wide range of requirements for students at all levels. Some schools may require 1 year of physical education, whereas other States or school districts may not require physical education beyond eighth grade.

Evidence suggests that adolescents may perceive vigorous physical activity as socially unacceptable.[7] The same research also suggests that adolescents—as they become more independent—reject adult-oriented health goals. These findings, in addition to diminished school-based physical education, provide possible explanations for the decrease in moderate and vigorous activity among this population group.

One initiative to increase physical activity among adolescents was "VERB™ It's what you do." VERB was a national, multicultural, social marketing campaign coordinated by the Centers for Disease Control and Prevention that helped influence the values of young people aged 9 to 13 years ("tweens") by encouraging them to be active every day. Begun in 2002 and concluded in 2006, the VERB campaign combined paid advertising, marketing strategies, and partnership efforts to reach the distinct audiences of tweens and adults/influencers. VERB was successful in increasing physical activity levels among tweens.[8] As these youth become high school students in the latter half of the decade, the long-term effects of VERB may be measured by the youth physical activity objectives.

Objectives that could not be assessed. Trend data were not available for the objectives regarding physical education requirements in schools (22-8), access to school physical activity facilities (22-12), worksite physical activity and fitness (22-13), and walking (22-14) or bicycling (22-15) for transportation. Data sources were identified for all of these objectives, and data to establish baselines and assess progress are anticipated by the end of the decade.

Progress Toward Elimination of Health Disparities

The following discussion highlights progress toward the elimination of health disparities. The disparities are illustrated in the Disparities Table (see Figure 22-2), which displays information about disparities among select populations for which data were available for assessment.

Of all the physical activity objectives examined, disparities were similar over time, with one exception: From 1999 to 2003, the disparity in the lack of participation in leisure-time physical activity (22-1) between high school graduates and persons with at least some college education increased. The population with at least some college had the best rate. In 2003, high school graduates had a rate of no leisure-time physical activity that was 50 percent to 99 percent higher than persons with at least some college, while the rate for those with less than a high school education was at least 100 percent higher.

The remaining objectives had similar changes from the baseline in all populations, which resulted in no change in disparities. For most objectives in this focus area, the best group rates were observed in the white non-Hispanic population, persons with at least some college education, urban dwellers, males, and adults without disabilities.

Significant gender differences were observed for several objectives. Men had a more favorable rate than women for participation in leisure-time physical activity (22-1). Boys in grades 9 through 12 had better rates of engaging in vigorous physical activity (22-7) and physical activity in physical education class (22-10). In addition, boys aged 5 to 15 years had a better rate for walking for transportation (22-14b) than did girls. Multiple programs exist that attempt to address these differences. The "Pick Your Path to Health" campaign, sponsored by the Office on Women's Health within the U.S. Department of Health and Human Services (HHS), encourages local communities to promote practical, culturally appropriate steps to wellness and targets minority women. Young women can also receive updated, science-based, plain language information sources at a website sponsored by the National Women's Health Information Center.[9]

The white non-Hispanic population had the best rates for no leisure-time physical activity (22-1) and regular physical activity (22-2 and 22-3). Persons of two or more races had the best rates for muscular strength and endurance (22-4) and flexibility (22-5). Hispanic students in grades 9 through 12 had the best rates for participation in daily physical activity in school and in physical education classes (22-9 and 22-10, respectively). However, disparities for Hispanic and black non-Hispanic populations were seen among adolescents engaging in vigorous physical activity (22-7). Television viewing (22-11) was associated with persistent disparities of 50 percent or more among Hispanic and black non-Hispanic youth, compared with the best rate.

Adults with at least some college had more favorable rates for physical activity participation (22-1 through 22-5) than persons with a high school education or less. Walking for transportation (22-14a) was less common among adults aged 18 years and older living in rural or nonmetropolitan areas than urban areas. Adults with disabilities were more likely to report less overall activity than adults without disabilities (22-1, 22-2, and 22-3).

Initiatives to combat disparities within the realm of physical activity and fitness exist at Federal, State, and local levels in many different and innovative forms. For example, REACH 2010 (Racial and Ethnic Approaches to Community Health 2010) is a collaborative Federal initiative aimed at eliminating disparities in health status experienced by select populations.[10] The VERB campaign targeted American Indian or Alaska Native adolescents and Hispanic adolescents with multicultural media messages about physical activity.[11] I Can Do It, You Can Do It! is an initiative supported by the HHS Office on Disability, the President's Council on Physical Fitness and Sports, the National Institutes of Health, and numerous community and nonprofit organizations to improve and evaluate the activity and nutrition of people with disabilities.[12] The *National Blueprint: Increasing Physical Activity Among Adults Aged 50 and Older* identifies organizations and strategies to help combat inactivity and improve the quality of life for older Americans.[13] Through these and other programs, persisting disparities are being addressed.

Opportunities and Challenges

Historically, physical activity and fitness were integral to daily life and culture as a means of transportation, occupation, and maintaining a home.[1] During the 20th century, most physical activity was engineered out of daily living by the emergence of automobiles and labor-saving devices.[14, 15] Thus, an active lifestyle for many people became one that included yard work and frequent trips to the gym during discretionary time. By the end of the century, physical inactivity was recognized as a risk factor for many chronic diseases and poor mental health, and active lifestyles were associated with overall health and well-being of individuals and communities. The restoration of physical activity to daily life increasingly has been considered by employers, school administrators, park and recreation managers, urban planners, transportation engineers, and public health practitioners. Intervention strategies are guided by recent science showing that multidisciplinary environmental interventions can improve physical activity levels and benefit local communities.[2]

Two Federal memorandums of understanding (MOUs) define future collaborations among Federal departments, including agencies within HHS. The Healthier Children and Youth MOU between HHS and the U.S. Departments of Agriculture (USDA) and Education synthesizes interagency activities in nutrition and physical activity that target young people. It provides an opportunity to widely shape the physical activity message to audiences, including school officials, parents, and children. The Public Health and Recreation MOU brings together the Federal land management agencies within USDA, the U.S. Departments of Interior and Transportation, the U.S. Army Corps of Engineers, and agencies in HHS. Together, they promote the use of public lands for public health and help ensure that all Americans understand the benefits of being physically active and the location of public spaces available to them for their active pursuits.

Also reflecting the role of public lands and recreational facilities in health promotion was a collaboration between the National Heart, Lung, and Blood Institute and the National Recreation and Park Association. Together, they developed Hearts N' Parks,[16] a community-based initiative designed to encourage all Americans to maintain a healthy weight by improving nutrition and increasing physical activity. Local park and recreation departments were instrumental in implementing the 3-year program. The collaboration was successful in improving healthy eating and physical activity knowledge and behaviors among adults and children through community-based programs.

Opportunities for professional development, communication, and collaboration among physical activity practitioners in public health are increasing. Emerging public health organizations, programs, journals, and institutions, with a focus on physical activity in partnership with nongovernmental organizations, will continue to provide opportunities to collaborate, share ideas, and obtain technical assistance.[17]

The population-based interventions recommended in the *Community Guide to Preventive Services* provide public health professionals with approaches that are effective in influencing physical activity behavior.[2] Evidence-based activities or interventions include the following:

- Informational approaches: communitywide campaigns and point-of-decision prompts.
- Behavioral approaches: school-based physical education, individually adapted health behavior-change programs, and social support interventions in community settings.
- Environmental and policy approaches: access to places offering physical activity combined with informational outreach, street-scale and community-scale urban design and land-use policies and practices, and point-of-decision prompts.

The lack of evidence-based practices for physical activity programs targeting select populations continues to challenge public health practitioners trying to affect physical activity behaviors. Program planners need to strategically target select populations. REACH 2010 uses evidence-based strategies toward that end. In contrast, among people with disabilities, a variety of challenges diminish physical activity participation. These challenges include limited research and recommendations for physical activity programming that is appropriate for individuals with specific disabilities[12] and physical barriers (for example, lack of access to changing rooms in fitness facilities).[13]

Emerging Issues

Since the beginning of the decade, opportunities for future objectives have emerged. The technology to measure individual physical activity levels has advanced to include additional types of devices (for example, pedometers, motion detectors, and heart rate monitors). Since their introduction in the National Health and Nutrition Examination Survey in 2003, motion detectors have been used for population assessment. These and similar technologies provide the opportunity to track population progress in physical activity and fitness measures that augment health surveys.

Increasing opportunities for physical activity through multidisciplinary environmental and policy interventions has emerged as a priority for public health. For example, the *Community Guide to Preventive Services*[2] recommends increasing access to and promoting public awareness of suitable locations for physical activity, such as walking or biking trails or recreational facilities, and reducing barriers associated with facilities' operating hours and usage fees. An example of a multidisciplinary method to increase physical activity is the Safe Routes to School initiative.[18] The project facilitates walking and bicycling to school by involving partners such as traffic engineers, public works officials, local school boards and school staff members, community planners, and parents.

At the midcourse of Healthy People 2010, progress was made toward increasing physical activity and fitness-related activities. However, many of the challenges present in 2000 still exist. Looking ahead to the future, public health practitioners increasingly view physical activity as a pillar of chronic disease prevention and mental health initiatives. The benefits of this status will be realized as interventions and programs that began between 2000 and 2005 come to fruition during the second half of the decade.

Figure 22-1. Progress Quotient Chart for Focus Area 22: Physical Activity and Fitness

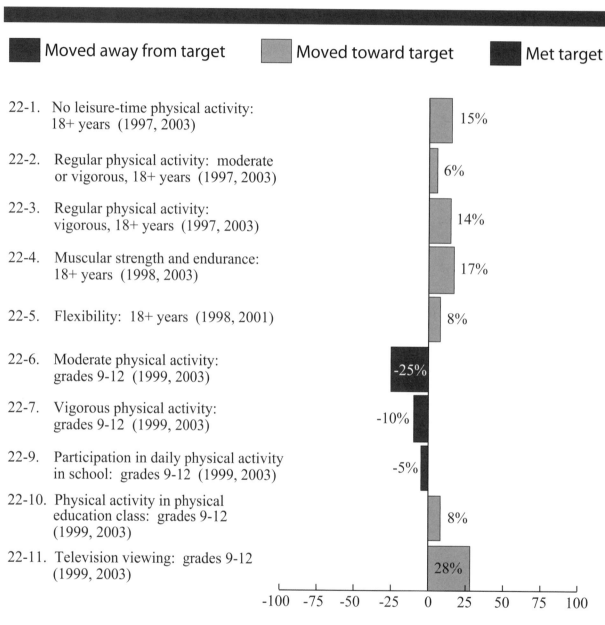

■ Moved away from target   ■ Moved toward target   ■ Met target

22-1. No leisure-time physical activity: 18+ years (1997, 2003) — 15%

22-2. Regular physical activity: moderate or vigorous, 18+ years (1997, 2003) — 6%

22-3. Regular physical activity: vigorous, 18+ years (1997, 2003) — 14%

22-4. Muscular strength and endurance: 18+ years (1998, 2003) — 17%

22-5. Flexibility: 18+ years (1998, 2001) — 8%

22-6. Moderate physical activity: grades 9-12 (1999, 2003) — -25%

22-7. Vigorous physical activity: grades 9-12 (1999, 2003) — -10%

22-9. Participation in daily physical activity in school: grades 9-12 (1999, 2003) — -5%

22-10. Physical activity in physical education class: grades 9-12 (1999, 2003) — 8%

22-11. Television viewing: grades 9-12 (1999, 2003) — 28%

-100 -75 -50 -25 0 25 50 75 100

Percent of targeted change achieved

Notes: Tracking data for objectives 22-8a and b, 22-12, 22-13, 22-14a and b, and 22-15a and b are unavailable.

Years in parentheses represent the baseline data year and the most recent data year used to compute the percent of the Healthy People 2010 target achieved.

$$\text{Percent of targeted change achieved} = \left(\frac{\text{Most recent value} - \text{baseline value}}{\text{Year 2010 target} - \text{baseline value}} \right) \times 100$$

Figure 22-2. Disparities Table for Focus Area 22: Physical Activity and Fitness

Disparities from the best group rate for each characteristic at the most recent data point and changes in disparity from the baseline to the most recent data point.

Population-based objectives	American Indian or Alaska Native	Asian	Native Hawaiian or other Pacific Islander	Two or more races	Hispanic or Latino	Black non-Hispanic	White non-Hispanic	Summary index	Female	Male	Less than high school	High school graduate	At least some college	Summary index	Urban or metropolitan	Rural or nonmetropolitan	Persons with disabilities	Persons without disabilities
	Race and ethnicity								Gender		Education				Location		Disability	
22-1. No leisure-time physical activity: 18+ years (1997, 2003) * [1]				b			B			B		↑	B		B			B
22-2. Regular physical activity: moderate or vigorous, 18+ years (1997, 2003) * [1]							B			B			B		B			B
22-3. Regular physical activity: vigorous, 18+ years (1997, 2003) * [1]							B			B			B		B			B
22-4. Muscular strength and endurance: 18+ years (1998, 2003) * [1]				B						B			B		B			B
22-5. Flexibility: 18+ years (1998, 2001) * [2]				B					B				B		B			B
22-6. Moderate physical activity: grades 9-12 (1999, 2003) *							B		B									
22-7. Vigorous physical activity: grades 9-12 (1999, 2003) *							B		B									
22-9. Participation in daily physical activity in schools: grades 9-12 (1999, 2003) *					B				B									
22-10. Physical activity in physical education class: grades 9-12 (1999, 2003) *					B				B									
22-11. Television viewing: grades 9-12 (1999, 2003) *						B			B									
22-14a. Walking for transportation: 18+ years (1995) †									B		B				B			
22-14b. Walking for transportation: 5-15 years (1995) †												B			B			
22-15a. Bicycling for transportation: 18+ years (1995) †										B	B		B		B			
22-15b. Bicycling for transportation: 5-15 years (1995) †												B			B			

Notes: Data for objectives 22-8a and b, 22-12, and 22-13 are unavailable or not applicable.

Years in parentheses represent the baseline data year and the most recent data year (if available).

Disparity from the best group rate is defined as the percent difference between the best group rate and each of the other group rates for a characteristic (for example, race and ethnicity). The summary index is the average of these percent differences for a characteristic. Change in disparity is estimated by subtracting the disparity at baseline from the disparity at the most recent data point. Change in the summary index is estimated by subtracting the summary index at baseline from the summary index at the most recent data point. See Technical Appendix for more information.

(continued)

Figure 22-2. *(continued)*

The **best group rate** at the most recent data point.	B	The group with the best rate for specified characteristic.	b	Most favorable group rate for specified characteristic, but reliability criterion not met.		Best group rate reliability criterion not met.

Disparity from the best group rate at the most recent data point.	**Percent difference from the best group rate**			
	Less than 10 percent or not statistically significant	10-49 percent	50-99 percent	100 percent or more

Changes in disparity over time are shown when the change is greater than or equal to 10 percentage points and statistically significant, or when the change is greater than or equal to 10 percentage points and estimates of variability were not available.	**Increase** in disparity (percentage points)		
	↑ 10-49	↑↑ 50-99	↑ 100 or more ↑↑
	Decrease in disparity (percentage points)		
	↓ 10-49	↓↓ 50-99	↓↓ 100 or more ↓

Availability of data.	Data not available.	Characteristic not selected for this objective.

* The variability of best group rates was assessed, and disparities of ≥ 10% are statistically significant at the 0.05 level. Changes in disparity over time, noted with arrows, are statistically significant at the 0.05 level. See Technical Appendix.

† Measures of variability were not available. Thus, the variability of best group rates was not assessed, and the statistical significance of disparities and changes in disparity over time could not be tested. See Technical Appendix.

[1] Baseline data by race and ethnicity are for 1999.

[2] Baseline data by race and ethnicity are for 2001.

Objectives and Subobjectives for Focus Area 22: Physical Activity and Fitness

Goal: Improve health, fitness, and quality of life through daily physical activity.

As a result of the Healthy People 2010 Midcourse Review, changes were made to the Healthy People 2010 objectives and subobjectives. These changes are specific to the following situations:

- Changes in the wording of an objective to more accurately describe what is being measured.
- Changes to reflect a different data source or new science.
- Changes resulting from the establishment of a baseline and a target (that is, when a formerly developmental objective or subobjective became measurable).
- Deletion of an objective or subobjective that lacked a data source.
- Correction of errors and omissions in *Healthy People 2010.*

Revised baselines and targets for measurable objectives and subobjectives do not fall into any of the above categories and, thus, are not considered a midcourse review change.[1]

When changes were made to an objective, three sections are displayed:

1. In the Original Objective section, the objective as published in *Healthy People 2010* in 2000 is shown.
2. In the Objective With Revisions section, strikethrough indicates text deleted, and underlining is used to show new text.
3. In the Revised Objective section, the objective appears as revised as a result of the midcourse review.

Details of the objectives and subobjectives in this focus area, including any changes made at the midcourse, appear on the following pages.

---

[1] See Technical Appendix for more information on baseline and target revisions.

Physical Activity in Adults

NO CHANGE IN OBJECTIVE

22-1. **Reduce the proportion of adults who engage in no leisure-time physical activity.**

Target: 20 percent.

Baseline: 40 percent of adults aged 18 years and older engaged in no leisure-time physical activity in 1997 (age adjusted to the year 2000 standard population).

Target setting method: Better than the best.

Data source: National Health Interview Survey (NHIS), CDC, NCHS.

NO CHANGE IN OBJECTIVE
(Data updated and footnoted)

22-2. **Increase the proportion of adults who engage in moderate physical activity for at least 30 minutes per day 5 or more days per week or vigorous physical activity for at least 20 minutes per day 3 or more days per week.[1]**

Target: 50[2] percent.

Baseline: 32[3] percent of adults aged 18 years and older engaged in moderate physical activity for at least 30 minutes per day or vigorous physical activity for at least 20 minutes per day[1] in 1997 (age adjusted to the year 2000 standard population).

Target setting method: Better than the best.

Data source: National Health Interview Survey (NHIS), CDC, NCHS.

[1] In 2001, the language of objective 22-2 was changed after November 2000 publication to include adults who met the definition for vigorous physical activity.
[2] Target revised from 30 because of baseline revision after November 2000 publication.
[3] Baseline revised from 15 after November 2000 publication.

NO CHANGE IN OBJECTIVE

22-3. **Increase the proportion of adults who engage in vigorous physical activity that promotes the development and maintenance of cardiorespiratory fitness for at least 20 minutes per day 3 or more days per week.**

Target: 30 percent.

Baseline: 23 percent of adults aged 18 years and older engaged in vigorous physical activity 3 or more days per week for 20 or more minutes per occasion in 1997 (age adjusted to the year 2000 standard population).

NO CHANGE IN OBJECTIVE *(continued)*

Target setting method: Better than the best.

Data source: National Health Interview Survey (NHIS), CDC, NCHS.

Muscular Strength/Endurance and Flexibility

NO CHANGE IN OBJECTIVE

22-4.   **Increase the proportion of adults who perform physical activities that enhance and maintain muscular strength and endurance.**

Target: 30 percent.

Baseline: 18 percent of adults aged 18 years and older performed physical activities that enhance and maintain strength and endurance 2 or more days per week in 1998 (age adjusted to the year 2000 standard population).

Target setting method: Better than the best.

Data source: National Health Interview Survey (NHIS), CDC, NCHS.

NO CHANGE IN OBJECTIVE

22-5.   **Increase the proportion of adults who perform physical activities that enhance and maintain flexibility.**

Target: 43 percent.

Baseline: 30 percent of adults aged 18 years and older did stretching exercises in the past 2 weeks in 1998 (age adjusted to the year 2000 standard population).

Target setting method: Better than the best.

Data source: National Health Interview Survey (NHIS), CDC, NCHS.

Physical Activity in Children and Adolescents

ORIGINAL OBJECTIVE

22-6.   **Increase the proportion of adolescents who engage in moderate physical activity for at least 30 minutes on 5 or more of the previous 7 days per week.**

Target: 35 percent.

ORIGINAL OBJECTIVE *(continued)*

Baseline: 27 percent of students in grades 9 through 12 engaged in moderate physical activity for at least 30 minutes on 5 or more of the previous 7 days in 1999.

Target setting method: Better than the best.

Data source: Youth Risk Behavior Surveillance System (YRBSS), CDC, NCCDPHP.

OBJECTIVE WITH REVISIONS

22-6. **Increase the proportion of adolescents who engage in moderate physical activity for at least 30 minutes <u>per day</u> ~~on~~ 5 or more ~~of the previous 7~~ days per week.**

Target: 35 percent.

Baseline: 27 percent of students in grades 9 through 12 engaged in moderate physical activity for at least 30 minutes on 5 or more of the previous 7 days in 1999.

Target setting method: Better than the best.

Data source: Youth Risk Behavior Surveillance System (YRBSS), CDC, NCCDPHP.

REVISED OBJECTIVE

22-6. **Increase the proportion of adolescents who engage in moderate physical activity for at least 30 minutes per day 5 or more days per week.**

Target: 35 percent.

Baseline: 27 percent of students in grades 9 through 12 engaged in moderate physical activity for at least 30 minutes on 5 or more of the previous 7 days in 1999.

Target setting method: Better than the best.

Data source: Youth Risk Behavior Surveillance System (YRBSS), CDC, NCCDPHP.

NO CHANGE IN OBJECTIVE

22-7. **Increase the proportion of adolescents who engage in vigorous physical activity that promotes cardiorespiratory fitness 3 or more days per week for 20 or more minutes per occasion.**

Target: 85 percent.

Baseline: 65 percent of students in grades 9 through 12 engaged in vigorous physical activity for at least 20 minutes on 3 or more of the previous 7 days in 1999.

NO CHANGE IN OBJECTIVE *(continued)*

Target setting method: Better than the best.

Data source: Youth Risk Behavior Surveillance System (YRBSS), CDC, NCCDPHP.

NO CHANGE IN OBJECTIVE
(Data updated and footnoted)

22-8. **Increase the proportion of the Nation's public and private schools that require daily physical education for all students.**

Target and baseline:

Objective	Increase in Schools Requiring Daily Physical Activity for All Students	2000 Baseline	2010 Target
		Percent	
22-8a.	Middle and junior high school	6.4[1]	9.4[2]
22-8b.	Senior high schools	5.8[3]	14.5[4]

Target setting method: 47 percent improvement for middle and junior high schools; 150 percent improvement for senior high schools.

Data source: School Health Policies and Programs Study (SHPPS), CDC, NCCDPHP.

[1] Baseline and baseline year revised from 17 and 1994 after November 2000 publication.
[2] Target revised from 25 because of baseline revision after November 2000 publication.
[3] Baseline and baseline year revised from 2 and 1994 after November 2000 publication.
[4] Target revised from 5 because of baseline revision after November 2000 publication.

NO CHANGE IN OBJECTIVE

22-9. **Increase the proportion of adolescents who participate in daily school physical education.**

Target: 50 percent.

Baseline: 29 percent of students in grades 9 through 12 participated in daily school physical education in 1999.

Target setting method: Better than the best.

Data source: Youth Risk Behavior Surveillance System (YRBSS), CDC, NCCDPHP.

NO CHANGE IN OBJECTIVE

22-10. Increase the proportion of adolescents who spend at least 50 percent of school physical education class time being physically active.

Target: 50 percent.

Baseline: 38 percent of students in grades 9 through 12 were physically active in physical education class more than 20 minutes 3 to 5 days per week in 1999.

Target setting method: Better than the best.

Data source: Youth Risk Behavior Surveillance System (YRBSS), CDC, NCCDPHP.

NO CHANGE IN OBJECTIVE

22-11. Increase the proportion of adolescents who view television 2 or fewer hours on a school day.

Target: 75 percent.

Baseline: 57 percent of students in grades 9 through 12 viewed television 2 or fewer hours per school day in 1999.

Target setting method: Better than the best.

Data source: Youth Risk Behavior Surveillance System (YRBSS), CDC, NCCDPHP.

Access

ORIGINAL OBJECTIVE

22-12. (Developmental) Increase the proportion of the Nation's public and private schools that provide access to their physical activity spaces and facilities for all persons outside of normal school hours (that is, before and after the school day, on weekends, and during summer and other vacations).

Potential data source: School Health Policies and Programs Study (SHPPS), CDC, NCCDPHP.

OBJECTIVE WITH REVISIONS

22-12. (Developmental) Increase the proportion of the Nation's public and private schools that provide access to their physical activity spaces and facilities for all persons outside of normal school hours (that is, before and after the school day, on weekends, and during summer and other vacations).

Target: 50 percent.

OBJECTIVE WITH REVISIONS *(continued)*

Baseline: <u>35 percent of public and private elementary, middle/junior high, and senior high schools provided community access to their physical activity or athletic facilities in 2000.</u>

Target setting method: <u>43 percent improvement.</u>

~~Potential d~~Data source: School Health Policies and Programs Study (SHPPS), CDC, NCCDPHP.

REVISED OBJECTIVE

22-12. **Increase the proportion of the Nation's public and private schools that provide access to their physical activity spaces and facilities for all persons outside of normal school hours (that is, before and after the school day, on weekends, and during summer and other vacations).**

Target: 50 percent.

Baseline: 35 percent of public and private elementary, middle/junior high, and senior high schools provided community access to their physical activity or athletic facilities in 2000.

Target setting method: 43 percent improvement.

Data source: School Health Policies and Programs Study (SHPPS), CDC, NCCDPHP.

NO CHANGE IN OBJECTIVE

22-13. **Increase the proportion of worksites offering employer-sponsored physical activity and fitness programs.**

Target: 75 percent.

Baseline: 46 percent of worksites with 50 or more employees offered physical activity and/or fitness programs at the worksite or through their health plans in 1998–1999.

Worksite Size	Worksite or Health Plan	Health Plan	Worksite
	Percent		
Total (50 or more employees)	46	22	36
50 to 99 employees	38	21	24
100 to 249 employees	42	20	31
250 to 749 employees	56	25	44

NO CHANGE IN OBJECTIVE *(continued)*

750 or more employees	68	27	61
Less than 50 employees	Developmental		

Target setting method: Better than the best.

Data source: National Worksite Health Promotion Survey (NWHPS), Partnership for Prevention and OPHS, ODPHP.

NO CHANGE IN OBJECTIVE
(Data updated and footnoted)

22-14. Increase the proportion of trips made by walking.

Target and baseline:

Objective	Increase in Trips Made by Walking	Length of Trip	1995 Baseline*	2010 Target
			Percent	
22-14a.	Adults aged 18 years and older	Trips of 1 mile or less	17	25
22-14b.	Children and adolescents aged 5 to 15 years	Trips to school of 1 mile or less	31	50

* Age adjusted to the year 2000 standard population.

Target setting method: 47 percent improvement for 22-14a and 61[1] percent improvement for 22-14b. (Better than the best will be used when data are available.)

Data source: Nationwide Personal Transportation Survey (NPTS), DOT.

[1] Target setting method corrected from 68 percent after November 2000 publication.

NO CHANGE IN OBJECTIVE

22-15. Increase the proportion of trips made by bicycling.

Target and baseline:

Objective	Increase in Trips Made by Bicycling	Activity	1995 Baseline*	2010 Target
			Percent	
22-15a.	Adults aged 18 years and older	Trips of 5 miles or less	0.6	2.0

NO CHANGE IN OBJECTIVE *(continued)*

22-15b.	Children and adolescents aged 5 to 15 years	Trips to school of 2 miles or less	2.4	5.0

* Age adjusted to the year 2000 standard population.

Target setting method: 233 percent improvement for 22-15a and 108 percent improvement for 22-15b. (Better than the best will be used when data are available.)

Data source: Nationwide Personal Transportation Survey (NPTS), DOT.

References

[1] U.S. Department of Health and Human Services (HHS). *Physical Activity and Health: A Report of the Surgeon General.* Atlanta, GA: HHS, Centers for Disease Control and Prevention (CDC), National Center for Chronic Disease Prevention and Health Promotion, 1996.

[2] CDC. Increasing physical activity: A report on the recommendations of the Task Force on Community Preventive Services. *Morbidity and Mortality Weekly Report* 50(RR-18):1–16, 2001.

[3] More information available at www.cdc.gov/nccdphp/dnpa/obesity/state_programs/index.htm, www.cdc.gov/dhdsp/state_program/index.htm, www.cdc.gov/cancer/ncccp/, and www.cdc.gov/healthyyouth/; accessed October 31, 2006.

[4] More information available at www.ed.gov/pubs/EPTW/eptw9/eptw9f.html; accessed October 31, 2006.

[5] More information available at www.cdc.gov/prc/tested-interventions/adoptable-interventions/catch-improved-physical-activity-diet-elementary-school.htm; accessed October 31, 2006.

[6] Roberts, D.F., et al. *Generation M: Media in the Lives of 8–18 Year-Olds.* Menlo Park, CA: The Henry J. Kaiser Family Foundation, 2005. More information available at www.kff.org/entmedia/entmedia030905pkg.cfm; accessed October 31, 2006.

[7] Rowland, T. Adolescence: A 'risk factor' for physical inactivity. President's Council on Physical Fitness and Sports. *Research Digest* 3(6):1999.

[8] Huhman, M., et al. Effects of a mass media campaign to increase physical activity among children: Year 1 results of the VERB campaign. *Pediatrics* 116:277–284, 2005.

[9] More information available at www.4girls.gov; accessed October 31, 2006.

[10] Giles, W.H., et al. Racial and ethnic approaches to community health (REACH 2010): An overview. *Ethnic Disparities* 14(3 Suppl 1):S5–S8, 2004.

[11] Wong, F., et al. VERB™—A social marketing campaign to increase physical activity among youth. *Preventing Chronic Disease* 1(3):2004.

[12] More information available at www.hhs.gov/od/physicalfitness.html#1; accessed October 31, 2006.

[13] More information available at www.agingblueprint.org/; accessed October 31, 2006.

[14] Peters, J.C. Combating obesity: Challenges and choices. *Obesity Research* (Suppl 11):7S–11S, 2003.

[15] Goran, M.I., and Treuth, M.S. Energy expenditure, physical activity, and obesity in children. *Pediatric Clinics of North America* 48(4):931–953, 2001.

[16] More information available at www.nhlbi.nih.gov/health/prof/heart/obesity/hrt_n_pk/index.htm; accessed October 31, 2006.

[17] More information on the National Society of Physical Activity Practitioners in Public Health available at the Physical Activity Collaborative website www.pacollaborative.org.

[18] More information on the Safe Routes to School initiative available at www.nhtsa.dot.gov/people/injury/pedbimot/bike/Safe-Routes-2004/index.html; accessed October 31, 2006.

Related Objectives From Other Focus Areas

1. Access to Quality Health Services
1-3.   Counseling about health behaviors

2. Arthritis, Osteoporosis, and Chronic Back Conditions
2-2.   Activity limitations due to arthritis
2-3.   Personal care limitations
2-8.   Arthritis education
2-9.   Cases of osteoporosis
2-11.   Activity limitations due to chronic back conditions

3. Cancer
3-5.   Colorectal cancer deaths
3-7.   Prostate cancer deaths
3-9.   Sun exposure and skin cancer
3-10.   Provider counseling about cancer prevention

4. Chronic Kidney Disease
4-8.   Medical evaluation and treatment for persons with diabetes and chronic kidney disease

5. Diabetes
5-1.   Diabetes education
5-2.   New cases of diabetes
5-3.   Overall cases of diagnosed diabetes
5-4.   Diagnosis of diabetes
5-5.   Diabetes deaths
5-6.   Diabetes-related deaths
5-7.   Cardiovascular disease deaths in persons with diabetes

6. Disability and Secondary Conditions
6-2.   Feelings and depression among children with disabilities
6-3.   Feelings and depression interfering with activities among adults with disabilities
6-4.   Social participation among adults with disabilities
6-9.   Inclusion of children and youth with disabilities in regular education programs
6-10.   Accessibility of health and wellness programs
6-12.   Environmental barriers affecting participation in activities
6-13.   Surveillance and health promotion programs

7. Educational and Community-Based Programs
7-2.   School health education
7-3.   Health-risk behavior information for college and university students
7-5.   Worksite health promotion programs
7-6.   Participation in employer-sponsored health promotion activities

7-10.   Community health promotion programs

7-11.   Culturally appropriate and linguistically competent community health promotion programs

7-12.   Older adult participation in community health promotion activities

8. Environmental Health

8-1.   Harmful air pollutants

8-2.   Alternative modes of transportation

8-9.   Beach closings

8-20.   School policies to protect against environmental hazards

9. Family Planning

9-11.   Reproductive health education

11. Health Communication

11-1.   Households with Internet access

11-4.   Quality of Internet health information sources

12. Heart Disease and Stroke

12-1.   Coronary heart disease (CHD) deaths

12-7.   Stroke deaths

12-9.   High blood pressure

12-10.   High blood pressure control

12-11.   Action to help control blood pressure

12-13.   Mean total blood cholesterol levels

12-14.   High blood cholesterol levels

12-16.   LDL-cholesterol level in CHD patients

15. Injury and Violence Prevention

15-1.   Nonfatal head injuries

15-2.   Nonfatal spinal cord injuries

15-13.   Deaths from unintentional injuries

15-14.   Emergency department visits for nonfatal unintentional injuries

15-16.   Pedestrian deaths

15-18.   Nonfatal pedestrian injuries

15-21.   Motorcycle helmet use

15-23.   Bicycle helmet use

15-24.   Bicycle helmet laws

15-27.   Deaths from falls

15-28.   Hip fractures

15-29.   Drownings

15-31.   Injury protection in school sports

16. Maternal, Infant, and Child Health

16-3.   Adolescent and young adult deaths

16-12.   Weight gain during pregnancy

17. Medical Product Safety
17-2. Use of information technology
17-5. Receipt of oral counseling about medications from prescribers and dispensers

18. Mental Health and Mental Disorders
18-5. Disordered eating behaviors
18-7. Treatment for children with mental health problems
18-9. Treatment for adults with mental disorders

19. Nutrition and Overweight
19-1. Healthy weight in adults
19-2. Obesity in adults
19-3. Overweight or obesity in children and adolescents
19-16. Worksite promotion of nutrition education and weight management

20. Occupational Safety and Health
20-1. Work-related injury deaths
20-2. Work-related injuries
20-3. Overextension or repetitive motion
20-9. Worksite stress reduction programs

23. Public Health Infrastructure
23-2. Public access to information and surveillance data
23-17. Population-based prevention research

24. Respiratory Diseases
24-1. Deaths from asthma
24-2. Hospitalizations for asthma
24-3. Hospital emergency department visits for asthma
24-4. Activity limitations
24-5. School or work days lost
24-6. Patient education
24-7. Appropriate asthma care

25. Sexually Transmitted Diseases
25-11. Responsible adolescent sexual behavior

26. Substance Abuse
26-9. Substance-free youth
26-14. Steroid use among adolescents
26-17. Perception of risk associated with substance abuse
26-23. Community partnerships and coalitions

27. Tobacco Use

27-1.   Adult tobacco use

27-2.   Adolescent tobacco use

27-3.   Initiation of tobacco use

27-4.   Age at first tobacco use

27-5.   Smoking cessation by adults

27-7.   Smoking cessation by adolescents

28. Vision and Hearing

28-9.   Protective eyewear

Physical Activity and Health

A Report of the Surgeon General
Executive Summary

U.S. DEPARTMENT OF HEALTH AND HUMAN SERVICES
Centers for Disease Control and Prevention
National Center for Chronic Disease Prevention and Health Promotion
The President's Council on Physical Fitness and Sports

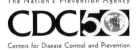
The Nation's Prevention Agency
Centers for Disease Control and Prevention

The President's
Council on
Physical Fitness
and Sports

Message from Donna E. Shalala
Secretary of Health and Human Services

The United States has led the world in understanding and promoting the benefits of physical activity. In the 1950s, we launched the first national effort to encourage young Americans to be physically active, with a strong emphasis on participation in team sports. In the 1970s, we embarked on a national effort to educate Americans about the cardiovascular benefits of vigorous activity, such as running and playing basketball. And in the 1980s and 1990s, we made breakthrough findings about the health benefits of moderate-intensity activities, such as walking, gardening, and dancing.

Now, with the publication of this first Surgeon General's report on physical activity and health, which I commissioned in 1994, we are poised to take another bold step forward. This landmark review of the research on physical activity and health—the most comprehensive ever—has the potential to catalyze a new physical activity and fitness movement in the United States. It is a work of real significance, on par with the Surgeon General's historic first report on smoking and health published in 1964.

This report is a passport to good health for all Americans. Its key finding is that people of all ages can improve the quality of their lives through a lifelong practice of moderate physical activity. You don't have to be training for the Boston Marathon to derive real health benefits from physical activity. A regular, preferably daily regimen of at least 30–45 minutes of brisk walking, bicycling, or even working around the house or yard will reduce your risks of developing coronary heart disease, hypertension, colon cancer, and diabetes. And if you're already doing that, you should consider picking up the pace: this report says that people who are already physically active will benefit even more by increasing the intensity or duration of their activity.

This watershed report comes not a moment too soon. We have found that 60 percent—well over half—of Americans are not regularly active. Worse yet, 25 percent of Americans are not active at all. For young people—the future of our country—physical activity declines dramatically during adolescence. These are dangerous trends. We need to turn them around quickly, for the health of our citizens and our country.

We will do so only with a massive national commitment—beginning now, on the eve of the Centennial Olympic Games, with a true fitness Dream Team drawing on the many forms of leadership that make up our great democratic society. Families need to weave physical activity into the fabric of their daily lives. Health professionals, in addition to being role models for healthy behaviors, need to encourage their patients to get out of their chairs and start fitness programs tailored to their individual needs. Businesses need to learn from what has worked in the past and promote worksite fitness, an easy option for workers. Community leaders need to reexamine whether enough resources have been devoted to the maintenance of parks, playgrounds, community centers, and physical education. Schools and universities need to reintroduce daily, quality physical activity as a key component of a comprehensive education. And the media and entertainment industries need to use their vast creative abilities to show all Americans that physical activity is healthful and fun—in other words, that it is attractive, maybe even glamorous!

We Americans always find the will to change when change is needed. I believe we can team up to create a new physical activity movement in this country. In doing so, we will save precious resources, precious futures, and precious lives. The time for action—and activity—is now.

Foreword

This first Surgeon General's report on physical activity is being released on the eve of the Centennial Olympic Games—the premiere event showcasing the world's greatest athletes. It is fitting that the games are being held in Atlanta, Georgia, home of the Centers for Disease Control and Prevention (CDC), the lead federal agency in preparing this report. The games' 100-year celebration also coincides with the CDC's landmark 50th year and with the 40th anniversary of the President's Council on Physical Fitness and Sports (PCPFS), the CDC's partner in developing this report. Because physical activity is a widely achievable means to a healthier life, this report directly supports the CDC's mission—to promote health and quality of life by preventing and controlling disease, injury, and disability. Also clear is the link to the PCPFS; originally established as part of a national campaign to help shape up America's younger generation, the Council continues today to promote physical activity, fitness, and sports for Americans of all ages.

The Olympic Games represent the summit of athletic achievement. The Paralympics, an international competition that will occur later this summer in Atlanta, represents the peak of athletic accomplishment for athletes with disabilities. Few of us will approach these levels of performance in our own physical endeavors. The good news in this report is that we do not have to scale Olympian heights to achieve significant health benefits. We can improve the quality of our lives through a lifelong practice of moderate amounts of regular physical activity of moderate or vigorous intensity. An active lifestyle is available to all.

Many Americans may be surprised at the extent and strength of the evidence linking physical activity to numerous health improvements. Most significantly, regular physical activity greatly reduces the risk of dying from coronary heart disease, the leading cause of death in the United States. Physical activity also reduces the risk of developing diabetes, hypertension, and colon cancer; enhances mental health; fosters healthy muscles, bones and joints; and helps maintain function and preserve independence in older adults.

The evidence about what helps people incorporate physical activity into their lives is less clear-cut. We do know that effective strategies and policies have taken place in settings as diverse as physical education classes in schools, health promotion programs at worksites, and one-on-one counseling by health care providers. However, more needs to be learned about what helps individuals change their physical activity habits and how changes in community environments, policies, and social norms might support that process.

Support is greatly needed if physical activity is to be increased in a society as technologically advanced as ours. Most Americans today are spared the burden of excessive physical labor. Indeed, few occupations today require significant physical activity, and most people use motorized transportation to get to work and to perform routine errands and tasks. Even leisure time is increasingly filled with sedentary behaviors, such as watching television, "surfing" the Internet, and playing video games.

Increasing physical activity is a formidable public health challenge that we must hasten to meet. The stakes are high, and the potential rewards are momentous: preventing premature death, unnecessary illness, and disability; controlling health care costs; and maintaining a high quality of life into old age.

David Satcher, M.D., Ph.D.   Philip R. Lee, M.D.
Director   Assistant Secretary
Centers for Disease Control   for Health
and Prevention

Florence Griffith Joyner
Tom McMillen
Co-Chairs
President's Council on
Physical Fitness and Sports

Preface

from the Surgeon General
U.S. Public Health Service

I am pleased to present the first report of the Surgeon General on physical activity and health. For more than a century, the Surgeon General of the Public Health Service has focused the nation's attention on important public health issues. Reports from Surgeons General on the adverse health consequences of smoking triggered nationwide efforts to prevent tobacco use. Reports on nutrition, violence, and HIV/AIDS—to name but a few—have heightened America's awareness of important public health issues and have spawned major public health initiatives. This new report, which is a comprehensive review of the available scientific evidence about the relationship between physical activity and health status, follows in this notable tradition.

Scientists and doctors have known for years that substantial benefits can be gained from regular physical activity. The expanding and strengthening evidence on the relationship between physical activity and health necessitates the focus this report brings to this important public health challenge. Although the science of physical activity is a complex and still-developing field, we have today strong evidence to indicate that regular physical activity will provide clear and substantial health gains. In this sense, the report is more than a summary of the science—it is a national call to action.

We must get serious about improving the health of the nation by affirming our commitment to healthy physical activity on all levels: personal, family, community, organizational, and national. Because physical activity is so directly related to preventing disease and premature death and to maintaining a high quality of life, we must accord it the same level of attention that we give other important public health practices that affect the entire nation. Physical activity thus joins the front ranks of essential health objectives, such as sound nutrition, the use of seat belts, and the prevention of adverse health effects of tobacco.

The time for this emphasis is both opportune and pressing. As this report makes clear, current levels of physical activity among Americans remain low, and we are losing ground in some areas. The good news in the report is that people can benefit from even moderate levels of physical activity. The public health implications of this good news are vast: the tremendous health gains that could be realized with even partial success at improving physical activity among the American people compel us to make a commitment and take action. With innovation, dedication, partnering, and a long-term plan, we should be able to improve the health and well-being of our people.

This report is not the final word. More work will need to be done so that we can determine the most effective ways to motivate all Americans to participate in a level of physical activity that can benefit their health and well-being. The challenge that lies ahead is formidable but worthwhile. I strongly encourage all Americans to join us in this effort.

Audrey F. Manley, M.D., M.P.H.
Surgeon General (Acting)

CHAPTER 1
INTRODUCTION, SUMMARY, AND CHAPTER CONCLUSIONS

Contents

CHAPTER 1
INTRODUCTION, SUMMARY, AND CHAPTER CONCLUSIONS

Introduction

This is the first Surgeon General's report to address physical activity and health. The main message of this report is that Americans can substantially improve their health and quality of life by including moderate amounts of physical activity in their daily lives. Health benefits from physical activity are thus achievable for most Americans, including those who may dislike vigorous exercise and those who may have been previously discouraged by the difficulty of adhering to a program of vigorous exercise. For those who are already achieving regular moderate amounts of activity, additional benefits can be gained by further increases in activity level.

This report grew out of an emerging consensus among epidemiologists, experts in exercise science, and health professionals that physical activity need not be of vigorous intensity for it to improve health. Moreover, health benefits appear to be proportional to amount of activity; thus, every increase in activity adds some benefit. Emphasizing the amount rather than the intensity of physical activity offers more options for people to select from in incorporating physical activity into their daily lives. Thus, a moderate amount of activity can be obtained in a 30-minute brisk walk, 30 minutes of lawn mowing or raking leaves, a 15-minute run, or 45 minutes of playing volleyball, and these activities can be varied from day to day. It is hoped that this different emphasis on moderate amounts of activity, and the flexibility to vary activities according to personal preference and life circumstances, will encourage more people to make physical activity a regular and sustainable part of their lives.

The information in this report summarizes a diverse literature from the fields of epidemiology, exercise physiology, medicine, and the behavioral sciences. The report highlights what is known about physical activity and health, as well as what is being learned about promoting physical activity among adults and young people.

Development of the Report

In July 1994, the Office of the Surgeon General authorized the Centers for Disease Control and Prevention (CDC) to serve as lead agency for preparing the first Surgeon General's report on physical activity and health. The CDC was joined in this effort by the President's Council on Physical Fitness and Sports (PCPFS) as a collaborative partner representing the Office of the Surgeon General. Because of the wide interest in the health effects of physical activity, the report was planned collaboratively with representatives from the Office of the Surgeon General, the Office of Public Health and Science (Office of the Secretary), the Office of Disease Prevention (National Institutes of Health [NIH]), and the following institutes from the NIH: the National Heart, Lung, and Blood Institute; the National Institute of Child Health and Human Development; the National Institute of Diabetes and Digestive and Kidney Diseases; and the National Institute of Arthritis and Musculoskeletal and Skin Diseases. CDC's nonfederal partners—including the American Alliance for Health, Physical Education, Recreation, and Dance; the American College of Sports Medicine; and the American Heart Association—provided consultation throughout the development process.

The major purpose of this report is to summarize the existing literature on the role of physical activity in preventing disease and on the status of interventions to increase physical activity. Any report on a topic this broad must restrict its scope to keep its message clear. This report focuses on disease prevention and therefore does not include the considerable body of evidence on the benefits of physical activity for treatment or

Physical Activity and Health

rehabilitation after disease has developed. This report concentrates on endurance-type physical activity (activity involving repeated use of large muscles, such as in walking or bicycling) because the health benefits of this type of activity have been extensively studied. The importance of resistance exercise (to increase muscle strength, such as by lifting weights) is increasingly being recognized as a means to preserve and enhance muscular strength and endurance and to prevent falls and improve mobility in the elderly. Some promising findings on resistance exercise are presented here, but a comprehensive review of resistance training is beyond the scope of this report. In addition, a review of the special concerns regarding physical activity for pregnant women and for people with disabilities is not undertaken here, although these important topics deserve more research and attention.

Finally, physical activity is only one of many everyday behaviors that affect health. In particular, nutritional habits are linked to some of the same aspects of health as physical activity, and the two may be related lifestyle characteristics. This report deals solely with physical activity; a Surgeon General's Report on Nutrition and Health was published in 1988.

Chapters 2 through 6 of this report address distinct areas of the current understanding of physical activity and health. Chapter 2 offers a historical perspective: after outlining the history of belief and knowledge about physical activity and health, the chapter reviews the evolution and content of physical activity recommendations. Chapter 3 describes the physiologic responses to physical activity—both the immediate effects of a single episode of activity and the long-term adaptations to a regular pattern of activity. The evidence that physical activity reduces the risk of cardiovascular and other diseases is presented in Chapter 4. Data on patterns and trends of physical activity in the U.S. population are the focus of Chapter 5. Lastly, Chapter 6 examines efforts to increase physical activity and reviews ideas currently being proposed for policy and environmental initiatives.

Major Conclusions

1. People of all ages, both male and female, benefit from regular physical activity.

2. Significant health benefits can be obtained by including a moderate amount of physical activity (e.g., 30 minutes of brisk walking or raking leaves, 15 minutes of running, or 45 minutes of playing volleyball) on most, if not all, days of the week. Through a modest increase in daily activity, most Americans can improve their health and quality of life.

3. Additional health benefits can be gained through greater amounts of physical activity. People who can maintain a regular regimen of activity that is of longer duration or of more vigorous intensity are likely to derive greater benefit.

4. Physical activity reduces the risk of premature mortality in general, and of coronary heart disease, hypertension, colon cancer, and diabetes mellitus in particular. Physical activity also improves mental health and is important for the health of muscles, bones, and joints.

5. More than 60 percent of American adults are not regularly physically active. In fact, 25 percent of all adults are not active at all.

6. Nearly half of American youths 12–21 years of age are not vigorously active on a regular basis. Moreover, physical activity declines dramatically during adolescence.

7. Daily enrollment in physical education classes has declined among high school students from 42 percent in 1991 to 25 percent in 1995.

8. Research on understanding and promoting physical activity is at an early stage, but some interventions to promote physical activity through schools, worksites, and health care settings have been evaluated and found to be successful.

Summary

The benefits of physical activity have been extolled throughout western history, but it was not until the second half of this century that scientific evidence supporting these beliefs began to accumulate. By the 1970s, enough information was available about the beneficial effects of vigorous exercise on cardiorespiratory fitness that the American College of Sports Medicine (ACSM), the American Heart Association (AHA), and other national organizations began issuing physical activity recommendations to the public. These recommendations generally focused on cardiorespiratory endurance and specified sustained periods of vigorous physical activity involving large muscle groups and lasting at least 20 minutes on 3 or more days per week. As understanding of the benefits of less vigorous activity grew, recommendations followed suit. During the past few years, the ACSM, the CDC, the AHA, the PCPFS, and the NIH have all recommended regular, moderate-intensity physical activity as an option for those who get little or no exercise. The *Healthy People 2000* goals for the nation's health have recognized the importance of physical activity and have included physical activity goals. The 1995 *Dietary Guidelines for Americans*, the basis of the federal government's nutrition-related programs, included physical activity guidance to maintain and improve weight—30 minutes or more of moderate-intensity physical activity on all, or most, days of the week.

Underpinning such recommendations is a growing understanding of how physical activity affects physiologic function. The body responds to physical activity in ways that have important positive effects on musculoskeletal, cardiovascular, respiratory, and endocrine systems. These changes are consistent with a number of health benefits, including a reduced risk of premature mortality and reduced risks of coronary heart disease, hypertension, colon cancer, and diabetes mellitus. Regular participation in physical activity also appears to reduce depression and anxiety, improve mood, and enhance ability to perform daily tasks throughout the life span.

The risks associated with physical activity must also be considered. The most common health problems that have been associated with physical activity are musculoskeletal injuries, which can occur with excessive amounts of activity or with suddenly beginning an activity for which the body is not conditioned. Much more serious associated health problems (i.e., myocardial infarction, sudden death) are also much rarer, occurring primarily among sedentary people with advanced atherosclerotic disease who engage in strenuous activity to which they are unaccustomed. Sedentary people, especially those with preexisting health conditions, who wish to increase their physical activity should therefore gradually build up to the desired level of activity. Even among people who are regularly active, the risk of myocardial infarction or sudden death is somewhat increased during physical exertion, but their overall risk of these outcomes is lower than that among people who are sedentary.

Introduction, Summary, and Chapter Conclusions

Research on physical activity continues to evolve. This report includes both well-established findings and newer research results that await replication and amplification. Interest has been developing in ways to differentiate between the various characteristics of physical activity that improve health. It remains to be determined how the interrelated characteristics of amount, intensity, duration, frequency, type, and pattern of physical activity are related to specific health or disease outcomes.

Attention has been drawn recently to findings from three studies showing that cardiorespiratory fitness gains are similar when physical activity occurs in several short sessions (e.g., 10 minutes) as when the same total amount and intensity of activity occurs in one longer session (e.g., 30 minutes). Although, strictly speaking, the health benefits of such intermittent activity have not yet been demonstrated, it is reasonable to expect them to be similar to those of continuous activity. Moreover, for people who are unable to set aside 30 minutes for physical activity, shorter episodes are clearly better than none. Indeed, one study has shown greater adherence to a walking program among those walking several times per day than among those walking once per day, when the total amount of walking time was kept the same. Accumulating physical activity over the course of the day has been included in recent recommendations from the CDC and ACSM, as well as from the NIH Consensus Development Conference on Physical Activity and Cardiovascular Health.

Despite common knowledge that exercise is healthful, more than 60 percent of American adults are not regularly active, and 25 percent of the adult population are not active at all. Moreover, although many people have enthusiastically embarked on vigorous exercise programs at one time or another, most do not sustain their participation. Clearly, the processes of developing and maintaining healthier habits are as important to study as the health effects of these habits.

The effort to understand how to promote more active lifestyles is of great importance to the health of this nation. Although the study of physical activity determinants and interventions is at an early stage, effective programs to increase physical activity have been carried out in a variety of settings, such as schools, physicians' offices, and worksites. Determining the most effective and cost-effective intervention

Physical Activity and Health

approaches is a challenge for the future. Fortunately, the United States has skilled leadership and institutions to support efforts to encourage and assist Americans to become more physically active. Schools, community agencies, parks, recreational facilities, and health clubs are available in most communities and can be more effectively used in these efforts.

School-based interventions for youth are particularly promising, not only for their potential scope—almost all young people between the ages of 6 and 16 years attend school—but also for their potential impact. Nearly half of young people 12–21 years of age are not vigorously active; moreover, physical activity sharply declines during adolescence. Childhood and adolescence may thus be pivotal times for preventing sedentary behavior among adults by maintaining the habit of physical activity throughout the school years. School-based interventions have been shown to be successful in increasing physical activity levels. With evidence that success in this arena is possible, every effort should be made to encourage schools to require daily physical education in each grade and to promote physical activities that can be enjoyed throughout life.

Outside the school, physical activity programs and initiatives face the challenge of a highly technological society that makes it increasingly convenient to remain sedentary and that discourages physical activity in both obvious and subtle ways. To increase physical activity in the general population, it may be necessary to go beyond traditional efforts. This report highlights some concepts from community initiatives that are being implemented around the country. It is hoped that these examples will spark new public policies and programs in other places as well. Special efforts will also be required to meet the needs of special populations, such as people with disabilities, racial and ethnic minorities, people with low income, and the elderly. Much more information about these important groups will be necessary to develop a truly comprehensive national initiative for better health through physical activity. Challenges for the future include identifying key determinants of physically active lifestyles among the diverse populations that characterize the United States (including special populations, women, and young people) and using this information to design and disseminate effective programs.

Chapter Conclusions

Chapter 2: Historical Background and Evolution of Physical Activity Recommendations

1. Physical activity for better health and well-being has been an important theme throughout much of western history.

2. Public health recommendations have evolved from emphasizing vigorous activity for cardiorespiratory fitness to including the option of moderate levels of activity for numerous health benefits.

3. Recommendations from experts agree that for better health, physical activity should be performed regularly. The most recent recommendations advise people of all ages to include a minimum of 30 minutes of physical activity of moderate intensity (such as brisk walking) on most, if not all, days of the week. It is also acknowledged that for most people, greater health benefits can be obtained by engaging in physical activity of more vigorous intensity or of longer duration.

4. Experts advise previously sedentary people embarking on a physical activity program to start with short durations of moderate-intensity activity and gradually increase the duration or intensity until the goal is reached.

5. Experts advise consulting with a physician before beginning a new physical activity program for people with chronic diseases, such as cardiovascular disease and diabetes mellitus, or for those who are at high risk for these diseases. Experts also advise men over age 40 and women over age 50 to consult a physician before they begin a vigorous activity program.

6. Recent recommendations from experts also suggest that cardiorespiratory endurance activity should be supplemented with strength-developing exercises at least twice per week for adults, in order to improve musculoskeletal health, maintain independence in performing the activities of daily life, and reduce the risk of falling.

Chapter 3: Physiologic Responses and Long-Term Adaptations to Exercise

1. Physical activity has numerous beneficial physiologic effects. Most widely appreciated are its effects on the cardiovascular and musculoskeletal systems, but benefits on the functioning of metabolic, endocrine, and immune systems are also considerable.

2. Many of the beneficial effects of exercise training—from both endurance and resistance activities—diminish within 2 weeks if physical activity is substantially reduced, and effects disappear within 2 to 8 months if physical activity is not resumed.

3. People of all ages, both male and female, undergo beneficial physiologic adaptations to physical activity.

Chapter 4: The Effects of Physical Activity on Health and Disease

Overall Mortality

1. Higher levels of regular physical activity are associated with lower mortality rates for both older and younger adults.

2. Even those who are moderately active on a regular basis have lower mortality rates than those who are least active.

Cardiovascular Diseases

1. Regular physical activity or cardiorespiratory fitness decreases the risk of cardiovascular disease mortality in general and of coronary heart disease mortality in particular. Existing data are not conclusive regarding a relationship between physical activity and stroke.

2. The level of decreased risk of coronary heart disease attributable to regular physical activity is similar to that of other lifestyle factors, such as keeping free from cigarette smoking.

3. Regular physical activity prevents or delays the development of high blood pressure, and exercise reduces blood pressure in people with hypertension.

Cancer

1. Regular physical activity is associated with a decreased risk of colon cancer.

2. There is no association between physical activity and rectal cancer. Data are too sparse to draw conclusions regarding a relationship between physical activity and endometrial, ovarian, or testicular cancers.

3. Despite numerous studies on the subject, existing data are inconsistent regarding an association between physical activity and breast or prostate cancers.

Non–Insulin-Dependent Diabetes Mellitus

1.) Regular physical activity lowers the risk of developing non–insulin-dependent diabetes mellitus.

Osteoarthritis

1. Regular physical activity is necessary for maintaining normal muscle strength, joint structure, and joint function. In the range recommended for health, physical activity is not associated with joint damage or development of osteoarthritis and may be beneficial for many people with arthritis.

2. Competitive athletics may be associated with the development of osteoarthritis later in life, but sports-related injuries are the likely cause.

Osteoporosis

1. Weight-bearing physical activity is essential for normal skeletal development during childhood and adolescence and for achieving and maintaining peak bone mass in young adults.

2. It is unclear whether resistance- or endurance-type physical activity can reduce the accelerated rate of bone loss in postmenopausal women in the absence of estrogen replacement therapy.

Falling

1. There is promising evidence that strength training and other forms of exercise in older adults preserve the ability to maintain independent living status and reduce the risk of falling.

Obesity

1. Low levels of activity, resulting in fewer kilocalories used than consumed, contribute to the high prevalence of obesity in the United States.

2. Physical activity may favorably affect body fat distribution.

Physical Activity and Health

Mental Health

1. Physical activity appears to relieve symptoms of depression and anxiety and improve mood.

2. Regular physical activity may reduce the risk of developing depression, although further research is needed on this topic.

Health-Related Quality of Life

1. Physical activity appears to improve health-related quality of life by enhancing psychological well-being and by improving physical functioning in persons compromised by poor health.

Adverse Effects

1. Most musculoskeletal injuries related to physical activity are believed to be preventable by gradually working up to a desired level of activity and by avoiding excessive amounts of activity.

2. Serious cardiovascular events can occur with physical exertion, but the net effect of regular physical activity is a lower risk of mortality from cardiovascular disease.

Chapter 5: Patterns and Trends in Physical Activity

Adults

1. Approximately 15 percent of U.S. adults engage regularly (3 times a week for at least 20 minutes) in vigorous physical activity during leisure time.

2. Approximately 22 percent of adults engage regularly (5 times a week for at least 30 minutes) in sustained physical activity of any intensity during leisure time.

3. About 25 percent of adults report no physical activity at all in their leisure time.

4. Physical inactivity is more prevalent among women than men, among blacks and Hispanics than whites, among older than younger adults, and among the less affluent than the more affluent.

5. The most popular leisure-time physical activities among adults are walking and gardening or yard work.

Adolescents and Young Adults

1. Only about one-half of U.S. young people (ages 12–21 years) regularly participate in vigorous physical activity. One-fourth report no vigorous physical activity.

2. Approximately one-fourth of young people walk or bicycle (i.e., engage in light to moderate activity) nearly every day.

3. About 14 percent of young people report no recent vigorous or light-to-moderate physical activity. This indicator of inactivity is higher among females than males and among black females than white females.

4. Males are more likely than females to participate in vigorous physical activity, strengthening activities, and walking or bicycling.

5. Participation in all types of physical activity declines strikingly as age or grade in school increases.

6. Among high school students, enrollment in physical education remained unchanged during the first half of the 1990s. However, daily attendance in physical education declined from approximately 42 percent to 25 percent.

7. The percentage of high school students who were enrolled in physical education and who reported being physically active for at least 20 minutes in physical education classes declined from approximately 81 percent to 70 percent during the first half of this decade.

8. Only 19 percent of all high school students report being physically active for 20 minutes or more in daily physical education classes.

Chapter 6: Understanding and Promoting Physical Activity

1. Consistent influences on physical activity patterns among adults and young people include confidence in one's ability to engage in regular physical activity (e.g., self-efficacy), enjoyment of physical activity, support from others, positive beliefs concerning the benefits of physical activity, and lack of perceived barriers to being physically active.

2. For adults, some interventions have been successful in increasing physical activity in communities, worksites, and health care settings, and at home.

3. Interventions targeting physical education in elementary school can substantially increase the amount of time students spend being physically active in physical education class.

Superintendent of Documents Publications Order Form

To fax your orders:
(202)512–2250

Order Processing Code
7895

☐ Yes, please send me _____ copies of the 1996 Surgeon General's Report on

Physical Activity and Health (S/N 017–023–00196–5) at $19 each.

The total cost of my order is $_____. (International customers please add 25%.) Prices include regular domestic postage and handling and are subject to change.

Please type or print

_____
(Company or personal name)

_____
(Additional address/attention line)

_____
(Street address)

_____
(City, state, ZIP Code)

_____
(Daytime phone including area code)

_____
(Purchase order number)

Please indicate method of payment

☐ Check payable to the Superintendent of Documents

☐ GPO Deposit Account ☐☐☐☐☐☐–☐

☐ VISA, Choice, or MasterCard Account

☐☐☐☐☐☐☐☐☐☐☐☐☐☐☐☐☐☐☐☐

☐☐☐☐ (Credit card expiration date)

_____
(Authorizing Signature)   7/96

Thank you for
your order!

Mail to: Superintendent of Documents, P.O. Box 371954, Pittsburgh, PA 15250–7954

Resources

Selected Organizations for Promoting Physical Activity

AARP

www.aarp.org

AARP is a nonprofit, nonpartisan membership organization for people age 50 and older. AARP focuses on many issues to advance the health, quality of life, and economic status of older adults, including dedicating efforts to promoting physical activity to enhance health and quality of life for all as we age. AARP aims to lead positive social change and deliver value to members through information, advocacy, and service.

The AARP Web site includes a section on physical activity: www.aarp.org/health/fitness

American Alliance for Health, Physical Education, Recreation and Dance (AAHPERD)

www.aahperd.org

The American Alliance for Health, Physical Education, Recreation and Dance is the largest organization of professionals supporting and assisting those involved in physical education, leisure, fitness, dance, health promotion, and education and all specialties related to achieving a healthy lifestyle.

AAHPERD is an alliance of five national associations and six district associations and is designed to provide members with a comprehensive and coordinated array of resources, support, and programs to help practitioners improve their skills and further the health and well-being of the American public.

American Cancer Society (ACS)

www.cancer.org

The American Cancer Society is a nationwide, community-based voluntary health organization. Its Web site includes information on prevention and early detection that includes a section on staying active: www.cancer.org/docroot/PED/ped_6.asp?sitearea=PED

American College of Sports Medicine (ACSM)

www.acsm.org

ACSM's mission is to promote and integrate scientific research, education, and practical applications of sports medicine and exercise science to maintain and enhance physical performance, fitness, health, and quality of life. Certifications are offered in personal trainer, health/fitness instructor, exercise specialist, physical activity in public health specialist, and clinical exercise physiologist areas, accredited by the National Commission for Certifying Agencies (NCCA).

Publications

- *Medicine & Science in Sports & Exercise* features original investigations, clinical studies, and comprehensive reviews.
- *Exercise and Sport Sciences Review* is a quarterly review of emerging scientific, medical, and research topics.
- *ACSM's Health & Fitness Journal* contains articles about products and trends in the health and fitness industry; it is geared toward fitness instructors, personal trainers, exercise leaders, program managers, and other frontline health and fitness professionals.
- *ACSM Fit Society Page* is a quarterly electronic newsletter written for the general public on a variety of popular health and fitness topics.

American Council on Exercise (ACE)

www.acefitness.org

Established in 1985, ACE is a nonprofit, educational organization committed to enriching quality of life through safe and effective physical activity. Certifications are offered for personal trainer, group fitness instructor, lifestyle and weight management, and clinical exercise specialist areas and are NCAA accredited (National Commission for Certifying Agencies).

Publications

- *ACE FitnessMatters* is a bimonthly publication that provides fitness enthusiasts with health and fitness information. The magazine accepts no advertising in order to remain unbiased.
- *ACE Certified News* is a bimonthly publication geared exclusively to ACE-certified professionals that provides industry-related news and tools to help fitness professionals build and maintain successful careers.
- *ACE Fit Facts* is a one-page, consumer-friendly article available for distribution to clients.
- Operation FitKids provides educational materials and professional training to those working to promote youth fitness: educators, fitness professionals, health professionals, and parents.

American Heart Association (AHA)

www.americanheart.org

The American Heart Association is a national voluntary health agency whose mission is to reduce disability and death from cardiovascular diseases and stroke.

Its Web site includes a section on exercise and fitness: www.americanheart.org/presenter.jhtml?identifier=1200013

Boys and Girls Clubs of America

www.bgca.org

The mission of the Boys and Girls Clubs of America is to inspire and enable all young people, especially those from disadvantaged circumstances, to realize their full potential as productive, responsible, and caring citizens.

Several programs are dedicated to sports, fitness, and recreation: www.bgca. org/programs/sportfitness.asp

The Cooper Institute for Aerobics Research
www.cooperinst.org

The Cooper Institute is dedicated to advancing the understanding of the relationship between living habits and health and to providing leadership in implementing these concepts to enhance the physical and emotional well-being of individuals. The Cooper Institute promotes physical activity through research, fitness programs, and continuing education opportunities.

Human Kinetics Publishers
www.humankinetics.com

Human Kinetics describes itself as "the information leader on physical activity" and publishes an array of books and journals on the topic.

National Association for Health and Fitness (NAHF)
www.physicalfitness.org

The National Association for Health and Fitness is a nonprofit organization to improve the quality of life for individuals in the United States through the promotion of physical fitness, sports, and healthy lifestyles. NAHF accomplishes this work by fostering and supporting governor's and state councils and coalitions that promote and encourages regular physical activity.

NAHF is also the national sponsor of National Employee Health and Fitness Day, the largest work-site health and fitness event in North America (the third Wednesday in May). The Web site is www.physicalfitness.org/nehf.html.

National Coalition for Promoting Physical Activity (NCPPA)
www.ncppa.org

The National Coalition for Promoting Physical Activity's mission is to unite the strengths of public, private, and industry efforts into collaborative partnerships that inspire and empower all Americans to lead more physically active lifestyles.

National Recreation and Park Association (NRPA)
www.nrpa.org

For more than 100 years, NRPA has advocated the significance of making parks, open space, and recreational opportunities available to all Americans. NRPA's mission is to advance parks, recreation, and environmental conservation efforts that enhance the quality of life for all people.

NRPA's programs and partnerships promote physical activity: www.nrpa.org/content/default.aspx?documentId=28

National Senior Games Association (NSGA)
www.nsga.com/

The National Senior Games Association is the national organization that spearheads the senior games movement, sanctioning and coordinating efforts of senior games organizations across the country. The organization serves 50 member state organizations, located in 49 states (excluding Oregon) and the District of Columbia.

A community-based member of the United States Olympic Committee (USOC) since 1988, the NSGA serves as the USOC's official arm to the senior population.

National Society of Physical Activity Practitioners in Public Health (NSPAPPH)

www.nspapph.org

The National Society of Physical Activity Practitioners in Public Health is a professional organization dedicated to growing the capacity of physical activity practitioners in public health. Those who work in this emerging field come from various academic backgrounds and professions, including health promotion and education, public health, exercise science and exercise physiology, and physical education. NSPAPPH intends to elevate physical activity in public health practice at national, state, and local levels through professional development. The mission of NSPAPPH is to make physical activity a public health priority through engagement, education, expansion of partnerships, and physical activity in public health specialist certification.

Arnold School of Public Health Prevention Research Center (PRC), University of South Carolina

http://prevention.sph.sc.edu

The PRC is committed to conducting research that benefits the public's health and to translating research into practice. The PRC works to ensure that research findings are put to work for individuals, families, and communities to promote physical activity through community intervention, training, dissemination, and applied research.

- The *USC Prevention Research Center Notes* is an e-mail newsletter with current information about physical activity and public health.
- The Physical Activity and Public Health On-Line Network is a listserv advancing public health approaches to promoting physical activity by creating a national network of public health practitioners, researchers, and interested others.

Training and education are core activities provided by the PRC. Physical activity and public health courses are offered annually and are cosponsored by the PRC and the Centers for Disease Control and Prevention. The courses consist of an 8-day postgraduate course on research directions and strategies and a 6-day practitioner's course on community interventions. The long-term goal of the training program is to improve the public's health by increasing the number of public health researchers and practitioners who have expertise in the promotion of physical activity in populations. The Web site for the training courses is http://prevention.sph.sc.edu/seapines/index.htm.

Wellness Council of America (WELCOA)

www.welcoa.org

WELCOA is a national nonprofit membership organization dedicated to promoting healthier lifestyles for all Americans, especially through health promotion initiatives in the workplace. WELCOA links communities and coalitions together into a supportive network that includes locally affiliated wellness councils, well city initiatives, well workplaces, and individual and corporate members throughout the United States.

Specifically, WELCOA focuses on building Well Workplaces—organizations that are dedicated to the health of their employees. The Well Workplace process provides business leaders and members with a structure or blue print to help their organizations build results-oriented wellness programs.

WELCOA serves as a national clearinghouse and information center on worksite wellness.

YMCA and YWCA of the USA

www.ymca.net

www.ywca.org

The nation's more than 2,500 YMCAs make up the largest not-for-profit community service organization in America, working to meet the health and social service needs of 18.9 million men, women, and children in 10,000 communities in the United States. YMCAs are for people of all faiths, races, abilities, ages, and incomes.

The Y's mission is to put Christian principles into practice through programs that build healthy spirit, mind, and body for all.

Selected U.S. Federal Web Sites and Publications for Promoting Physical Activity

Centers for Disease Control and Prevention (CDC)

Division of Nutrition, Physical Activity and Obesity (DNPAO)

www.cdc.gov/nccdphp/dnpao

The CDC's Division of Nutrition, Physical Activity and Obesity (DNPAO) pursues a public health approach to the prevention and management of physical inactivity, poor dietary practices, and obesity across the life span by conducting surveillance, epidemiologic and behavioral research, applied social marketing and consumer research, intervention research and design, training and education, health promotion and leadership, policy and environmental change, health communication, and partnership development.

A section of the Web site is dedicated to physical activity in the general public: www.cdc.gov/nccdphp/DNPAO/index.html

Selected Publications and Resources From DNPAO and DNPAO's Partners

- National Physical Activity Plan (launch planned for May 2010).

- *2008 Physical Activity Guidelines for Americans*. The federal government has issued its first-ever *Physical Activity Guidelines for Americans*. They describe the types and amounts of physical activity that offer substantial health benefits to Americans: www.health.gov/paguidelines/

- *The Guide to Community Preventive Services*. See information in part II and www.thecommunityguide.org/index.html.

- *KidsWalk-to-School* is a guide that promotes collaboration within communities to identify and create safe walking routes to school: www.cdc.gov/nccdphp/dnpa/kidswalk/

■ *Growing Stronger: Strength Training for Older Adults* is a resource book for older adults developed by scientists at the CDC and Tufts University. The book outlines a program that has been proven to increase muscle strength, maintain bone density, and improve balance, coordination, and mobility. The book can be downloaded free of charge at http://growingstronger.nutrition.tufts.edu/growing stronger/book.html.

■ *The Physical Activity Evaluation Handbook.* This handbook outlines the six basic steps of program evaluation and illustrates each step with examples of physical activity programs. Appendixes provide information about physical activity indicators, practical case studies, and additional evaluation resources. The Web site is www.cdc.gov/nccdphp/dnpa/physical/handbook/pdf/handbook.pdf.

■ *Reference Guide of Physical Activity Programs for Older Adults: A Resource for Planning Intervention.* This guide describes multiple programs for promoting physical activity among older adults that may have potential to help prevent or delay type 2 diabetes: www.cdc.gov/diabetes.

■ *Community-Wide Campaign to Promote Physical Activity Among Mid-Life and Older Adults: Lessons Learned from AARP's Active for Life Campaign and a Synopsis of Evidence-Based Interventions.* A guide that describes lessons learned from two community intervention demonstration studies (one in Madison, Wisconsin, and one in Richmond, Virginia) conducted by AARP with Robert Wood Johnson Foundation funding. The two community interventions were designed to increase physical activity among adults 50 years and older. The guide articulates the key findings from these projects to help translate the research for use by communities other than Richmond and Madison. Physical activity interventions identified by the *Community Guide for Preventive Services* are also described.

■ *National Blueprint: Increasing Physical Activity Among Adults Aged 50 and Older* brought together more than 50 national organizations, including representatives from the CDC, Administration on Aging (AOA), National Institute on Aging (NIA), and President's Council on Physical Fitness and Sports (PCPFS). Eighteen high-priority strategies were ultimately identified and key organizations selected to play a lead role in the planning and implementation of programs or initiatives to help combat inactivity and improve the quality of life for older Americans. The Environmental Protection Agency, PCPFS, and CDC serve as coleaders of one of the marketing strategies and are charged with developing a national program that provides incentives for communities to increase physical activity among the 50 and older population: www.agingblueprint.org.

■ *The Healthy Brain Initiative: A National Public Health Road Map to Maintaining Cognitive Health* is a national public health action plan to address healthy brain issues including the relationship between physical activity and brain health. The plan is intended to focus the nation's resources on addressing risk and protective factors for promoting cognitive health. See www.cdc.gov/Aging/healthybrain/roadmap.htm.

Division of Adolescent and School Health (DASH)
www.cdc.gov/nccdphp/dash

The CDC's Division of Adolescent and School Health works to prevent the most serious health risks among children, adolescents, and young adults. The division collaborates with other federal agencies, national nongovernmental organizations, and state and local departments of education, health, and social services to plan and implement four interrelated strategies. These strategies include (a) identifying and monitoring critical health related events and interventions designed to influence those events, (b) synthesizing and applying research to increase the effectiveness of interventions, (c) enabling relevant constituents to plan and implement effective interventions, and (d) evaluating the impact of interventions over time.

A list of physical activity resources has been compiled: www.cdc.gov/HealthyYouth/physicalactivity/publications.htm

Selected Publications and Resources

- Provided support to the National Association of State Board of Education for the development of *Fit, Healthy, and Ready to Learn*: www.nasbe.org/index.php/shs/53-shs-resources/396-fit-healthy-and-ready-to-learn-a-school-health-policy-guide

- *School Health Index: A Self-Assessment and Planning Guide* helps schools identify strengths and weaknesses in physical activity and nutrition policies and involves teachers, parents, students and the community in developing action plans for improving student health. The School Health Improvement Plan: www.cdc.gov/healthyyouth/SHI/training/03-Orientation/docs/Orientation-Slides.pdf

- The *Physical Education Curriculum Analysis Tool (PECAT)* helps school districts conduct clear, complete, and consistent analyses of written physical education curricula, based on national physical education standards. The PECAT is customizable to include local standards. The results from the analysis can help school districts enhance existing curricula, develop their own curricula, or select a published curriculum for the delivery of quality physical education in schools: www.cdc.gov/healthyyouth/pecat.

Other CDC Web Sites

- Exemplary state programs focusing on nutrition and physical activity: www.cdc.gov/nccdphp/exemplary/physical_activity.htm

- Designing and Building Healthy Places: www.cdc.gov/healthyplaces/default.htm

President's Council on Physical Fitness and Sports (PCPFS)

The PCPFS advises the President on opportunities and initiatives to improve the health, physical activity, and fitness of all Americans. The PCPFS council members approved the following recommendations on June 20, 2002: the creation and launch of www.presidentschallenge.org, a new interactive Web site for the President's Challenge; a revamped government Web site (www.fitness.gov); and increased partnerships and collaborative endeavors with the public, private, and nonprofit sectors. These efforts have enhanced the office's grassroots outreach.

The goals and objectives of the PCPFS are addressed through professional consultation, technical assistance, public information, and program development and evaluation. These services are provided to school systems, government agencies, professional organizations, private businesses and industry, recreation and parks departments, and national sport governing bodies and others who wish to introduce or improve physical activity and sports programs.

Selected Publications and Resources

- *PCPFS Research Digest* is a quarterly publication focusing on selected aspects of the science of physical activity, physical fitness, and sports medicine. The digest is a synthesis of the latest scientific information translated into lay language and disseminated free of charge to practitioners, educators, and other interested parties. Used as a basis for many university classes, the digest is updated by the author and made available as a monograph. Digests are also available on the PCPFS and President's Challenge Web sites.

- PCPFS partnered with the American Academy of Clinical Endocrinologists (AACE) on the *Rx for Physical Activity* pamphlet, which is delivered via AACE volunteer members to sixth graders across the country. The postcard-sized pamphlet, with both English and Spanish translations, shows how kids can get their 60 minutes of physical activity each day.

- *Kids in Action Fitness for Children Birth to Age Five* is the product of a partnership between the PCPFS, National Association for Sport and Physical Education, and Kellogg's. The booklet was updated and rereleased in 2003.

- The *Nolan Ryan Fitness Guide* is a basic fitness primer and has been distributed free of charge to more than 1.5 million Americans since its publication.

National Institutes of Health (NIH)

Selected Publications and Resources

- *Energize Yourself! Stay Physically Active* is one of a package of seven booklets designed to reduce cardiovascular disease and stroke among African Americans: http://win.niddk.nih.gov/publications/energize.htm
- Weight Control Information Network (WIN) publications: www.niddk.nih.gov/health/nutrit/winbro/winbro1.html
  - *Active at Any Size*
  - *Energize Yourself and Your Family* (contains information on *Sisters Together, Move More, Eat Better,* a program that raises the awareness about the health benefits of healthy eating and regular physical activity among Black women).
  - *Fit and Fabulous as You Mature*
  - *Fit for Two: Tips for Pregnancy*
  - *Healthy Eating and Physical Activity Across the Lifespan: Tips for Adults and Healthy Eating and Physical Activity Across the Lifespan* and *Helping Your Child: Tips for Parents*
  - *Walking: A Step in the Right Direction*
  - *Young at Heart: Tips for Older Adults*
- *Exercise:* This book and video from the National Institute on Aging show older adults how to start and continue an exercise program in a safe and effective manner. The video provides demonstrations of stretching, strength training, and balancing exercises and features the companion book *Exercise and Physical Activity: Your Everyday Guide from the National Institute on Aging.*

Other NIH Web Sites

- NIH Senior Health Web site: http://nihseniorhealth.gov/exercise/toc.html
- *Maintaining a Healthy Back with Exercise and Rest:* http://dohs.ors.od.nih.gov/industrial.htm (scroll down to lower part of this Web page to locate this information)
- *Aim for a Healthy Weight:* www.nhlbi.nih.gov/health/public/heart/obesity/lose_wt/index.htm
- This Web page from the National Heart, Lung, and Blood Institute has both "Information for Health Professionals," which includes clinical guidelines, and "Information for Patients and the Public," available from the Obesity Education Initiative. It contains a body mass index calculator, food shopping and preparation tips, dining out and physical activity ideas, and low-calorie menu plans. The Web page includes an interactive quiz called "Portion Distortion" that illustrates the change over the past 20 years in the portion size of different foods for sale in restaurants, supermarkets, or other food outlets. The Web page features key findings, outcomes, and programs on obesity-related topics.

Office on Women's Health (OWH)

Selected Publications and Resources

- *A Lifetime of Good Health: Your Guide to Staying Healthy*—provides an approach to lifelong health and addresses healthy behaviors to prevent and manage the many health conditions that affect women: www.womenshealth.gov/pub/05prevguide.pdf

- BodyWise—A Toolkit for School Personnel on Eating Disorders. This campaign targets girls aged 8 to 12 with messages about healthy eating, self-esteem, and physical activity: See www.womenshealth.gov/pub/bodywise.cfm for valuable information; however, the BodyWise materials are not available at this site.

Web Sites

The site www.girlshealth.gov encourages adolescent girls to choose healthy behaviors. The site, part of the U.S. Department of Health and Human Services National Women's Health Information Center, provides girls ages 10 to 16 with information on several health topics, including nutrition and fitness, in an interactive, user-friendly format. The fitness section provides girls with the tools to develop an exercise plan that is enjoyable, safe, and long-lasting. Highlights include an online fitness questionnaire, tips on strength training, information on avoiding exercise-related injuries, and advice on keeping exercise interesting.

U.S. Department of Agriculture

Selected Publications and Resources

- *Dietary Guidelines for Americans 2005 [Dietary Guidelines]* provides science-based advice to promote health and to reduce risk for major chronic diseases through diet and physical activity: www.healthierus.gov/dietaryguidelines. New dietary guidelines will be released in 2010.

■ Power of Choice: A product of a partnership between the USDA Food and Nutrition Service and the Food and Drug Administration. This resource is for after-school program coordinators to use to help promote healthy eating and physical activity choices among adolescents: www.fns.usda.gov/tn/Resources/power_of_choice.html

Web Sites

■ The Interactive Healthy Eating Index and Physical Activity Tool (MyPyramid Tracker). The Physical Activity Tool, one portion of this interactive Web site, assesses physical activity status and provides related energy expenditure information and educational messages. Use of this tool enhances the link between good nutrition and the health benefits of regular physical activity: www.mypyramidtracker.gov/

U.S. Department of Transportation

Selected Publications and Resources

■ Stepping Out—Mature Adults: Be Healthy, Walk Safely is an information resource available at www.nhtsa.dot.gov/people/injury/olddrive/SteppingOut/index.html or through a printable 26-page booklet (www.nhtsa.dot.gov/people/injury/olddrive/SteppingOut/pdf_version/stepping_out.pdf).

■ *Safe Routes to School: Promise and Practice* is available at www.nhtsa.dot.gov/people/injury/pedbimot/bike/Safe-Routes-2004.

Web Sites

Safe Routes to School: www.nhtsa.dot.gov/people/injury/pedbimot/bike/Safe-Routes-2002/toc.html

GLOSSARY

active transportation—Walking and bicycling as a means of travel.

accessibility—Buildings, structures, programs, and transportation services are designed or modified to enable persons with activity limitations or disabilities to use them without undue difficulty.

adaptation—Modifying an activity, equipment, or technique so that an individual with a limitation or disability can participate in an activity.

aerobic capacity—Maximum amount of oxygen that can be transported from the lungs to the tissues during exercise. Aerobic capacity is influenced by age, sex, exercise habits, heredity factors, and clinical cardiovascular status. It is used as an index of an individual's capacity for sustained work performance and is commonly used to measure cardiovascular fitness. It is also referred to as maximal oxygen consumption ($\dot{V}O_2$max).

aerobic exercise—Exercise in which aerobic (oxidative) metabolism is used to generate the energy required to perform an activity. Regular aerobic exercise increases the functional capacity of the cardiovascular system. Aerobic exercises include activities such as running, jogging, brisk walking, cycling, and swimming.

association—Simple relationship between factors, often expressed as Pearson's product moment correlation (r) and Spearman's rank correlation (r).

baseline data—Data reflecting the initial status or interests of the participants or data from a needs assessment before the implementation of a program or intervention that can be used for comparison with the follow-up data collected from program participants.

BMI—Body mass index can be calculated using pounds and inches with the following non-metric conversion equation: [weight (in pounds) ÷ height (in inches)^2 x 704.5]. For example, a person who weighs 220 pounds and is 6 feet 3 inches tall has a BMI of 27. A metric conversion can also be done using the equation [weight (in kilograms) ÷ height (in meters)^2]. A person who weighs 100 kilograms and is 1.905 meters tall has a BMI of 27.

body composition—Relative amounts of muscle, fat, bone, and other anatomical components that contribute to a person's total body weight. Body composition differs markedly between men and women. Simple methods for determining body composition are often stated as percent body fat, pounds of fat, or lean body mass. Body composition is one of the five health-related components of physical fitness.

body fat—Total amount of fat deposited in the body as "storage fat" (which accumulates in adipose tissue) and "essential fat" (which is required for normal physiologic functioning and is stored in bone marrow as well as in major organs and tissues). Essential fat is about four times higher in women than in men.

built environment—The form and character of communities, made up of specific places (e.g., homes, streets, offices, parking lots, shopping malls, restaurants, parks, movie theaters) that constitute a city, town, or suburb.

calorie—measure of energy from food (3,500 kilocalories of food energy = 1 pound [.45 kg] of body weight). Also the amount of heat required to raise the temperature of 1 gram of water 1°C (1,000 calories = 1 kilocalorie). An interesting fact: The word *calories* on a food label actually refers to kilocalories.

campaign—A planned, organized, and integrated set of activities with a clearly defined purpose that uses multiple strategies and channels. Campaigns are waged during a defined time and are usually long (e.g., more than a year) and sustained. In addition to including mass communication activities, a campaign may consist of grassroots programming, community organization, and legislative advocacy.

cardiorespiratory fitness—Ability of the circulatory and respiratory systems to supply fuel during sustained physical activity. Cardiorespiratory fitness is one of the five health-related components of physical fitness.

coalition—An alliance of organizations to achieve a common purpose or joint action. The underlying concept behind coalitions is collaboration and resource sharing.

community—A social unit that usually encompasses a geographic region where residents live and interact socially, such as a political subdivision (e.g., a county, city, or town) or a smaller area (e.g., a section of town, a housing complex, or a neighborhood). A community may be a social organization (a formal or informal group of people who share common concerns or interests). Very often, a community is a composite of subgroups defined by a variety of factors, including age, sex, occupation, socioeconomic status, physical activity history, and current physical activity preferences.

community-wide campaigns—Interventions that are large scale, intense, and highly visible; messages are directed to large audiences through different types of media, including television, radio, newspapers, movie theaters, billboards, and mailings. Such campaigns are typically conducted as part of a multicomponent effort that includes strategies such as support or self-help groups, physical activity counseling, risk factor screening and education, community health fairs and other community events, and environmental or policy changes such as creating walking trails.

confidence interval—In statistics, a range of possible true values (within a given probability) of an estimated statistic. For example, in 2003, an estimated 48.8% of adults in Maryland met the physical activity recommendations. The confidence interval within which the true prevalence was likely to vary was 46.8% to 50.8%.

connectivity—Measured in terms of the degree to which the street network provides direct routes and facilities provide safe connections for pedestrians and bicyclists. Connectivity is determined by the speed and volume of automobile traffic, the width and condition of walking paths, the extent to which pathways are dedicated for pedestrian use and protected from automobile traffic, and the number of blocks and intersections per unit or area.

coronary heart disease—Condition in which blood flow is restricted through a coronary artery by the thickening of the arterial wall from deposits of plaque. It is also known as *coronary atherosclerosis*.

correlate—Factor that is associated with a second factor in an association.

density—Measure of the number of people residing or working in a given area. Density is thought to increase nonmotorized travel because of decreased trip lengths, reduced vehicle ownership, and increased choice of travel mode options. However, some researchers have suggested that density may serve as a proxy measure for other variables such as parking costs, traffic congestion, automobile ownership, and availability of transit service.

duration—The length of time in which an activity or exercise is preformed. Duration is generally expressed in minutes.

effective—The activity or set of activities leads to the desired outcome.

efficient—The activity or set of activities that uses resources in a responsible manner.

employment density—Land-use measure of the intensity of commercial development, the number of employees per land area.

enhanced access—Interventions that may involve the efforts of work sites, coalitions, agencies, and communities in attempts to change the local environment to create opportunities for physical activity. Changes may include creating walking trails, building exercise facilities, or providing access to existing nearby facilities.

evaluation framework—A skeleton of a plan that can be used to conduct an evaluation that places an order to the steps that are to be followed.

evaluation—The concept of determining the worth or value in the object of interest (health-promotion program) against a standard of acceptability. The type of evaluation reflects whether the results are needed to improve a program before or during implementation, to assess the effectiveness of a program, or to determine whether the program met the goals and objectives.

exercise—Physical activity that is planned or structured. It involves repetitive bodily movement done to improve or maintain one or more of the components of physical fitness: cardiorespiratory endurance (aerobic fitness), muscular strength, muscular endurance, flexibility, and body composition.

flexibility—Range of motion available at a joint. The length of the muscles, ligaments, and tendons largely determines the amount of movement possible at each joint. Flexibility is one of the five health-related components of physical fitness.

focus group—A small group of people (8-10) who together respond to a set of questions and undertake a discussion on a selected topic. All participants represent the target audience and are encouraged to express their views related to the topic.

formal evaluation—A process characterized by a systematic, well-planned procedure that is designed to control a variety of extraneous variables that could produce evaluation outcomes that are not correct. Evaluation is the driving force for planning new, effective health-promotion programs, improving existing programs, and demonstrating the results of resource investments.

formative assessment— Formative assessment is conducted during the developmental stages of a project. It may include identification of barriers and resources and pilot-testing on a small scale before full implementation. It's purpose is to maximize the likelihood of effective intervention

formative research—Research conducted during the developmental stages of a project or campaign. It may include reviews, pretesting messages or materials, and pilot testing programs on a small scale before full implementation. The primary purpose of formative research is to maximize the likelihood of effective intervention; it can suggest improvements in message or program content and delivery as well as identify potentially misleading or misunderstood messages and intervention strategies before more costly implementation occurs.

frequency—The number of times an exercise or activity is preformed. Frequency is generally expressed in sessions, episodes, or bouts per week.

gatekeeper—Someone to work with or through to reach the intended audience or accomplish a task. These individuals stand "at the gate" between the health-promotion planner and the target audience and often determine whether the health-promotion planner gains access to others. Examples are policy makers, decision makers, homemakers, and heads of households.

goal—A future event toward which a committed endeavor is directed and representing a long-range program purpose.

health belief model—One of the most frequently used theories in health behavior applications. It hypothesizes that health-related action depends on the simultaneous occurrence of three classes of factors: existence of sufficient motivation (or health concern) to make issues salient or relevant, belief that one is susceptible to a serious health problem or to the sequelae of that illness or condition (perceived threat,), and belief that following a particular health recommendation will be beneficial in reducing the perceived threat and at an acceptable cost (perceived barrier). These costs must be overcome to follow the health recommendation and can include financial outlays, time, and lack of self-efficacy.

incidence—Occurrence of new cases of a disease during a specified time period, often expressed as a rate per thousand population or as a percentage of the population. For example, in 1980, 541,000 new cases of diabetes were diagnosed, or 2.5 new cases per 1,000 population.

indicators—Measures of specific environments and policies related to physical activity and healthy eating on which information is systematically and routinely collected and used to monitor changes in these environments and policies over time.

individually adapted health behavior change—Programs that are tailored to an individual's specific interests, preferences, and readiness for change. In addition, they are designed to teach behavioral skills to help participants incorporate physical activity into their daily routines, including: setting goals for physical activity and self-monitoring of progress toward goals, building social support for new behavioral patterns, reinforcing behavior through self-reward and positive self-talk, problem-solving geared to maintenance of the behavior change, and preventing relapse into sedentary behaviors.

intensity—Level of energy required to perform a specific activity. It is often described as maximum oxygen consumption ($\dot{V}O_2$max), percent maximum heart rate reserve, or multiples of resting metabolism (metabolic equivalents).

intermediaries—Organizations (such as professional, industrial, civic, social, or fraternal groups) that serve as a channel for distributing program messages and materials to members of the target audience.

intervention—The activity or experience to which those in the target population will be exposed or in which they will take part. Activities may be communication, educational, behavior modification, environmental change, or regulatory.

kilocalorie—Amount of heat required to raise the temperature of 1 kilogram of water 1°C. Kilocalorie is the ordinary calorie discussed in food and exercise energy-expenditure tables and food labels.

land use—Degree to which different types of activities (i.e., residential, commercial, industrial) exist together in a specific geographic area. An example of a high land-use area is the downtown area of a city where high-rises offer shopping, residential, and office spaces within the same building. A suburban community is an example of a low land-use area because residential spaces are located separately from commercial and business spaces.

leisure-time physical activity—Exercise, sports, recreation, and hobbies that are not associated with activities as part of one's regular job duties, household, and transportation. Synonymous with *discretionary-time physical activity*.

logic model—A logic model describes the sequence of events for bringing about change and synthesizes the main program elements into a picture of how the program is supposed to work. Often, this model is displayed in a flow chart, map, or table to portray the sequence of steps leading to program results.

MET (metabolic equivalent) —The standard metabolic equivalent, or MET, level. This unit is used to estimate the amount of oxygen used by the body during physical activity.

- 1 MET = energy (oxygen) used by the body as you sit quietly, perhaps while talking on the phone or reading a book. The harder your body works during an activity, the higher the MET.
- Any activity that burns 3 to 5.9 METs is considered moderate-intensity physical activity.
- Any activity that burns 6 METs and above is considered vigorous-intensity physical activity.

mixed-use development—Built environment in an area characterized by buildings that contain commercial, residential, and industrial spaces.

model—Subclass of a theory as they draw on theories to help people understand a specific problem in a particular setting or context.

moderate-intensity physical activity—A level of effort in which a person should experience some increase in breathing or heart rate or a "perceived exertion" of 11 to 14 on the Borg scale. It is the effort a healthy individual might expend while walking briskly, mowing the lawn, dancing, swimming, or bicycling on level terrain, for example. This level of activity requires 3 to 5.9 metabolic equivalents (METs) and burns 3.5 to 7 calories per minute

muscular endurance—Ability of muscle groups to exert external force through repetitive motion or sustained exertion. It is one of the five health-related components of physical fitness.

muscular strength—Amount of external force a muscle can exert against resistance in a single effort (i.e., how much weight a person can lift or how much tension can be exerted). It is one of the five health-related components of physical fitness.

nonmotorized travel—Walking, bicycling, skating, and riding a nonmotorized scooter.

objectives—Precise steps that are taken in pursuit of a goal and outlined in measurable terms that will reflect specific changes that are to occur in the target population at a given point in time as the result of the program that, if completed, will reach program goals.

organic street network—Unplanned street network resulting from gradual, unplanned changes made to street systems over many centuries. Typically narrow, winding streets bounded by the city's defensive wall with an important civic, religious, commercial, or political structure at the center.

outcome evaluation—Focuses on the ultimate goal or product of a program or treatment, generally measured in the health field by morbidity or mortality statistics in a population, vital measures, symptoms, signs, or physiological indicators on individuals.

partnership—A group of individuals or organizations that work together on a common task or goal. This may include key contacts, community-based organizations, county agencies, policy makers, and advocacy groups.

physical activity—Bodily movement produced by skeletal muscles that results in energy expenditure and that is positively correlated with physical fitness.

physical fitness—Set of attributes that people have or achieve relating to their ability to perform physical activity. The health-related components of physical fitness include the following: body composition, cardiovascular endurance, flexibility, muscular endurance, and muscular strength.

pilot test—Also known as piloting or a pilot study, a set of procedures used by planners and evaluators to try out various processes during program development on a small group of subjects before implementation with the purpose of identifying and, if necessary, correcting problems before implementation.

point-of-decision prompt—Item that encourages people to make a certain decision, for example, a sign placed by elevators and escalators that encourage people to use nearby stairs for health benefits or weight loss. These signs tell people about a health benefit from taking the stairs and remind people who already want to be more active that an opportunity to do so is at hand.

policy change—A modification to laws, regulations, formal and informal rules, and standards of practice. Policy change may occur at the organizational, community, or societal level.

policy—Laws, regulations, and rules (both formal and informal) within a setting.

predisposing factors—Factors that influence an action; include knowledge and affective traits such as a person's attitude, values, beliefs, and perceptions.

preparation stage—A Transtheoretical Model stage at which people intend to take action in the next month and or have unsuccessfully taken action in the past year.

prevalence—Existing cases of a disease, often expressed as a percentage of the population or as a rate per thousand population. For example, in 2003, 45.9 percent of adults aged 18 years and older in the United States, Puerto Rico, Guam, and the U.S. Virgin Islands met the physical activity recommendations.

primary prevention—Activities intended to prevent the onset of disease in the first place.

process evaluation—A combination of measurements obtained during implementation of program activities to control, ensure, or improve the quality of performance or delivery. Added to preprogram studies, this makes up formative evaluation.

program—A set of planned activities often beyond the scope of a single intervention designed to lead toward a given mission. A program may include multiple interventions.

proximity—Measured through the mix of homes, shops, schools, and other destinations.

random assignment—Obtained by taking a list of participants and choosing the sample by following a table of random numbers, giving each individual an equal chance of being selected.

reach—In communications, an estimation of the number of people or households exposed to a specific media message during a specific period of time. When describing a program, it is the number of people attending or exposed to an intervention, program, or message.

regular physical activity—Regular, weekly participation in at least 150 minutes of moderate-intensity aerobic physical activity (e.g., five days a week, 30 minutes per day), 75 minutes of vigorous-intensity aerobic physical activity (e.g., three days a week, 25 minutes per day), or an equivalent combination of both. Activity should be performed in episodes of at least 10 minutes, and preferably spread throughout the week.

reinforcement—An event that follows a behavior, which in turn increases the probability that the same behavior will be repeated in the future.

residential density—Land use measure, total number of residents per land area.

safe environment—Surroundings that are physically safe (i.e., that minimize the potential for bodily injury or harm) as well as emotionally safe (i.e., free from ridicule or harassment). In the process of behavior change, people need opportunities to practice newly acquired behaviors or skills in an environment that allows them to perform imperfectly, free from the potential danger of physical or emotional harm.

self-efficacy—A construct of the social cognitive theory that refers to an individual's belief in his competence to perform certain desired tasks or behavior and that changes with regard to the specific behavior or action being addressed (i.e., may be competent in performing aerobic exercise but not in reducing fat in the diet).

settings—Describe the site where the interventions occur. Also includes what was formerly called "channel" (e.g., community, faith, schools, childcare, work site).

smart growth—Development that serves the economy, community, and natural environment by providing healthy communities, economic development and jobs, strong neighborhoods, and transportation choices.

social cognitive theory—Previously known as social learning theory, combines the stimulus response and cognitive theories and belief that although reinforcement is an integral part of learning, it emphasizes the role of subjective hypotheses or expectations held by the individual.

social marketing—Applying advertising and marketing principles and techniques (i.e., applying the planning variables of product, promotion, place, and price) to health or social issues with the intent of bringing about behavior change. Similar to the commercial marketing principles, the process offers benefits the audience wants, reduces barriers the audience faces, and uses persuasion to influence intentions to act favorably.

sprawl—Any environment characterized by a population that is widely dispersed in low-density residential development; rigid separation of homes, shops, and workplaces; a lack of distinct, thriving activity centers, such as strong downtowns or suburban town centers; and a network of roads characterized by large block size and poor access from one place to another.

stakeholder—An individual or organization that has something to gain or lose as a result of health-promotion program efforts or ideas. This person or group has a stake in the outcome of the program and a unique appreciation of the issues and problems involved.

surveillance—The systematic, ongoing assessment of the health of a community, based on the collection, interpretation, and use of health data and information. National health, transportation, school policy, and work-site policy surveys are used for physical activity surveillance to monitor trends and generate research hypotheses.

survey—A standard list of questions to obtain information, either directly or indirectly, from a selected group of individuals about their opinions, attitudes, knowledge, and practices.

target audience or target population—A group of individuals or an organization, community, subpopulation, or society that is the focus of a specific health promotion effort.

Task Force on Community Preventive Services—Group that makes recommendations for the use of various interventions based on the evidence gathered through the rigorous and systematic scientific reviews of published studies conducted by the review teams of the *Community Guide*. The findings from the reviews are published in peer-reviewed journals and also made available on www.thecommunityguide.org.

The Guide to Community Preventive Services (aka the *Community Guide*)—Publication that serves as a filter for scientific literature on specific health problems that can be large, inconsistent, uneven in quality, and even inaccessible. The *Community Guide* summarizes what is known about the effectiveness, economic efficiency, and feasibility of interventions to promote community health and prevent disease.

theory of planned behavior—An extension of the theory of reasoned action that addresses the problem of incomplete volitional control (as in a smoker who intends to quit) but has the additional determinant of intention, which refers to the perceived ease or difficulty of performing the behavior and is assumed to reflect past experiences as well as future impediments and obstacles.

theory—Systematic interpretations to help health educators better understand what influences health (relevant individual, group, and institutional behaviors) and to thereupon plan effective interventions directed at health-beneficial results.

transtheoretical model—An integrative framework for understanding how individuals and populations progress toward adopting and maintaining health behavior change for optimal health. This model uses stages of change (precontemplation, contemplation, preparation, action, and maintenance stages) to integrate processes and principles of change from across major theories of interventions. The core constructs of the model include the stages of change, the processes of change, the pros and cons of changing, self-efficacy, and temptation. In addition, this model is based on critical assumptions about the nature of behavior change and interventions that can best facilitate change.

universal design—An architectural approach to accessibility that focuses on making all aspects of an environment accessible to all people, regardless of physical ability or disability. It increases the overall usability of the environment, accommodates a wide range of individual preferences and abilities, minimizes hazards and adverse consequences, is easy to understand, and communicates necessary information effectively. Examples include a power door at a facility entrance, uncluttered fitness space, and multistation exercise equipment.

urban form—A composite of several characteristics such as connectivity, density, land use, and transportation systems (e.g., bikeways, bus systems).

vigorous-intensity physical activity—Hard or very hard physical activity requiring sustained, rhythmic movements and 6 or more METs of energy expenditure or 7 calories per minute (i.e., performed at 70 percent or more of maximum heart rate according to age (220 minus a person's age). Vigorous activity is intense enough to represent a substantial physical challenge to an individual and results in

- a large increase in breathing or heart rate (conversation is difficult or "broken") and
- a perceived exertion of 15 or greater on the Borg scale.

Vigorous activity, for example, is the effort a healthy individual might expend while jogging, mowing the lawn with a nonmotorized push mower, participating in high-impact aerobic dancing, swimming continuous laps, bicycling uphill, carrying more than 25 pounds (11 kg) up a flight of stairs, or standing or walking with more than 50 pounds (22 kg).

zoning—A legal tool of local government to specify how land is to be used based on health, safety, and welfare considerations.

REFERENCES

Preface

U.S. Department of Health & Human Services. 1996. *Physical Activity and Health: A Report of the Surgeon General.* Atlanta: U.S. Department of Health & Human Services, Centers for Disease Control and Prevention, National Center for Chronic Disease Prevention and Health Promotion.

U.S. Department of Health & Human Services, Public Health Service, Centers for Disease Control and Prevention, National Center for Chronic Disease Prevention and Health Promotion, Division of Nutrition and Physical Activity. 1999. *Promoting Physical Activity: A Guide for Community Action.* Champaign, IL: Human Kinetics.

Introduction

U.S. Department of Health & Human Services. 1996. *Physical Activity and Health: A Report of the Surgeon General.* Atlanta: U.S. Department of Health & Human Services, Centers for Disease Control and Prevention, National Center for Chronic Disease Prevention and Health Promotion.

U.S. Department of Health & Human Services, Public Health Service, Centers for Disease Control and Prevention, National Center for Chronic Disease Prevention and Health Promotion, Division of Nutrition and Physical Activity. 1999. *Promoting Physical Activity: A Guide for Community Action.* Champaign, IL: Human Kinetics.

U.S. Department of Health & Human Services. 2000. *Healthy People 2010*, 2nd edition. With *Understanding and Improving Health* and *Objectives for Improving Health*. 2 volumes. Washington, DC: U.S. Government Printing Office.

U.S. Public Health Service. 1964. *Smoking and Health: Report of the Advisory Committee to the Surgeon General of the Public Health Service.* U.S. Department of Health, Education, and Welfare, Public Health Service, Center for Disease Control. PHS Publication No.1103.

Zaza S, Briss PA, Harris KW (Eds). Task Force on Community Preventive Services. 2005. *The Guide to Community Preventive Services: What Works to Promote Health?* New York: Oxford University Press.

Chapter 1

Abbott RD, White LR, Ross GW, Masaki KH, Curb JD, Petrovich H. 2004. Walking and dementia in physically capable elderly men. *Journal of the American Medical Association* 292(12):1447-1453.

Ainsworth BE, Haskell WL, Whitt MC, Irwin ML, Swartz AM, Strath SJ, et al. 2000. Compendium of physical activities: an update of activity codes and MET intensities. *Medicine and Science in Sports and Exercise* 32(9 suppl):s498-s4504.

American Psychiatric Association. 1994. *Diagnostic and Statistical Manual of Mental Disorders, Fourth Edition (DSM-IV).* Washington DC: American Psychiatric Association, 320-327.

Biddle SJH, Fox KR, Boutcher SH (Eds). 2000. *Physical Activity and Psychological Well-Being.* New York: Routledge.

Binder EF, Schechtman KB, Ehsani AA, Steger-May K, Brown M, Sinacore KE, Yarasheski KE, Holloszy JO. 2002. Effects of exercise training on frailty in community-dwelling older adults: results of a randomized controlled trial. *Journal of the American Geriatrics Society* 50:1921-1928.

Brown DR, Raglin JS, Morgan WP. 1993. Effects of exercise and rest on the state anxiety and blood pressure of physically challenged college students. *Journal of Sports Medicine and Physical Fitness* 33:300-305.

Butcher LR, Thomas A, Backx K, Roberts A, Webb R, Morris K. 2008. Low-intensity exercise exerts beneficial effects on plasma lipids via PPARgamma. *Medicine & Science in Sports & Exercise* 40(7):1263-1270.

Campbell A, Robertson M, Gardner M, Norton R, Tilyard M, Buchner D. 1997. Randomized controlled trial of a general practice programme of home based exercise to prevent falls in elderly women. *British Medical Journal* 315:1065-1069.

Centers for Disease Control and Prevention. 2009. *Cancer Prevention and Control.* www.cdc.gov/cancer.

Centers for Disease Control and Prevention. n.d. *United States Cancer Statistics.* http://apps.nccd.cdc.gov/uscs/.

Commonwealth Department of Health and Aged Care. 1999. National physical activity guidelines for Australians. Sydney: Active Australia.

deVries HA. 1987. Tension reduction with exercise. In: Morgan WP, Goldstein SE (Eds), *Exercise and Mental Health.* Washington, DC: Hemisphere; pp. 99-104.

deVries HA, Adams GM. 1972. Electromyographic comparison of single doses of exercise and meprobanmate as to effects on muscular relaxation. *American Journal of Physical Medicine* 51:130-141.

DiPietro L, Kohl HW III, Barlow CE, Blair SN. 1998. Improvements in cardiorespiratory fitness attenuate age-related weight gain in healthy men and women: the Aerobics Center Longitudinal Study. *International Journal of Obesity and Related Metabolic Disorders* 22(1):55-62.

Dishman RK, Washburn RA, Heath GW. 2004. Mental health. In: Dishman RK, Washburn RA, Heath GW (Eds), *Physical Activity Epidemiology.* Champaign, IL: Human Kinetics.

Durstine JL. 1997. *ACSM's Exercise Management for Persons With Chronic Diseases and Disabilities.* Champaign, IL: Human Kinetics.

Felson DT, Niu J, Clancy M, Sack B, Aliabadi P. 2007. Effect of recreational physical activities on the development of knee osteoarthritis in older adults of different weights: the Framingham Study. *Arthritis and Rheumatism* 57(1):6-12.

Frontera WR, Slovik DM, Dawson DM (Eds). 2006. *Exercise in Rehabilitation Medicine.* Champaign, IL: Human Kinetics.

Goodwin RD. 2003. Association between physical activity and mental disorders among adults in the United States. *Preventive Medicine* 36:698-703.

Goodman LR, Warren MP. 2005. The female athlete and menstrual function. *Obstetrics and Gynecology* 17(5):466-470.

Guilleminault C, Clerk A, Black J, Labanowski M, Pelayo R, Claman D. 1995. Nondrug treatment trials in psychophysiologic insomnia. *Archives of Internal Medicine* 155(8):838-844.

Hamman RF, Wing RR, Edelstein SL, Lachin JM, Bray GA, Delahanty L, Hoskin M, Kriska AM, Mayer-Davis EJ, Pi-Sunyer X, Regensteiner J, Venditti B, Wylie-Rosett J. 2006. Effect of weight loss with lifestyle intervention on risk of diabetes. *Diabetes Care* 29(9):2102-2107.

Hart DJ, Doyle DV, Spector TD. 1999. Incidence and risk factors for radiographic knee osteoarthritis in middle-aged women: the Chingford Study. *Arthritis and Rheumatism* 42(1):17-24.

Haskell WL, Lee I-M, Pate RR, Powell KE, Blair SN, Franklin BA, et al. 2007. Physical activity and public health: updated recommendation for adults from the American College of Sports Medicine and the American Heart Association. *Medicine & Science in Sports & Exercise* 39(8):1423-1434.

Heyn P, Abreu BC, Ottenbacher KJ. 2004. The effects of exercise training on elderly persons with cognitive impairment and dementia: a meta-analysis. *Archives of Physical Medicine and Rehabilitation* 85(10):1694-1704.

Hillsdon MM, Brunner EJ, Guralnik JM, Marmot MG. 2005. Prospective study of physical activity and physical function, in early old age. *American Journal of Preventive Medicine* 28:245-250.

Hootman JM, Macera CA, Ainsworth BE, Addy CL, Marin M, Blair SN. 2002. Epidemiology of musculoskeletal injuries among sedentary and physically active adults. *Medicine & Science in Sports & Exercise* 34:838-844.

Hootman JM, Macera CA, Helmick CG, Blair SN. 2003. Influence of physical activity-related joint stress on the risk of self-reported hip/knee osteoarthritis: a new method to quantify physical activity. *Preventive Medicine* 36:636-644.

Huang Y, Macera CA, Blair SN, Brill PA, Kohl HW III, Kronenfeld JJ. 1998. Physical fitness, physical activity, and functional limitation in adults age 40 and older. *Medicine & Science in Sports & Exercise* 30:1430-1435.

Karper WB, Hopewell R. 1998. Exercise, immunity, acute respiratory infections, and homebound older adults. *Home Care Provider* 3(1):41-46.

Katzmarzyk PT, Janssen I. 2004. The economic costs associated with physical activity and obesity in Canada: an update. *Canadian Journal of Applied Physiology* 29(1):90-115.

King AC, Baumann K, O'Sullivan P, Wilcox S, Castro C. 2002. Effects of moderate-intensity exercise on physiological, behavioral, and emotional responses to family caregiving: a randomized controlled trial. *Journals of Gerontology, Series A, Biological Sciences and Medical Sciences* 57(1):M26-M36.

King AC, Oman RF, Brassington GS, Bliwise DL, Haskell WL. 1997. Moderate-intensity exercise and self-rated quality of sleep in older adults: a randomized controlled trial. *Journal of the American Medical Association* 277(1):32-37.

Kramer AF, Colcombe SJ, McAuley E, Eriksen KI, Scalf P, Jerome GJ, Marquez DX, Elavsky S, Webb AG. 2003. Enhancing brain and cognitive function of older adults through fitness training. *Journal of Molecular Neuroscience* 20:213-221.

Kostka T, Berthouze SE, Lacour J, Bonnefoy M. 2000. The symptomatology of upper respiratory tract infections and exercise in elderly people. *Medicine & Science in Sports & Exercise* 32(1):46-51.

Knowler WC, Barrett-Connor E, Fowler SE, Hamman RF, Lachin JM, Walker EA, Nathan DM; Diabetes Prevention Program Research Group. 2002. Reduction in the incidence of type 2 diabetes with lifestyle intervention or metformin. *New England Journal of Medicine* 346(6):393-403.

Larson EB, Wang L, Bowen JD, McCormick WC, Teri L, Crane P, Kukull W. 2006. Exercise is associated with reduced risk for incident dementia among persons 65 years of age and older. *Annals of Internal Medicine* 144(2):73-81.

Lee I-M, Oguma Y. 2006. Physical activity. In Schottenfeld D, Fraumeni JF Jr (Eds), *Cancer Epidemiology and Prevention,* 3rd edition. New York: Oxford University Press; pp. 449-467.

Leveille SG, Guralnik JM, Ferrucci L, Langlois JA. 1999. Aging successfully until death in old age: opportunities for increasing active life expectancy. *American Journal of Epidemiology* 149:654-664.

Lewis CE, Smith DE, Wallace DD, Williams OD, Bild DE, Jacobs DR Jr. 1997. Seven-year trends in body weight and associations with lifestyle and behavioral characteristics in black and white young adults: the CARDIA study. *American Journal of Public Health* 87(4):635-642.

Lindsay J, Laurin D, Verreault R, Hebert R, Helliwell B, Hill GB, McDowell I. 2002. Risk factors for Alzheimer's disease: a prospective analysis from the Canadian Study of Health and Aging. *American Journal of Epidemiology* 156(5):445-453.

Lord SR, Castell S, Corcoran J, Dayhew J, Matters B, Shan A, Williams P. 2003. The effect of group exercise on physical functioning and falls in frail older people living in retirement villages: a randomized controlled trial. *Journal of the American Geriatrics Society* 51:1685-1692.

Luukinen H, Lehtola S, Jokelainen J, Vaananen-Sainio R, Lotvonen S, Koistinen P. 2006. Prevention of disability by exercise among the elderly: a population-based, randomized controlled trial. *Scandinavian Journal of Primary Health Care* 24:199-205.

Mackinnon LT. 2000. Chronic exercise training effects on immune function. *Medicine & Science in Sports & Exercise* 32(7 suppl):s369-s376.

Manson JE, Greenland PHP, LaCroix AZ, Stefanick ML, Mouton, CP, Oberman A, Perri MG, Sheps DS, Pettinger MB, Siscovick DS. 2002. Walking compared with vigorous exercise for the prevention of cardiovascular events in women. *New England Journal of Medicine* 347:716-725.

Martinsen EW, Morgan WP. 1997. Antidepressant effects of physical activity. In: Morgan WP (Ed), *Physical Activity and Mental Health*. Washington, DC: Taylor and Francis; pp. 93-126.

Matthews CE, Ockene IS, Freedson PS, Rosal MC, Merriam PA, Hebert JR. 2002. Moderate to vigorous physical activity and risk of upper-respiratory tract infection. *Medicine & Science in Sports & Exercise* 34(8):1242-1248.

McAuley E, Konopack JF, Motl RW, Morris KS, Doerksen SE, Rosengren KR. 2006. Physical activity and quality of life in older adults: influence of health status and self-efficacy. *Annals of Behavioral Medicine* 31(1):99-103.

Morgan WP (Ed). 1997. *Physical Activity and Mental Health*. Washington, DC: Taylor and Francis.

Morris JN, Heady JA, Raffle PAB, Roberts CG, Parks JW. 1953. Coronary heart disease and physical activity of work. *Lancet* 2:1111-1120.

Myers J, Prakash M, Froelicher V, Do D, Partington S, Atwood JE. 2002. Exercise capacity and mortality among men referred for exercise testing. *New England Journal of Medicine* 346:793-801.

National Academy of Sciences, Institute of Medicine. 2002. Dietary reference intakes for energy, carbohydrate, fiber, fat, fatty acids, cholesterol, protein, and amino acids. Washington, DC: National Academies Press.

Nattiv A, Loucks AB, Manore MM, Sanborn CF, Sundgot-Borgen J, Warren MP. 2007. The female triad: special communication American College of Sports Medicine position stand. *Medicine & Science in Sports & Exercise* 39(10):1867-1882.

Netz Y, Wu MJ, Beck BJ, Tenenbaum G. 2005. Physical activity and psychological well-being in advanced age: a meta-analysis of intervention studies. *Psychology and Aging* 20(2):272-284.

Ostbye T, Taylor DH, Jung SH. 2002. A longitudinal study of the effects of tobacco smoking and other modifiable risk factors on ill health in middle-aged and old Americans: results from the Health and Retirement Study and Asset and Health Dynamics among the Oldest Old survey. *Preventive Medicine* 34:334-345.

Paffenbarger RS, Hyde RT, Wing AL, Hsieh CC. 1986. Physical activity, all-cause mortality, and longevity of college alumni. *New England Journal of Medicine* 314:605-613.

Paffenbarger RS, Wing AL, Hyde RT. 1978. Physical activity as an index of heart attack risk in college alumni. *American Journal of Epidemiology* 108(3):161-175.

Pate RR, Pratt M, Blair SN, Haskell WL, Macera CA, Bouchard C, et al. 1996. Physical activity and public health: a recommendation from the Centers for Disease Control and Prevention and the American College of Sports Medicine, *Journal of the American Medical Association* 273:402-407.

Physical Activity Guidelines Advisory Committee. 2008. Physical Activity Guidelines Advisory Committee Report, 2008. Washington, DC: U.S. Department of Health and Human Services.

Puetz TW, O'Connor PJ, Dishman RK. 2006. Effects of chronic exercise on feelings of energy and fatigue: a quantitative synthesis. *Psychological Bulletin* 132:866-876.

Raglin JS. 1997. Anxiolytic effects of physical activity. In Morgan WP (Ed), *Physical Activity and Mental Health*. Washington, DC: Taylor and Francis; pp. 107-126.

Raglin JS, Morgan WP. 1987. Influence of exercise and quiet rest on state anxiety and blood pressure. *Medicine & Science in Sports & Exercise* 19:456-463.

Robertson C, Campbell AJ, Gardner MM, Devlin N. 2002. Preventing injuries in older people by preventing falls: a meta-analysis of individual-level data. *Journal of the American Geriatrics Society* 50:905-911.

Rogers LQ, Macera CA, Hootman JM, Ainsworth BE, Blair SN. 2002. The association between joint stress from physical activity and self-reported osteoarthritis: an analysis of the Cooper Clinic data. *Osteoarthritis and Cartilage* 10:617-622.

Rogers RL, Meyer JS, Mortel KF. 1990. After reaching retirement age physical activity sustains cerebral perfusion and cognition. *Journal of the American Geriatrics Society* 38:123-128.

Rozanski A, Blumenthal JA, Kaplan J. 1999. Impact of psychological factors on the pathogenesis of cardiovascular disease and implications for therapy. *Circulation* 99:2192-2217.

Sjosten N, Sivela S. 2006. The effects of physical exercise on depressive symptoms among the aged: a systematic review. *International Journal of Geriatric Psychiatry* 21(5):410-418.

Strong WB, Malina RM, Bumkie CJR, Daniels SR, Dishman RK, Gutin B, Hergenroeder AC, Must A, Nixon PA, Pivarnik JM, Rowland T, Trost S, Trudeau F. 2005. Evidence based physical activity for school-age youth. *Journal of Pediatrics* 146:732-737.

Taaffe, DR, Irie F, Masaki KH, Abbott RD, Petrovitch H, Ross GW, White LR. 2008. Physical activity, physical function, and incident dementia in elderly men: the Honolulu–Asia Aging Study. *Journal of Gerontology* 63:529-535.

Taylor AH. 2000. Physical activity, anxiety, and stress. In: Biddle SJH, Fox K., Boutcher SH (Eds), *Physical Activity and Psychological Well-being.* New York: Routledge; pp. 10-45.

Thompson PD, Franklin BA, Balady GJ, Blair SN, Corrado D, Estes NAM III, Fulton JE, Gordon NF, Haskell WL, Link MS, Maron BJ, Mittleman MA, Pelliccia A, Wenger NK, Willich SN, Costa F. 2007. Exercise and acute cardiovascular events: placing the risks into perspective: a scientific statement from the American Heart Association, Council on Nutrition, Physical Activity, and Metabolism and the Council on Clinical Cardiology. *Circulation* 115:2358-2368.

Tworoger SS, Yasui Y, Vitiello MV, Schwartz RS, Ulrich CM, Aiello EJ, Irwin ML, Bowen D, Potter JD, McTiernan A. 2003. Effects of a year long moderate-intensity exercise and stretching intervention on sleep quality in postmenopausal women. *Sleep* 26(7): 830-836.

U.S. Department of Health & Human Services. 2004. *Bone Health and Osteoporosis: A Report of the Surgeon General.* Rockville, MD: U.S. Department of Health & Human Services, Office of the Surgeon General.

U.S. Department of Health & Human Services. 1998. *Clinical Guidelines on the Identification, Evaluation, and Treatment of Overweight and Obesity in Adults: The Evidence Report.* Bethesda, MD: National Institutes of Health, National Heart, Lung, and Blood Institute; p. x.

U.S. Department of Health & Human Services. 2008. *2008 Physical Activity Guidelines for Americans.* www.health.gov/PAGuidelines/guidelines/default.aspx

U.S. Department of Health and Human Services. 1999. *Mental Health: A Report of the Surgeon General.* Rockville, MD: U.S. Department of Health and Human Services, Substance Abuse and Mental Health Services Administration, Center for Mental Health Services, National Institute of Mental Health.

Weuve J, Kang JH, Manson JE, Breteler MMB, Ware JH, Grodstein F. 2004. Physical activity including walking, and cognitive function in older women. *Journal of the American Medical Association* 292(12):1454-1461.

Williams PT, Wood PD. 2006. The effects of changing exercise levels on weight and age-related weight gain. *International Journal of Obesity (London)* 30(3):543-551.

Wong PC, Chia MY, Tsou IY, Wansaicheong GK, Tan B, Wang JC, Tan J, Kim CG, Boh G, Lim D. 2008. Effects of a 12-week exercise training programme on aerobic fitness, body composition, blood lipids and c-reactive protein in adolescents with obesity. *Annals of the Academy of Medicine, Singapore* 37(4):286-288.

Woolf-May K, Kearney EM, Owen A, Jones DW, Davison RCR, Bird SR. 1999. The efficacy of accumulated short bouts versus single daily bouts of brisk walking in improving aerobic fitness and blood lipid profiles. *Health Education Research* 14(6):803-815.

Xuemei S, LaMonte MJ, Laditka JN, Hardin JW, Chase N, Hooker SP, Blair SN. 2007. Cardio-respiratory fitness and adiposity as mortality predictors in older adults. *Journal of the American Medical Association* 298 (21):2507-2516.

Yaffe K, Barnes D, Nevitt M, Lui L-Y, Covinsky K. 2001. A prospective study of physical activity and cognitive decline in elderly women: women who walk. *Archives of Internal Medicine* 161:1703-1708.

Yiannis TE, Amalia YE, Dimitrios B, Stavros KA, Labros SS. 2007. A single bout of brisk walking increases basal very low-density lipoprotein triacylglycerol clearance in young men. *Metabolism* 56(8):1037-1043.

Youngstedt SD, O'Connor PJ, Dishman RK. 1997. The effects of acute exercise on sleep: a quantitative synthesis. *Sleep* 20(3):203-214.

Zhang JQ, Ji LL, Nunez G, Feathers S, Hart CL, Yao WX. 2004. Effect of exercise timing on postprandial lipemia in hypertriglyceridemic men. *Canadian Journal of Applied Physiology* 590-603.

Chapter 2

Agency for Healthcare Research and Quality, U.S. Department of Health & Human Services. 1998. *Clinician's Handbook of Preventive Services,* 2nd edition.

American Academy of Pediatrics. 1994. Assessing physical activity and fitness in the office setting. *Pediatrics* 93 686-689.

American College of Sports Medicine. 2000. Exercise testing and prescription for children, the elderly, and pregnant women. In: Franklin BA, Whaley MH, Howley ET (Eds), *ACSM's Guidelines for Exercise Testing and Prescription,* 6th edition. Baltimore: Lippincott Williams & Wilkins; pp. 217-234.

American College of Sports Medicine position statement on the recommended quantity and quality of exercise for developing and maintaining fitness in healthy adults. 1978. *Medicine & Science in Sports & Exercise* 10(3):vii-x.

American College of Sports Medicine position stand. 1990 The recommended quantity and quality of exercise for developing and maintaining cardiorespiratory and muscular fitness in healthy adults. *Medicine & Science in Sports & Exercise* 22(2):265-274.

American College of Sports Medicine Position Stand. 1998 Exercise and physical activity for older adults. *Medicine & Science in Sports & Exercise* 30(6):992-1008.

American College of Sports Medicine. 2009. Position stand: exercise and physical activity for older adults. *Medicine & Science in Sports & Exercise* 41(7):1510-1530.

American Heart Association. 1972. *Exercise Testing and Training of Apparently Healthy Individuals: A Handbook for Physicians*. Dallas: American Heart Association.

American Heart Association. 1975. *Exercise Testing and Training of Individuals With Heart Disease or at High Risk for Its Development: A Handbook for Physicians*. Dallas: American Heart Association.

American Medical Association. 1996. *Guidelines for Adolescent Preventive Services (GAPS): Recommendations Monograph,* 2nd edition. Chicago: American Medical Association.

Byers T, Nestle M, McTiernan A, et al. 2002. American Cancer Society guidelines on nutrition and physical activity for cancer prevention: reducing the risk of cancer with healthy food choices and physical activity. *CA: A Cancer Journal for Clinicians* 52:92-119.

Health Canada. 2002a. *Canada's Physical Activity Guide for Children*. Ottawa, Canada: Minister of Public Works and Government Services.

Health Canada. 2002b. *Canada's Physical Activity Guide for Youth*. Ottawa, Canada: Minister of Public Works and Government Services.

Centers for Disease Control and Prevention. 1997. Guidelines for school and community programs to promote lifelong physical activity among young people. *Morbidity and Mortality Weekly Report* 46(No. RR-6):1-36.

Corbin CB, Pangrazi RP. 1998. *Physical Activity for Children: A Statement of Guidelines.* Reston, VA: National Association for Sport and Physical Education.

Cress ME, Buchner DM, Prohaska T, Rimmer J, Brown M, Macera C, et al. 2004. Physical activity programs and behavior counseling in older adult populations. *Medicine & Science in Sports & Exercise* 36(11):1997-2003.

Duncan JJ, Gordon NF, Scott CB. 1991 Women walking for health and fitness. How much is enough? *Journal of the American Medical Association* 266(23):3295-3299.

Fletcher GF. 1997. How to implement physical activity in primary and secondary prevention: a statement for healthcare professionals from the Task Force on Risk Reduction, American Heart Association. *Circulation* 96:355-357.

Fulton JE, Garg M, Galuska DA, Rattay KT, Caspersen CJ. 2004. Public health and clinical recommendations for physical activity and physical fitness: special focus on overweight youth. *Sports Medicine* 34(9):581-599.

Haskell WL, Lee IM, Pate RR, Powell KE, Blair SN, Franklin BA, Macera CA, Heath GW, Thompson PD, Bauman A. 2007. Physical activity and public health: updated recommendation for adults from the American College of Sports Medicine and the American Heart Association. *Medicine & Science in Sports & Exercise* 39(8):1423-1434.

Morris JN, Heady JA, Raffle PAB, Roberts CG, Parks JW 1953. Coronary heart disease and physical activity of work. *Lancet* 2:1111-1120.

National Academy of Sciences, Institute of Medicine. 2002. *Dietary Reference Intakes for Energy, Carbohydrate, Fiber, Fat, Fatty Acids, Cholesterol, Protein, and Amino Acids.* Washington, DC: National Academy Press.

National Association for Sport and Physical Education. 2000. *Active Start: A Statement of Physical Activity Guidelines for Children Birth to Five Years.* Reston, VA: NASPE.

National Association for Sport and Physical Education. 2004. *Physical Activity for Children: A Statement of Guidelines for Children ages 5-12,* 2nd edition. Reston, VA: NASPE.

Nelson ME, Rejeski WJ, Blair SN, Duncan PW, Judge JO, King AC, Macera CA, Castaneda-Sceppa C. 2007. Physical activity and public health in older adults: recommendation from the American College of Sports Medicine and the American Heart Association. *Medicine & Science in Sport & Exercise* 39(8):1435-1445.

NIH Consensus Development Panel on Physical Activity and Cardiovascular Health. 1996 Physical activity and cardiovascular health. NIH Consensus Conference. *Journal of the American Medical Association* 1996 Jul 17:276(3):241-246.

Commonwealth Department of Health and Aged Care. 1999. *National Physical Activity Guidelines for Australians.* Sydney: Active Australia.

Paffenbarger RS Jr, Wing AL, Hyde RT. 1978. Physical activity as an index of heart attack risk in college alumni. *American Journal of Epidemiology* 108(3):161-175.

Paffenbarger RS, Hale WE. 1975. Work activity and coronary heart mortality. *New England Journal of Medicine* 292(11):545-550.

Pate RR, Pratt M, Blair SN, et al. 1995. Physical activity and public health: a recommendation from the Centers for Disease Control and Prevention and the American College of Sports Medicine. *Journal of the American Medical Association* 273:402-407.

Pate RR, Trost SM, Williams C. 1998. Critique of existing guidelines for physical activity in young people. In: Biddle S, Sallis J, Cavill N (Eds), *Young and Active? Young People and Health Enhancing Physical Activity: Evidence and Implications.* London: Health Education Authority; pp. 162-176.

Patrick K, Spear B, Holt K, et al. (Eds). 2001. *Bright Futures in Practice: Physical Activity.* Arlington, VA: National Center for Education in Maternal and Child Health.

Physical Activity Guidelines Advisory Committee. 2008. *Physical Activity Guidelines Advisory Committee Report, 2008.* Washington, DC: U.S. Department of Health & Human Services.

Powell KE, Thompson PD, Caspersen CJ, et al. 1987. Physical activity and the incidence of coronary heart disease. *Annual Review of Public Health* 8:253-287.

Robert Wood Johnson Foundation. 2001. National blueprint: increasing physical activity among adults age 50 and older. *Journal of Aging and Physical Activity* 9(suppl):s1-s28.

Sallis JF, Patrick K. 1994. Physical activity guidelines for adolescents: consensus statement. *Pediatric Exercise Science* 6:302-314.

Strong WB, Malina RM, Blimkie CJ, Daniels SR, Dishman RK, Gutin B, Hergenroeder AC, Must A, Nixon PA, Pivarnik JM, Rowland T, Trost S, Trudeau F. 2005. Evidence based physical activity for school-age youth. *Journal of Pediatrics* 146(6):732-737. www.healthysd.gov/Documents/Youth%20PA%20recs.pdf.

Taylor HL, Kleptar E, Keys A, Parlin W, Blackburn H, Puchner T. 1962. Death rates among physically active and sedentary employees of the railroad industry. *American Journal of Public Health* 52:1697-1707.

U.S. Department of Agriculture, U.S. Department of Health & Human Services. 2000. *Nutrition and Your Health: Dietary Guidelines for Americans*, 5th edition. Washington, DC: U.S. Government Printing Office.

U.S. Department of Health & Human Services and U.S. Department of Agriculture. 2005. *Dietary Guidelines for Americans,* 6th edition, Washington, DC: U.S. Government Printing Office.

U.S. Department of Health & Human Services. 2008. *2008 Physical Activity Guidelines for Americans*. Washington, DC: U.S. Government Printing Office, October 2008. www.health.gov/paguidelines

U.S. Department of Health & Human Services. 2000. Physical Activity and Fitness. In: *Healthy People 2010,* 2nd edition. With *Understanding and Improving Health* and *Objectives for Improving Health*. 2 vols. Washington, DC: U.S. Government Printing Office 122-1 to 22-39. www.healthypeople.gov/Document/HTML/Volume2/22Physical.htm#_Toc490380800.

U.S. Department of Health & Human Services. 1996. *Physical Activity and Health: A Report of the Surgeon General.* Atlanta: U.S. Department of Health & Human Services, Centers for Disease Control and Prevention, National Center for Chronic Disease Prevention and Health Promotion.

U.S. Preventive Services Task Force. 1996. *Guide to Clinical Preventive Services,* 2nd edition. Alexandria, VA: International Medical Publishing.

Williams CL, Hayman LL, Daniels SR, et al. 2002. Cardiovascular health in childhood: a statement for health professionals from the Committee on Atherosclerosis, Hypertension, and Obesity in the Young (AHOY) of the Council on Cardiovascular Disease in the Young, American Heart Association. *Circulation* 106:143-160.

Part II

Brownson RC, Baker EA, Housemann RA, Brennan LK, Bacak SJ. 2001. Environmental and policy determinants of physical activity in the United States. *American Journal of Public Health* 91:1995-2003.

Frank LD, Engelke PO. 2001. The built environment and human activity patterns: exploring the impacts of urban form on public health. *Journal of Planning Literature* 16(2):202-218.

Green, LW, Richard, L, Potvin, L. 1996. Ecological foundations of health promotion. *American Journal of Health Promotion* 10:270-281.

Handy SL, Boarnet MG, Ewing R, Killingsworth RE. 2002. How the built environment affects physical activity: views from urban planning. *American Journal of Preventive Medicine* 23(2S):64-73.

Hann NE, Kean TJ Matulionis RM, Russell CM, Sterling TD. 2004. Policy and environmental change: new directions for public health. *Health Promotion Practice* 5(4):377-381.

Heath GW, Brownson RC, Kruger JK, Miles R, Powell KE, Ramsey LT. 2006. The effectiveness of urban design and land use policies and practices to increase physical activity: a systematic review. *Journal of Physical Activity and Health* 3(suppl 1):s55-s76.

Humpel N, Owen N, Leslie E. 2002. Environmental factors associated with adults' participation in physical activity: a review. *American Journal of Preventive Medicine* 22:188-199.

Kahn EB, Ramsey LT, Brownson RC, Heath GW, Howze EH, Powell KE, Stone EJ, Rajab MW, Corso P; Task Force on Community Preventive Services. 2002. The effectiveness of interventions to increase physical activity: a systematic review. *American Journal of Preventive Medicine* 22(4S):73-96.

King AC, Stokols D, Talen E, Brassington GS, Killingsworth R. 2002. Theoretical approaches to the promotion of physical activity: forging a transdisciplinary paradigm. *American Journal of Preventive Medicine* 23(2S):15-25.

McLeroy KR, Bibeau D, Steckler A, Glanz K. 1988. An ecological perspective on health promotion programs. *Health Education Quarterly* 15:351-377.

Saelens BE, Sallis JF, Frank LD. 2003. Environmental correlates of walking and cycling: findings from the transportation, urban design, and planning literatures. *Annals of Behavioral Medicine* 25:80-91.

Sallis JF, Bauman A, Pratt M. 1998. Environmental and policy interventions to promote physical activity. *American Journal of Preventive Medicine* 15(4):379-397.

Sallis JF, Owen N. 1996. Ecological models. In: Glanz K, Lewis FM, Rimer BK (Eds), *Health Behavior and Health Education: Theory, Research, and Practice,* 2nd edition. San Francisco: Jossey-Bass; pp. 403-424.

Schmid TL, Pratt M, Witmer L. 2006. A framework for physical activity policy research. *Journal of Physical Activity & Health* Volume 3 (supplement 1):S20-S29.

U.S. Department of Health & Human Services. 2000. *Healthy People 2010.* Washington, DC: U.S. Government Printing Office.

Zaza S, Briss PA, Harris KW (Eds). Task Force on Community Preventive Services. 2005. *The Guide to Community Preventive Services: What Works to Promote Health?* New York: Oxford University Press.

Chapter 3 Subsection 1

Berkowitz JM, Huhman M, Nollin MJ. 2008. Did augmenting the VERB campaign advertising in select communities have an effect on awareness, attitudes, and physical activity? *American Journal of Preventive Medicine* 34(6 suppl):S257-S266.

Bjaras G, Harberg LK, Sydhoff J, Ostenson CG. 2001. Walking campaign: a model for developing participation in physical activity? Experiences from three campaign periods of the Stockholm Diabetes Prevention Program (SDPP). *Patient Education and Counseling* 42(1):9-14.

Bretthauer-Mueller, R, Berkowitz, JM, Thomas, M, McCarthy, S, Green, LA, Melancon, H, Courtney, AH, Bryant, CA, Dodge, K. 2008. Catalyzing community action within a national campaign: community and national partnerships. *American Journal of Preventive Medicine* 34(6S):S210-S221.

Brown WJ, Mummery K, Eakin E, Schofield G. 2006. 10,000 Steps Rockhampton: evaluation of a whole community approach to improving population levels of physical activity. *Journal of Physical Activity and Health* 3(1):1-14.

Cochrane T, Davey RC. 2008. Increasing uptake of physical activity: a social ecological approach. *Journal of the Royal Society for the Promotion of Health* 128(1):31-40.

De Cocker KA, De Bourdeaudhuij IM, Brown WJ, Cardon GM. 2008. The effect of a pedometer-based physical activity intervention on sitting time. *Preventive Medicine* 47(2):179-181.

De Cocker KA, De Bourdeaudhuij IM, Brown WJ, Cardon GM. 2007. Effects of "10,000 Steps Ghent" a whole-community intervention. *American Journal of Preventive Medicine* 33(6):455-463.

Goodman RM, Wheeler FC, Lee PR. 1995. Evaluation of the Heart To Heart Project: lessons from a community-based chronic disease prevention project. *American Journal of Health Promotion* 9(6):443-455.

Huhman M, Heitzler C, Wong F. 2005. The VERB campaign logic model: a tool for planning and evaluation. *Preventing Chronic Disease [serial online]* 1(3): 1-6.

Huhman ME, Potter LD, Duke JC, Judkins DR, Heitzler CD, Wong FL. 2007. Evaluation of a national physical activity intervention for children: VERB campaign, 2002-2004. *American Journal of Preventive Medicine* 32(1):38-43.

Huhman M, Potter LD, Wong FL, et al. 2005. Effects of a mass media campaign to increase physical activity among children: year-1 results of the VERB campaign. *Pediatrics* 116(2):e277-e284.

Huhman, ME, Potter, LD, Nolin, MJ, Piesse, A, Judkins, DR, Banspach, SW, Wong, FL. 2009. The influence of the VERB campaign on children' physical activity in 2002 to 2006. *American Journal of Public Health* 2009:99(9)1-8.

Jason LA, Greiner BJ, Naylor K, et al. 1991. A large-scale, short-term, media-based weight loss program. *American Journal of Health Promotion* 5(6):432-437.

Jordan KC, Erickson ED, Cox R, et al. 2008. Evaluation of the gold medal schools program. *Journal of the American Dietetics Association* 108(11):1916-1920.

Jenum AK, Anderssen SA, Birkeland KI, et al. 2006. Promoting physical activity in a low-income multiethnic district: effects of a community intervention study to reduce risk factors for type 2 diabetes and cardiovascular disease: a community intervention reducing inactivity. *Diabetes Care* 29(7):1605-1612.

Kahn EB, Ramsey LT, Brownson RC, et al. 2002. The effectiveness of interventions to increase physical activity: a systematic review. *American Journal of Preventive Medicine* 22(4 suppl 1):73-107.

Lorentzen C, Ommundsen Y, Jenum AK, Holme I. 2007. The "Romsas in Motion" community intervention: program exposure and psychosocial mediated relationships to change in stages of change in physical activity. *International Journal of Behavioral Nutrition and Physical Activity* 4:15.

Luepker RV, Murray DM, Jacobs DR Jr, et al. 1994. Community education for cardiovascular disease prevention: risk factor changes in the Minnesota Heart Health Program. *American Journal of Public Health* 84(9):1383-1393.

Malmgren S, Andersson G. 1986. Who were reached by and participated in a one year newspaper health information campaign? *Scandinavian Journal of Public Health Supplement* 14(3):133-140.

Matsuda S, Matsudo V, Andrade D, et al. 2004. Physical activity promotion: experiences and evaluation of the Agita Sao Paulo Program using the ecological mobile model. *Journal of Physical Activity and Health* 1(2):81-97.

Matsudo V, Matsuda S, Andrade D, et al. 2002. Promotion of physical activity in a developing country: the Agita Sao Paulo experience. *Public Health Nutrition* 5(1A):253-261.

Meyer AJ, Nash JD, McAlister AL, et al. 1980. Skills training in a cardiovascular health education campaign. *Journal of Consulting and Clinical Psychology* 48(2):129-142.

Neiger BL, Thackeray R, Hanson CL, Rigby S, Hussey C, Anderson JW. 2008. A policy and environmental response to overweight in childhood: the impact of Gold Medal Schools. *Preventing Chronic Disease* 5(4):A132.

Osler M, Jespersen NB. 1993. The effect of a community-based cardiovascular disease prevention project in a Danish municipality. *Danish Medical Bulletin* 40(4):485-489.

Owen N, Bauman A, Booth M, et al. 1995. Serial mass-media campaigns to promote physical activity: reinforcing or redundant? *American Journal of Public Health* 85(2):244-248.

Pearson TA, Wall S, Lewis C, et al. 2001. Dissecting the "black box" of community intervention: lessons from community-wide cardiovascular disease prevention programs in the US and Sweden. *Scandinavian Journal of Public Health Supplement* 56: 69-78.

Reger B, Cooper L, Booth-Butterfield S, et al. 2002. Wheeling Walks: a community campaign using paid media to encourage walking among sedentary older adults. *Preventive Medicine* 35(3):285-292.

Reger-Nash B, Bauman A, Booth-Butterfield S, et al. 2005. Wheeling Walks: evaluation of a media-based community intervention. *Family and Community Health* 28(1):64-78.

Reger-Nash B, Bauman A, Cooper L, et al. 2008. WV Walks: replication with expanded reach. *Journal of Physical Activity and Health* 5(1):19-27.

Reger-Nash B, Fell P, Spicer D, et al. 2006. BC Walks: replication of a communitywide physical activity campaign. *Preventing Chronic Disease* 3(3):A90.

Task Force on Community Preventive Services. 2002. Recommendations to increase physical activity in communities. *American Journal of Preventive Medicine* 22 (4 suppl):67-72.

Tudor-Smith C, Nutbeam D, Moore L, Catford J. 1998. Effects of the Heartbeat Wales programme over five years on behavioural risks for cardiovascular disease: quasi-experimental comparison of results from Wales and a matched reference area. *British Medical Journal* 316(7134):818-822.

Wimbush E, Macgregor A, Fraser E. 1998. Impacts of a national mass media campaign on walking in Scotland. *Health Promotion International* 13(1):45-53.

Wong F, Huhman M, Heitzler C, et al. 2005. VERB—a social marketing campaign to increase physical activity among youth. *Preventing Chronic Disease [serial online]* 1(3):1-7.

Young DR, Haskell WL, Taylor CB, Fortmann SP. 1996. Effect of community health education on physical activity knowledge, attitudes, and behavior: the Stanford Five-City Project. *American Journal of Epidemiology* 144(3):264-274.

Zaza S, Briss PA, Harris KW (Eds). Task Force on Community Preventive Services. 2005. *The Guide to Community Preventive Services: What Works to Promote Health?* New York: Oxford University Press.

Chapter 3 Subsection 2

Adams J, White M. 2002. A systematic approach to the development and evaluation of an intervention promoting stair use. *Health Education Journal* 61(3):272-286.

Andersen RE, Franckowiak SC, Snyder J, et al. 1998. Can inexpensive signs encourage the use of stairs? Results from a community intervention [see comments]. *Annals of Internal Medicine* 129:363-369.

Andersen RE, Franckowiak SC, Zuzak KB, et al. 2000. Community intervention to encourage stair use among African American commuters [abstract]. *Medicine and Science in Sports and Exercise* 32:38.

van den Auweele Y, Boen F, Schapendonk W, Dornez K. 2005. Promoting stair use among females employees: the effects of a health sign followed by an e-mail. *Journal of Sport & Exercise Psychology* 27:188-196.

Blamey A, Mutrie N, Aitchison T. 1995. Health promotion by encouraged use of stairs. *British Medical Journal* 311:289-290.

Boutelle KN, Jeffery RW, Murray DM, Schmitz MK. 2001. Using signs, artwork, and music to promote stair use in a public building. *American Journal of Public Health* 91(12):2004-2006.

Brownell KD, Stunkard AJ, Albaum JM. 1980. Evaluation and modification of exercise patterns in the natural environment. *American Journal of Psychiatry* 137:1540-1545.

Centers for Disease Control and Prevention. 2007. *StairWELL to Better Health.* www.cdc.gov/nccdphp/dnpa/hwi/toolkits/stairwell/.

Coleman KJ, Gonzalez EC. 2001. Promoting stair use in a US-Mexico border community. *American Journal of Public Health* 91(12):2007-2009.

Dolan L, Weiss A, Lewis RA, Pietrobelli A, Heo H, Faith MS. 2006. Take the stairs instead of the escalator: effect of environmental prompts on community stair use and implications for a national "Small Steps" campaign. *Obesity Reviews* 7:25-32.

Eves FF, Masters RS. 2006. An uphill struggle: effects of a point-of-choice stair climbing intervention in a non-English speaking population. *International Journal of Epidemiology* 35:1286-1290.

Eves FF, Olander EK, Nicoll G, Puig-Ribera A, Griffin C. 2009. Increasing stair climbing in a train station: effects of contextual variables and visibility. *Journal of Environmental Psychology* 29(2):300-303.

Eves FF, Webb OJ. 2006. Worksite interventions to increase stair climbing: reasons for caution. *Preventive Medicine* 43:4-7.

Eves FF, Webb OJ, Mutrie N. 2006. A workplace intervention to promote stair climbing: greater effects in the overweight. *Obesity* 14:2210-2216.

Iversen MK, Händel MN, Jensen EN, Frederiksen P, Heitman BL. 2007. Effect of health-promoting posters placed on the platforms of two train stations in Copenhagen, Denmark, on the choice between taking the stairs or the escalator: a secondary publication. *International Journal of Obesity* 31:950-955.

Kahn, E.B., Ramsey, L.T., Brownson, R.C., et al. 2002. The effectiveness of interventions to increase physical activity: a systematic review. *American Journal of Preventive Medicine* 22(4 suppl):73-107.

Kerr J, Eves F, Carroll D. 2000. Posters can prompt less active people to use the stairs. *Journal of Epidemiology and Community Health* 54:942-943.

Kerr J, Eves F, Carroll D. 2001. Getting more people on the stairs: the impact of a new message format. *Journal of Health Psychology* 91(12):2007-2009.

Kerr NA, Yore MM, Ham SA, Dietz WH. 2004. Increasing stair use in a worksite through environmental changes. *American Journal of Health Promotion* 18(4):312-315.

Kwak L, Kremers SPJ, van Baak MA, Brug J. 2007. A poster-based intervention to promote stair use in blue- and white-collar worksites. *Preventive Medicine* 45:177-181.

Marshall AL, Bauman AC, Patch C, et al. 2002. Can motivational signs prompt increases in physical activity in an Australian health-care facility? *Health Educational Research* 17(6):743-749.

Olander EK, Eves FF, Puig-Ribera A. 2008. Promoting stair climbing: stair-riser banners are better than posters . . . sometimes. *Preventive Medicine* 46(4):308-310.

Russell W, Dzewaltowski D, Ryan G. 1999. The effectiveness of a point-of-decision prompt in deterring sedentary behavior. *American Journal of Health Promotion* 13:257-259.

Russell WD, Hutchison J. 2000. Comparison of health promotion and deterrent prompts in increasing use of the stairs over escalators. *Perceptive Motor Skills* 91(1):55-61.

Soler RE, Leeks KD, Buchanan RC, Brownson RC, Heath GW, Hopkins DH, Task Force on Community Preventive Services. 2010. Point-of-decision prompts to increase stair use: a systematic review update. *American Journal of Preventive Medicine*. 38(2S): s290-s300.

Soler RE, Leeks KD, Hopkins DH. 2005. Point-of-decision prompts to increase stair use: an update. A presentation to the Task Force on Community Preventive Services, Atlanta, GA.

Task Force on Community Preventive Services. 2001. Increasing physical activity: a report on recommendations of the Task Force on Community Preventive Services. *Morbidity and Mortality Weekly Report* 50(No. RR-18):1-16.

U.S. Department of Health and Human Services, Public Health Service, Centers for Disease Control and Prevention, National Center for Chronic Disease Prevention and Health Promotion, Division of Nutrition and Physical Activity. 1999. *Promoting Physical Activity: A Guide for Community Action.* Champaign, IL: Human Kinetics: p. 364.

Webb OJ, Eves FF. 2005. Promoting stair climbing: single vs. multiple messages. *American Journal of Public Health* 95:1543-1544.

Webb OJ, Eves FF. 2007. Promoting stair climbing: intervention effects generalize to a subsequent stair ascent. *American Journal of Health Promotion* 22:114-119.

Zaza S, Briss PA, Harris KW (Eds). Task Force on Community Preventive Services. 2005. *The Guide to Community Preventive Services: What Works to Promote Health?* New York: Oxford University Press.

Chapter 4 Subsection 1

Allegrante JP, Michela JL. 1990. Impact of a school-based workplace health promotion program on morale of inner-city teachers. *Journal of School Health* 60:25-28.

American Cancer Society. 1999. *Improving School Health: A Guide to School Health Councils.* Atlanta: American Cancer Society.

Centers for Disease Control and Prevention. 2006. Youth Risk Behavior Surveillance—United States, 2005. Surveillance Summaries, June 6, 2006. *Morbidity and Mortality Weekly Report* 55:No. SS-5.

Centers for Disease Control and Prevention, Division of Nutrition, Physical Activity and Obesity. State legislative database. http://apps.nccd.cdc.gov/DNPALeg/index.asp. Accessed August 31, 2007.

Coleman KJ, Tiller CL, Sanchez J, Heath EM, Sy O, Milliken G, Dzewaltowski DA. 2005. Prevention of the epidemic increase in child risk of overweight in low-income schools: the El Paso Coordinated Approach to Child Health. *Archives of Pediatrics and Adolescent Medicine* 159:217-224.

Cullen KW, Baranowski T, Herbert D, deMoor C, Hearn MD, Resnicow K. 1999. Influence of school organizational characteristics on the outcomes of a school health promotion program. *Journal of School Health* 69:376-380.

Donnelly JE, Jacobsen DJ, Whatley JE, et al. 1996. Nutrition and physical activity program to attenuate obesity and promote physical and metabolic fitness in elementary school children. *Obesity Research* 4(3):229-243.

Fardy PS, White RE, Haltiwanger-Schmitz K, et al. 1996. Coronary disease risk factor reduction and behavior modification in minority adolescents: the PATH Program. *Journal of Adolescent Health* 18:427-453.

Fetro JV. 1998. Implementing coordinated school health programs in local schools. In: Marx E, Wooley SF, Northrop D (Eds), *Health Is Academic*. New York: Teachers College Press; pp. 15-42.

Harrell JS, McMurray RG, Bangdiwala SI, et al. 1996. Effects of a school-based intervention to reduce cardiovascular disease risk factors in elementary-school children: the Cardiovascular Health in Children (CHIC) study. *Journal of Pediatrics* 128:797-805.

Heath EM, Coleman, KJ. 2003. Adoption and institutionalization of the Child and Adolescent Trail for Cardiovascular Health (CATCH) in El Paso, Texas. *Health Promotion Practice* 4:157-164.

Kahn EB, Ramsey LT, Brownson RC, et al. 2002. The effectiveness of interventions to increase physical activity: a systematic review. *American Journal of Preventive Medicine* 22(4 suppl):73-107.

Lee SM, Burgeson CR, Fulton JE, Spain C. 2007. Physical education and physical activity: results from the School Health Policies and Programs Study 2006. *Journal of School Health* 77(8):435-463.

Manios Y, Moschandreas J, Hatzis C, Kafatos A. 1999. Evaluation of a health and nutrition education program in primary school children of Crete over a three-year period. *Preventive Medicine* 28:149-159.

McKenzie TL, Nader PR, Strikmiller PK, et al. 1996. School physical education: effect of the child and adolescent trial for cardiovascular health. *Preventive Medicine* 25:423-431.

McKenzie TL, Feldman H, Woods SE, Romero KA, Dahlstrom V, Stone EJ, Strikmiller PK, Williston JM, Harsha DW. 1995. Student activity levels and lesson context during third-grade physical education. *Research Quarterly for Exercise and Sport* 66:184-193.

National Association for Sport and Physical Education. 2004. *Moving Into the Future: National Standards for Physical Education*, 2nd edition. Reston, VA: National Association for Sport and Physical Education.

Pate R, Ward DS, Saunders RP, Felton G, Dishman RK, Dowda M. 2005. Promotion of physical activity among high school girls: a randomized controlled trial. *American Journal of Public Health* 95:1582-1587.

Sallis JF, McKenzie TL, Alcaraz JE, et al. 1997. The effects of a 2-year physical education program (SPARK) on physical activity and fitness in elementary school students. *American Journal of Public Health* 87(8):1328-1334.

Simons-Morton BG, Parcel GS, Baranowski T, et al. 1991. Promoting physical activity and a healthful diet among children: results of a school-based intervention study. *American Journal of Public Health* 81(8):986-991.

U.S. Department of Health & Human Services. 2000. *Healthy People 2010*, 2nd edition. With *Understanding and Improving Health and Objectives for Improving Health*. 2 volumes. Washington, DC: U.S. Government Printing Office.

U.S. Department of Health & Human Services. 2008. *Physical Activity Guidelines for Americans.* Washington, DC: U.S. Government Printing Office.

Vandongen R, Jennfer DA, Thompson C, et al. 1995. A controlled evaluation of a fitness and nutrition intervention program on cardiovascular health in 10- to 12-year-old children. *Preventive Medicine* 24:9-22.

Zaza S, Briss PA, Harris KW (Eds). Task Force on Community Preventive Services. 2005. *The Guide to Community Preventive Services: What Works to Promote Health?* New York: Oxford University Press.

Chapter 4 Subsection 2

Brownson RC, Haire-Joshu D, Luke DA 2006. Shaping the context of health: a review of environmental and policy approaches in the prevention of chronic diseases. *Annual Review of Public Health* 27:17.1-17.30.

Castro CM, King AC. 2002. Telephone assisted counseling for physical activity. *Exercise and Sport Sciences Reviews* 30(2):64-68.

Chen AH, Sallis JF, Castro CM, et al. 1998. A home-based behavioral intervention to promote walking in sedentary ethnic minority women: Project WALK. *Women's Health* 4(1):19-39.

Coleman KJ, Raynor HR, Mueller DM, et al. 1999. Providing sedentary adults with choices for meeting their walking goals. *Preventive Medicine* 28:510-519.

Dunn, AL, Marcus BH, Kampert JB, et al. 1999. Comparison of lifestyle and structured interventions to increase physical activity and cardiorespiratory fitness: a randomized trial. *Journal of the American Medical Association* 281(4):327-334.

Etkin C et al. 2006. Feasibility of implementing the Strong for Life program in community settings. *Gerontologist* 46(2):284-292.

Foster C, Hillsdon M, Thorogood M. 2005. Interventions for promoting physical activity. *Cochrane Database of Systematic Reviews* (1):CD003180.

Humpel N, Marshall A, Iverson D, et al. 2004. Trial of print and telephone delivered interventions to influence walking. *Preventive Medicine* 39:635-641.

Jarvis KL, Friedman RH, Heeren T, Cullinane PM. 1997. Older women and physical activity: using the telephone to walk. *Women's Health Issues* 7(1):24-29.

Jette AM, Lachman M, Giorgetti MM, et al. 1999. Exercise—it's never too late: the Strong-for-Life Program. *American Journal of Public Health* 89(1):66-72.

Kahn EB, Ramsey LT, Brownson R, et al. 2002. Task Force on Community Preventive Services. The effectiveness of interventions to increase physical activity. *American Journal of Preventive Medicine* 22(4S):73-107.

King AC, Carl F, Birkel L, Haskell WL. 1988. Increasing exercise among blue-collar employees: the tailoring of worksite programs to meet specific needs. *Preventive Medicine* 17(3):357-365.

King AC, Haskell WL, Taylor CB, et al. 1991. Group vs. home-based exercise training in healthy older men and women: a community-based clinical trial. *Journal of the American Medical Association* 266(11):1535-1542.

King AC, Haskell WL, Young DR, et al. 1995. Long term effects of varying intensities and formats of physical activity on participation rates, fitness, and lipoproteins in men and women aged 50 to 65 years. *Circulation* 91(10):2596-2604.

King AC, Taylor CB, Haskell WL, DeBusk RF. 1988. Strategies for increasing early adherence to and long-term maintenance of home-based exercise training in healthy middle-aged men and women. *American Journal of Cardiology* 61(8):628-632.

Marcus BH, Bock BC, Pinto BM, et al. 1998. Efficacy of an individualized motivationally-tailored physical activity intervention. *Annals of Behavioral Medicine* 20(3):174-180.

Marcus BH, Forsyth LH. 2009. *Motivating People to be Physically Active.* Champaign, IL: Human Kinetics.

Marcus BH, Lewis BA, Williams DM, Dunsiger S, Jakcic JM, Whiteley JA, et al. 2007. A comparison of internet and print-based physical activity interventions. *Archives of Internal Medicine* 167 944-949.

Marcus BH, Nigg CR, Riebe D, Forsyth LAH. 2000. Interactive communication strategies: implications for population-based physical activity promotion. *American Journal of Preventive Medicine* 19(2):121-126.

Marcus BH, Owen N, Forsyth LAH., Cavill NA, Fridinger F. 1998. Physical activity interventions using mass media, print media, and information technology. *American Journal of Preventive Medicine* 15(4):362-378.

Marshall AL, Owen N, Bauman AE. 2004. Mediated approaches for influencing physical activity: update of the evidence on mass media, print, telephone and website delivery of interventions. *Journal of Science and Medicine in Sport* 7(1 suppl):74-80.

Mayer JA, Jermanovich A, Wright BL, et al. 1994. Changes in health behaviors of older adults: the San Diego Medicare Preventive Health Project. *Preventive Medicine* 23(2):127-133.

McAuley E, Courneya KS, Rudolph DL, Lox CL. 1994. Enhancing exercise adherence in middle-aged males and females. *Preventive Medicine* 23(4):498-506.

Napolitano MA, Marcus BH. 2002. Targeting and tailoring physical activity information using print and information technologies. *Exercise and Sport Sciences Reviews* 30(3):122-128.

Owen N, Christina L, Naccerella L, Haag K. 1987 Exercise by mail: a mediated behavior-change program for aerobic exercise. *Journal of Sport Psychology* 9:346-357.

Pinto B, Friedman R, Marcus B. 2002. Effects of a computer-based, telephone counseling system on physical activity. *American Journal of Preventive Medicine* 23(2):113-120.

U.S. Department of Health & Human Services, Public Health Service, Centers for Disease Control and Prevention, National Center for Chronic Disease Prevention and health Promotion, Division of Nutrition and Physical Activity. 1999. *Promoting Physical Activity: A Guide for Community Action.* Champaign, IL: Human Kinetics.

Vandelanotte C, Spathonis KM, Eakin EG, Owen N. 2007. Website-delivered physical activity interventions: a review of the literature. *American Journal of Preventive Medicine* 33(1):54-64.

Vandelanotte C, Bourdeaudhuij ID, Sallis JF, Spittaels H, Brug J. 2005. Efficacy of sequential or simultaneous interactive computer-tailored interventions for increasing physical activity and decreasing fat intake. *Annals of Behavioral Medicine* 29(2):138-146.

van den Berg MH, Schoones JW, Vliet Vlieland TPM. 2007. Internet-based physical activity interventions: A systematic review of the literature. *Journal of Medical Internet Research* 9(3):e26.

Zaza S, Briss PA, Harris KW (Eds). Task Force on Community Preventive Services. 2005. *The Guide to Community Preventive Services: What Works to Promote Health?* New York: Oxford University Press.

Chapter 4 Subsection 3

Avila P, Hovell M. 1994. Physical activity training for weight loss in Latinas: a controlled trial. *International Journal of Obesity and Related Metabolic Disorders* 18:476-482.

Baker E, Brennan L, et al. 2000. Measuring the determinants of physical activity in the community: current and future directions. *Research Quarterly for Exercise and Sport* 71:(2 suppl):S146-S158.

Briss PA, Zaza S, et al. 2000. Developing an evidence-based Guide to Community Preventive Services–methods. The Task Force on Community Preventive Services. *American Journal of Preventive Medicine* 18(1 suppl):35-43.

Briss PA, Brownson RC, et al. 2004. Developing and using the Guide to Community Preventive Services: lessons learned about evidence-based public health. *Annual Review of Public Health* 25:281-302.

Elliot DL, Goldberg L, et al. 2004. The PHLAME firefighters' study: feasibility and findings. *American Journal of Health Behavior* 28(1):13-23.

Gill A, Veigl V, et al. 1984. A well woman's health maintenance study comparing physical fitness and group support programs. *Occupational Therapy Journal of Research* 4:286-308.

Heaney CA, Israel BA. 2002. Social networks and social support. In: Glanz K, Rimer BK, Lewis FM (Eds), *Health Behavior and Health Education: Theory, Research and Practice*, 3rd edition. San Francisco: Jossey-Bass; pp. 185-209.

Heath GW, Brownson RC, et al. 2006) The effectiveness of urban design and land use and transport policies and practices to increase physical activity: a systematic review. *J Physical Activity and Health* 3(suppl 1):S55-S76.

Hillsdon M, Foster C, et al. 2005. Interventions for promoting physical activity. *Cochrane Database of Systematic Reviews* (1):CD003180.

Jason L, Greiner B, et al. 1991. A large-scale, short-term, media-based weight loss program. *American Journal of Health Promotion* 5:432-437.

Kahn EB, Ramsey LT, Brownson RC, Heath GW, Howze EH, Powell KE, Stone EJ, Rajab MW, Corso P, and the Task Force on Community Preventive Services. 2002. The effectiveness of interventions to increase physical activity: a systematic review. *American Journal of Preventive Medicine* 22(4S):73-96.

King A. 1988. Strategies for increasing early adherence to and long-term maintenance of home-base exercise training in healthy middle-aged men and women. *American Journal of Cardiology* 61:628-632.

King A, Frederiksen L. 1984. Low-cost strategies for increasing exercise behavior: relapse preparation training and social support. *Behavior Modification* 8:3-21.

Kriska A, Bayles C, et al. 1986. A randomized exercise trial in older women: increased activity over two years and the factors associated with compliance. *Medicine & Science in Sports & Exercise* 18:557-562.

Lombard D, Lombard T, et al. 1995. Walking to meet health guidelines: the effect of prompting frequency and prompt structure. *Health Psychology* 14:164-170.

Peterson JA, Yates BC, et al. 2005. Effects of a physical activity intervention for women. *Western Journal of Nursing Research* 27(1):93-110.

U.S. Department of Health & Human Services, Public Health Service, Centers for Disease Control and Prevention, National Center for Chronic Disease Prevention and health Promotion, Division of Nutrition and Physical Activity. 1999. *Promoting Physical Activity: A Guide for Community Action.* Champaign, IL: Human Kinetics p. 364.

Simmons D, Fleming C, et al. 1998. A pilot urban church-based program to reduce risk factors for diabetes among Western Samoans in New Zealand. *Diabetic Medicine* 15:136-142.

Wankel L, Yardley J, et al. 1985. The effects of motivational interventions upon the exercise adherence of high and low self-motivated adults. *Canadian Journal of Applied Sport Sciences/Journal canadien des sciences appliquées au sport* 10:147-156.

Williams DM, Matthews CE, et al. 2008. Interventions to increase walking behavior. *Medicine & Science in Sports & Exercise* 40(7 suppl):S567-S573.

Zaza S, Briss PA, Harris KW (Eds). Task Force on Community Preventive Services. 2005. *The Guide to Community Preventive Services: What Works to Promote Health?* New York: Oxford University Press.

Chapter 5 Subsection 1

Blair SN, Piserchia P, Wilbur C, Crowder J. 1986. A public health intervention model for worksite health promotion: impact on exercise and physical fitness in a health promotion plan after 24 months. *Journal of American Medical Association* 255:921-926.

Bowne DW, Russell M, Morgan J, Optenberg S, Clarke A. 1984. Reduced disability and health care costs in an industrial fitness program. *Journal of Occupational Medicine* 26(11):809-816.

Boarnet MG, Anderson C, Day K, McMillan T, Alfonzo M. 2005. Evaluation of the California Safe Routes to School legislation: urban form changes and children's active transportation to School. *American Journal of Preventive Medicine* 28(2S2):134-140.

Brownson RC, Hagood L, Lovegreen S, Britton B, Caito N, Elliott M, et al. 2005. A multilevel ecological approach to promoting walking in rural communities. *Preventive Medicine* 41:837-842.

Brownson RC, Houseman R, Brown D, Jackson-Thompson J, King A, Malone B, Sallis J. 2000. Promoting physical activity in rural communities: walking trail access, use, and effects. *American Journal of Preventive Medicine* 18(3):235-241.

Brownson RC, Smith C, Pratt M, et al. 1996. Preventing cardiovascular disease through community-based risk reduction: the Bootheel Heart Health Project. *American Journal of Public Health.* 86(2):206-213.

Carande-Kulis VG, Maciosek M, Briss P, et al. 2000. Methods for systematic reviews of economic evaluations for the *Guide to Community Preventive Services. American Journal of Preventive Medicine* 18(1 suppl)L75-91.

Cady LD Jr, Thomas P, Karwasky R. 1985. Program for increasing health and physical fitness of fire fighters. *Journal of Occupational Medicine* 27(2):110-114.

Eddy JM, Eynon D, Nagy S, Paradossi P. 1990. Impact of a physical fitness program in a bluecollar workforce. *Health Values* 14(6):14-23.

Eyler AA, Mayer J, Rafii R, Houseman R, Brownson R, King A. 1999. Key informant surveys as a tool to implement and evaluate physical activity interventions in the community. *Health Education Research* 14:289-298.

Giles-Corti B, Broomhall MH, Knuiman M, Collins C, Douglas K, Ng K, Lange A, Donovan RRJ. 2005. Increasing walking: How important is distance to, attractiveness, and size of public open space? *American Journal of Preventive Medicine* 28(2S2):169-176.

Godbey GC. Caldwell L, Floyd M, Payne L. 2005. Contributions of leisure studies and recreation and park management research to the active living agenda. *American Journal of Preventive Medicine* 28(2, suppl 2):150-158.

Golaszewski T, Snow D, Lynch W, Yen L, Solomita D. 1992. A benefit-to-cost analysis of a work-site health promotion program. *Journal of Occupational Medicine* 34(12):1164-1172.

Guide to Community Preventive Services. 2001. Economic evaluation abstraction form, version 3.0. www.thecommunityguide.org/index.html.

Heirich MA, Foote A, Erfurt J, Konopka B. 1993. Work-site physical fitness programs: comparing the impact of different program designs on cardiovascular risks. *Journal of Occupational Medicine* 35:510-517.

Henritze J, Brammell H, McGloin J. 1992. LIFECHECK: a successful, low touch, low tech, in-plant, cardiovascular disease risk identification and modification program. *American Journal of Health Promotion* 7(2):129-136.

Kahn EB, Ramsey L, Brownson R, Heath G, Howze E, Powell K, Stone E, Rajab M, Corso P. 2002. The effectiveness of interventions to increase physical activity: a systematic review. *American Journal of Preventive Medicine* 22(4 suppl):73-107.

King AC, Carl F, Birkel L, Haskell W. 1988. Increasing exercise among blue-collar employees: the tailoring of worksite programs to meet specific needs. *Preventive Medicine* 17(3):357-365.

Larsen P, Simons N. 1993. Evaluating a federal health and fitness program: indicators of improving health. *AAOHN Journal* 41(3):143-148.

Lewis CE, Raczynski J, Heath G, Levinson R, Hilyer J, Cutter G. 1993. Promoting physical activity in low-income African-American communities: the PARR project. *Ethnicity and Disease* 3(2):106-118.

Linenger JM, Chesson C, Nice D. 1991. Physical fitness gains following simple environmental change. *American Journal of Preventive Medicine* 7(5):298-310.

Moody JS, Prochaska J, Sallis J, McKenzie T, Brown M, Conway T. 2004. Viability for parks and recreation centers as sites for youth physical activity promotion. *Health Promotion and Practice* 5:438-443.

Sallis JF, Conway T, Prochaska J, McKenzie T, Marshall S, Brown M. 2001. The association of school environments with youth physical activity. *American Journal of Public Health* 91:618-620.

Staunton CE, Hubsmith D, Kallins W. 2003. Promoting safe walking and biking to school: the Marin County success story. *American Journal of Public Health* 93:1431-1434.

Wang G, Macera C, Scudder-Soucie B, Schmid T, Pratt M, Buchner D. 2004. Cost effectiveness of a bicycle/pedestrian trail development in health promotion. *Preventive Medicine* 38(2):237-242.

Wiggs I, Brownson R, Baker E. 2006. If you build it, they will come: lessons from developing walking trails in rural Missouri. *Health Promotion Practice* 10(10):1-8

Zaza S, Briss PA, Harris KW (Eds). Task Force on Community Preventive Services. 2005. *The Guide to Community Preventive Services: What Works to Promote Health?* New York: Oxford University Press.

Chapter 5 Subsection 2

Amarasinghe A, D'Sousa G, Brown, C, Borisova, T. 2006. The Impact of Socioeconomic and Spatial Differences on Obesity in West Virginia. Agricultural and Applied Economics Association, Annual Meeting, July 23-26, Long Beach, CA. http://purl.umn.edu.21159.

Bassett DR, Pucher J, Buehler R, Thompson DL, Crouter SE. 2008. Walking, cycling and obesity rates in Europe, North America and Australia. *Journal of Physical Activity and Health* 5:795-814.

Besser LM, Dannenberg AL. 2005. Walking to public transit: steps to help meet physical activity recommendations. *American Journal of Preventive Medicine* 29:273-280.

Boarnet MG, Anderson C, Day K, McMillan T, Alfonzo M. 2005. Evaluation of the California Safe Routes to School legislation: urban form changes and children's active transportation to school. *American Journal of Preventive Medicine* 28:134-140.

Centers for Disease Control and Prevention (CDC). 2004. KidsWalk-to-School: KidsWalk-to-School Encourages Pedestrian Safety 2004. www.cdc.gov/nccdphp/dnpa/kidswalk/.

Cervero, R. 1988. Land-use mixing and suburban mobility. *Transportation Quarterly* 42:429-446.

Cervero R, Radisch C. 1996. Travel choices in pedestrian versus automobile oriented neighborhoods. *Transport Policy* 3:127-141.

Cleary J, McClintock H. 2000. Evaluation of the cycle challenge project: A case study of the Nottingham cycle-friendly employers project. *Transport Policy* 7:117-125.

Cooper AR, Page AS, Foster LJ, Qahwaji D. 2003. Commuting to school: are children who walk more physically active? *American Journal of Preventive Medicine* 25: 273-276.

Craig C, Brownson R, Cragg S, Dunn A. 2002. Exploring the effect of the environment on physical activity: a study examining walking to work. *American Journal of Preventive Medicine* 23:S36-S43.

deVries SI, Bakker I, van Mechelen W, Hopman-Rock M. 2007. Determinants of activity-friendly neighborhoods for children: results from the SPACE study. *American Journal of Health Promotion* 27(suppl 4):312-316.

Ewing R, Schmid TL, Killingsworth R, Zlot A, Raudenbush S. 2003. Relationship between urban sprawl and physical activity, obesity and morbidity. *American Journal of Health Promotion* 18:47-57.

Frank LD, Andersen MA, Schmid TL. 2004. Obesity relationships with community design, physical activity, and time spent in cars. *American Journal of Preventive Medicine* 27(4): 87-96.

Frank LD, Engelke PO, Schmid TL. 2003. *Health and Community Design: The Impact of the Built Environment on Physical Activity*. Washington, DC: Island Press.

Frank LD, Sallis JF, Conway T L, Chapman J E, Saelens BE, Bachman W. 2006. Associations between neighborhood walkability and active transportation, body mass index, and air quality. *Journal of the American Planning Association* 72(1):75-87.

Frank LD, Saelens BE, Powell KE, Chapman JE. 2007. Stepping towards causation: Do built environments or neighborhood and travel preferences explain physical activity and driving behavior? *Social Science and Medicine* 65:1898-1914.

Li F, Fisher KJ, Brownson RC, Bosworth M. 2005. Multilevel modeling of built environment characteristics related to neighborhood walking activity in older adults. *Journal of Environmental and Community Health* 59:558-564.

Gomez LF, Jacoby E, Mosquera J. 2006. Urban Design, Transportation, Physical Activity and Quality of Life, Lessons from Bogota Columbia. Paper presented at the International Congress on Physical Activity and Health, Atlanta, April 18, 2006.

Gordon-Larsen P, Nelson MC, Page P, Popkin BM. 2006. Inequality in the built environment underlies key health disparities in physical activity and obesity. *Pediatrics* 117(2):417-424.

Greenberg M, Renne J, Lane R, Zupan J. 2005. Physical activity and the use of suburban train stations: an exploratory analysis. *Journal of Public Transportation* 8(3): 89-116.

Handy SL, Xinyu Cao, Mokhtarian P L. 2006. Self-selection in the relationship between the built environment and walking: empirical evidence from northern California. *Journal of the American Planning Association* 72(1):55-74.

Heath GW, Brownson RC, Kruger J, Miles R, Powell K, Ramsey LT, and the Task Force on Community Preventive Services. 2006. The Effects of Urban Design and Land Use and Transportation Policies and Practices to Increase Physical Activity: A Systematic Review *Journal of Physical Activity and Health* 3, Suppl 1, S55-S76.

Kerr J, Frank L, Sallis J, Chapman J. 2007. Urban form correlates of pedestrian travel in youth: differences by gender, race-ethnicity and household attributes. *Transportation Research Part D: Transportation and Environment* 12(3): 177-182.

Lawlor, DA, Ness AR, Cope AM, Davis A, Insall P, Riddoch C. 2003. The challenges of evaluating environmental interventions to increase population levels of physical activity: the case of the UK National Cycle Network. *Journal of Epidemiology and Community Health* 57; 96-101

Lee C, Moudon AV. 2006. Environmental and socio-demographic correlates of walking for transportation or recreation purposes. *Journal of Physical Activity and Health* 3(suppl 1) S77-S98.

Librett J, Yore, M, Schmid TL, Kohl HW III. 2007. Do physical activity levels predict demand for activity-friendly communities? *Health and Place* 13(3):767-733.

Mc Nally MG, Kulkarni A. 1996. Assessment of influence of land use-transportation system on travel behavior. *Transportation Research Record* 1607:105-115.

Moudon AV, Lee C, Cheadle A, Garvin C, Johnson D, Schmid T, Weathers R, Lin L. 2006. Operational definitions of walkable neighborhood: theoretical and empirical insights. *Journal of Physical Activity and Health* 3(suppl):S99-S117.

Mutrie N, Carney C, Blamey A, Crawford F, Aitchison T, Whitelaw A. 2002. "Walk in the Work Out": a randomized control trial of a self-help intervention to promote active commuting. *Journal of Epidemiology and Community Health* 56:407-412.

NICE. 2006. Physical Activity and the Environment: Transport Evidence Review. NICE Public Health Collaborating Centre—Physical Activity. *www.nice.org.uk/nicemedia/pdf/word/Transport%20evidence%20review.doc*

Oja P, Vuori I, Paronen O. 1998. Daily walking and cycling to work: their utility as health-enhancing physical activity. *Patient Education and Counseling* 33:S87-S94.

Pucher, J. 1997. Bicycling boom in Germany: a revival engineered by public policy. *Transportation Quarterly* 51:31-46.

Rutt CD, Coleman KJ. 2005a. Examining the impact of the built environment on body mass index (BMI) and vigorous physical activity along the U.S./Mexico border. *Preventive Medicine* 40:831-841.

Rutt CD, Coleman KJ. 2005b. The impact of the built environment on walking as a leisure time activity along the U.S./Mexico border. *Physical Activity and Health* 3:257-271.

Sallis JF, Hovell MF, Hofstetter CR. 1992. Predictors of adoption and maintenance of vigorous physical activity in men and women. *Preventive Medicine* 21:237-251.

Shaw SM, Bonen A, McCabe JF. 1991. Do more constraints mean less leisure? Examining the relationship between constraints and participation. *Journal of Leisure Research* 23:286-300.

Shriver K. 1997. Influence of environmental design on pedestrian travel behavior in four Austin neighborhoods. *Transportation Research Record* 1578:64-75.

Snow J. 1855. *On the Mode of Communication of Cholera*. New Burlington Street, England: John Churchill.

Staunton C, Hubsmith D, Kallins W. 2003 Promoting safe walking and biking to school: the Marin County success story. *American Journal of Public Health* 93:1431-1434.

Suminiski R, Poston W, Petosa R, Stevens E, Katzenmoyer L. 2005. Features of the neighborhood environment and walking in U.S. adults. *American Journal of Preventive Medicine* 28(2):149-155.

Transportation Research Board and Institute of Medicine. (2005). Does the Built Environment Influence Physical Activity? Examining the Evidence (Special Report 282). Washington, DC: National Academy Press.

Tudor-Locke C, Ainsworth BE, Adair LS, Popkin BM. 2003. Objective physical activity of Filipino youth stratified for commuting mode to school. *Medicine & Science in Sports & Exercise* 35:465-471.

Wardman M, Tight M, Page M. 2007. Factors influencing the propensity to cycle to work. *Transportation Research Part A* 41:339-350.

Werner RE, Evans GW. 2007. A morning stroll-Levels of physical activity in car and mass transit commuting. *Environment and Behavior* 39(1):62-74.

Wen LF, Orr N, Millett C, Rissel C. 2006. Driving to work and overweight and obesity: findings from the 2003 New South Wales Health Survey, Australia. *International Journal of Obesity* 30:782-786.

Chapter 6

American Heritage Dictionary, 4th edition. 2006. Boston: Houghton Mifflin.

Centers for Disease Control and Prevention. 2009. Active environments. www.cdc.gov/nccdphp/dnpa/physical/health_professionals/active_environments/index.htm.

Chrislip DD, Larson, CE. 1995. *Collaborative Leadership—How Citizens and Civic Leaders Can Make a Difference*. San Francisco: Jossey Bass.

Mattessich P, Murray-Close M, Monsey B. 2001. *Collaboration: What Makes It Work,* 2nd edition. St. Paul: Amherst H. Wilder Foundation.

Satcher D. 1996. CDC's first 50 years: lessons learned and relearned. *American Journal of Public Health* 86:1705-1708.

U.S. Department of Health & Human Services, Public Health Service, Centers for Disease Control and Prevention, National Center for Chronic Disease Prevention and health Promotion, Division of Nutrition and Physical Activity. 1999. *Promoting Physical Activity: A Guide for Community Action.* Champaign, IL: Human Kinetics.

Chapter 7

Andreasen AR. 1995. *Marketing Social Change: Changing Behavior to Promote Health, Social Development, and the Environment.* San Francisco: Jossey-Bass.

Centers for Disease Control and Prevention. 1999. Framework for program evaluation in public health. *MMWR Recommendations and Reports* 48(RR-11):1-40. www.cdc.gov/mmwr/preview/mmwrhtml/rr4811a1.htm.

Cook TD, Campbell DT. 1979. *Quasi-Experimentation: Design and Analysis Issues for Field Settings*. Boston: Houghton Mifflin.

Green LW, Kreuter MW. 1992. CDC's Planned Approach to Community Health as an application of PRECEDE and an inspiration for PROCEED. *Journal of Health Education* 23(3):140-147.

Heath GW, Brownson RC, Kruger J, Miles R, Powell KE, Ramsey LT; Task Force on Community Preventive Services. 2006. The effectiveness of urban design and land use and transport policies and practices to increase physical activity: a systematic review. *Journal of Physical Activity and Health* 3(suppl 1):S55-S76.

Kahn EB, Ramsey LT, Brownson RC, Heath GW, Howze EH, Powell KE, Stone EJ, Rajab MW, Corso P; Task Force on Community Preventive Services. 2002. The effectiveness of interventions to increase physical activity: a systematic review. *American Journal of Preventive Medicine* 22(4 suppl):73-107.

U.S. Department of Health & Human Services, Public Health Service, Centers for Disease Control and Prevention, National Center for Chronic Disease Prevention and Health Promotion, Division of Nutrition and Physical Activity. 1999. *Promoting Physical Activity: A Guide for Community Action.* Champaign, IL: Human Kinetics.

U.S. Department of Health & Human Services. Physical Activity Evaluation Handbook. 2002. Atlanta: U.S. Department of Health & Human Services, Centers for Disease Control and Prevention; www.cdc.gov/nccdphp/dnpa/physical/handbook/pdf/handbook.pdf

Warden B, Wong S. 2007. Introduction to Qualitative Analysis. Paper presented at the American Evaluation Association and Centers for Disease Control and Prevention 2007 Summer Evaluation Institute with support from the National Association of Chronic Disease Directors. Atlanta, GA, June 11-12.

Zaza S, Briss PA, Harris KW (Eds). Task Force on Community Preventive Services. 2005. *The Guide to Community Preventive Services: What Works to Promote Health?* New York: Oxford University Press.

Appendix A

Rimmer JH, Braddock D, Pitetti KH. 1996. Research on physical activity and disability: an emerging national priority. *Medicine & Science in Sports & Exercise* 28(8):1366-1372.

U.S. Department of Health & Human Services. 2000. *Healthy People 2010,* 2nd edition. With *Understanding and Improving Health* and *Objectives for Improving Health.* 2 volumes. Washington, DC: U.S. Government Printing Office.

ABOUT THE ORGANIZATION

The **Centers for Disease Control and Prevention** is the nation's premier public health agency, working to ensure healthy people in a healthy world.

The Centers for Disease Control and Prevention (CDC), a part of the U.S. Department of Health and Human Services, is the primary federal agency for conducting and supporting public health activities in the United States. CDC's focus is not only on scientific excellence but also on the essential spirit that is CDC—to protect the health of all people. CDC keeps humanity at the forefront of its mission to ensure health protection through promotion, prevention, and preparedness.

CDC's, Division of Nutrition, Physical Activity and Obesity (DNPAO) is part of the CDC's National Center for Chronic Disease Prevention and Health Promotion. DNPAO's vision, mission, and goals are:

- *DNPAO's vision*—a world where regular physical activity, good nutrition, and healthy weight are part of everyone's life.

- *DNPAO's mission*—to lead strategic public health efforts to prevent and control obesity, chronic disease, and other health conditions though regular physical activity and good nutrition.

DNPAO's goals:

- Increase health-related physical activity through population-based approaches.
- Improve those aspects of dietary quality most related to the population burden of chronic disease and unhealthy child development.
- Decrease prevalence of obesity through preventing excess weight gain and maintenance of healthy weight loss.

ABOUT THE EDITORS

David R. Brown, PhD, is a research behavioral scientist with the Centers for Disease Control and Prevention (CDC), National Center for Chronic Disease Prevention and Health Promotion, Division of Nutrition, Physical Activity and Obesity. He earned his PhD in Kinesiology with a major in Exercise and Sport Psychology from the University of Wisconsin-Madison, MA and PhD degrees in Educational Psychology from the University of Arizona, and a BS degree in Special Education from Western Michigan University. Before coming to CDC in 1992, he served as a special education teacher and then as school psychologist in a public school district in Tucson, Arizona; as assistant professor in the Department of Physical Education, Health, and Sport Studies at Miami University-Ohio; and as director of exercise and sport psychology in the Exercise Physiology and Nutrition Laboratory at the University of Massachusetts Medical School. His public health focus is on mental health outcomes associated with physical activity and promoting physical activity among older adults, persons with disabilities, and different racial and ethnic groups. He has authored numerous scientific articles and served on review and writing teams to develop *Physical Activity and Health: A Report of the Surgeon General* and the *2008 Physical Guidelines for Americans.* Dr. Brown is a fellow of the American College of Sports Medicine and vice-chair of the Executive Committee of CDC's Behavioral and Social Sciences Working Group.

Gregory W. Heath, DHSc, MPH, is the guerry professor and head of the Department of Health and Human Performance at the University of Tennessee at Chattanooga and director of research at the University of Tennessee College of Medicine, Chattanooga. Dr. Heath was formally the lead health scientist with the Division of Nutrition and Physical Activity at the Centers for Disease Control and Prevention (CDC). His training is in physiology, nutrition, and epidemiology. He received his Masters of Public Health and Doctor of Health Science degrees from Loma Linda University in California and completed his post-doctoral training in applied physiology at the Washington University School of Medicine in St. Louis, Missouri. A former epidemic intelligence service officer, he worked at CDC for over 20 years. Dr. Heath has spent most of his professional career devoted to understanding and promoting physical activity and exercise for the enhancement of health and the prevention and treatment of chronic diseases. He has published widely in scientific literature. Dr. Heath is a fellow in the American College of Sports Medicine and American Heart Association's Councils on Epidemiology and Prevention and Nutrition, Physical Activity, and Metabolism.

Sarah Levin Martin, PhD, is a research associate of the Maine Center for Public Health where she currently serves as the team leader for the evaluation of the Healthy Maine Partnerships Initiative of the Maine Center for Disease Control and Prevention. She has a doctoral degree in epidemiology from the School of Public Health at the University of South Carolina (1999), a master's degree in health education from the University of New Mexico, and bachelor's degree from Brown University. Dr. Martin has over 20 years of experience in the public health arena, beginning with the Pawtucket Heart Health Project in Rhode Island in the late 1980s. She specialized then in physical activity promotion, and now in program evaluation. Dr. Martin is the lead author of the *Physical Activity Evaluation Handbook* (DHHS, 2002; translated into 3 languages) which she wrote in her tenure as a health scientist for the CDC's Physical Activity and Health Branch. Her career spans health promotion and research projects with youth in the Northeast, Native Americans in the Southwest, African Americans in the Southeast, the Catawba Indian Tribe of the Carolinas, and the entire nation in her role with the federal government (2001-2006). Dr. Levin Martin is the lead author of over 25 peer-reviewed journal articles and has presented papers internationally.